Methods in Bioengineering

3D Tissue Engineering

François Berthiaume
Department of Biomedical Engineering, Rutgers University

Jeffrey Morgan
Department of Molecular Pharmacology, Physiology & Biotechnology, Brown University

Editors

ARTECH
HOUSE

BOSTON | LONDON
artechhouse.com

Library of Congress Cataloging-in-Publication Data
A catalog record for this book is available from the U.S. Library of Congress.

British Library Cataloguing in Publication Data
A catalogue record for this book is available from the British Library.

ISBN-13: 978-1-59693-458-0

Cover design by Vicki Kane

685 Canton Street
Norwood MA 02062

10 9 8 7 6 5 4 3 2 1

Contents

Preface

The emerging field of tissue engineering has great promise for the replacement and repair of tissues and organs that have been lost or compromised by disease or trauma. In fact, the first wave of new medical therapies based on the principles and methods of tissue engineering is currently available. Other tissue engineering therapies are under active clinical evaluation and still more are energetically under investigation in labs throughout the world. Far from being a mature and static field, the fundamental methods of tissue engineering are in an extraordinary creative phase of refinement, improvement, and innovation. These methods are tackling ever-increasing problems in the medical application of tissue engineering and will form the underpinnings of future medical therapies.

Concordant with this activity is a growing recognition that conventional in vitro cell culture (the growth of a single thin layer of living cells on flat rigid plastic dishes) does not adequately replicate the biological function and complexity found in vivo. Missing are cell-to-cell interactions, cell-to-matrix interactions, biomechanical effects, and the influence of the limitations of diffusion, to name just a few. Tissue engineering is offering new methods for the culture of cells in 3D, and these systems more accurately replicate the complex microenvironments and phenotypes found in vivo. In addition to being adopted as fundamental tools for basic science studies, such 3D cell culture systems are being used to reduce the cost and use of animals in research and are being used for toxicology testing and drug discovery.

In this volume of the Artech House Methods in Bioengineering Series, detailed protocols are provided for a wide spectrum of complementary tissue engineering methods. Covered in this volume are methods for the fabrication of scaffolds from synthetic polymers, peptides that self-assemble, and the quantitative methods to characterize the mechanical and chemical properties of these scaffolds. Scaffold fabrication and design have been an important part of the field of tissue engineering, and this field is advancing beyond the first generation of scaffolds. Methods are provided for the derivation of these scaffolds to increase their functionality via enhanced cell attachment or the ability to act as drug delivery systems for small molecules and bioactive peptides. Also covered are the formation of various forms of hydrogels and their functionalizations and characterizations. Such hydrogels offer new possibilities for the transplantation and encapsulation of cells. A method is provided for the scaffold-free self-assembly of 3D multicellular microtissues that maximize cell-to-cell interactions. These 3D microtissues can be formed in the shape of spheroids, toroids, and honeycombs, which open up new possibilities. Another method covers the use of chip-based design for making bioreactors of cells. Other methods are also covered that use these materials (scaffolds, hydrogels, and cells) as building blocks to create even larger structures with complex shapes using layer-by-layer deposition or macromolding approaches. In total, this is an impressive collection of methods for the tissue engineering toolbox that can be used singly or in combination to build complex 3D structures applicable to a variety of tissues. This book goes further by providing several chapters where these and additional tissue engineering methods are focussed on the challenges of specific tissues and organs, such as cartilage and the nervous system. Nearly all the chapters in this book provide valuable methods for the quantitative evaluation of cells and cell function via biochemical assays, immunostaining procedures, gene expression analysis, and various forms of microscopy that are often a challenge to perform in 3D cultures. In addition to detailed methods, all of the chapters are well referenced and provide guidance on anticipated results and troubleshooting, which are of value to beginners and experts alike. By providing the important details for experimental success along with the larger context, we hope that *Methods in Bioengineering: 3D Tissue Engineering* will be a source of creative innovation for the next phase in tissue engineering.

François Berthiaume
Massachusetts General Hospital
Boston, Massachusetts

Jeffrey Morgan
Brown University
Providence, Rhode Island
Editors
May 2010

CHAPTER

1

Chemical Modification of Porous Scaffolds Using Plasma Polymers

Paul Roach,[1†] Daniel Howard,[2] John J. A. Barry,[3] Kevin M. Shakesheff[2], Steven M. Howdle,[4] and Morgan R. Alexander[1]*

[1]Laboratory of Biophysics and Surface Analysis, School of Pharmacy, The University of Nottingham, University Park, Nottingham, NG7 2RD, United Kingdom, [2]Centre for Biomolecular Sciences, School of Pharmacy, The University of Nottingham, University Park, Nottingham, NG7 2RD, United Kingdom, [3]Baxter Biosurgery, Wagramer Strasse 17-19, A-1220 Vienna, Austria, [4]School of Chemistry, The University of Nottingham, University Park, Nottingham, NG7 2RD, United Kingdom, [†]Current Address: Institute of Science and Technology in Medicine, Guy Hilton Research Centre, Keele University, Hartshill Campus, Stoke-on-Trent, Staffordshire, ST4 7QB, United Kingdom, Corresponding author: Morgan R. Alexander, Laboratory of Biophysics and Surface Analysis, School of Pharmacy, The University of Nottingham, University Park, Nottingham, NG7 2RD, United Kingdom, e-mail: Morgan.Alexander@Nottingham.ac.uk

Abstract

Macroporous scaffolds are of utility in many tissue-engineering applications. For a given material, surface chemical modification of the scaffold can allow control over adsorbing species from the surrounding culture media, which subsequently affects cell adhesion and function. Here we present the use of plasma polymers to introduce nitrogen-containing functionality to enhance cell adhesion in the center of a porous 3D object, while decreasing cell adhesion using a hydrophobic hexane plasma polymer at the periphery. Critically, plasma polymerization allows a gradient in chemistry to be achieved using these two polymers to counteract the tendency of cells to adhere to the periphery of a porous object.

Key terms: cell penetration
plasma polymer
porous scaffold
tissue engineering

1.1 Introduction

Synthetic porous scaffolds are widely used as cellular supports in tissue engineering for regeneration of various tissues including bone [1], cartridge [2, 3], muscle [4], and nerve [5]. The chemistry at the material surface is key in dictating the initial cell-material interactions and consequently critical in the subsequent tissue growth. Scaffold materials are often chosen for their bulk properties such as degradation rate, mechanical properties and pore structure. Thus, to gain control over the cell adhesion to a given material, it is common to modify the surface chemistry.

The chemical modification of surfaces has generated much interest over the past decades as a means to control and understand cell attachment using a wide range of approaches. Specific ligands such as the RGD tripeptide derived from cell adhesive proteins have been shown to be useful at surfaces through mediation of cell attachment via integrin receptors on the cell surface [6]. Simple functionalities have also been shown to provide a good control over cell response at surfaces by control of the proteins adsorbed from the culture media [7]. Amine and carboxylic acid containing surfaces have been used to enhance adhesion of different cell types, and ethylene glycol and hydrophobic alkane groups have been used to reduce cell attachment in the form of self assembled monolayers (SAMs) [8–12]. Since SAMs are restricted to only a few metal/metal oxide surfaces they have not generally progressed on from model studies. Preadsorption of proteins to surfaces is a common strategy to control cell adhesion to a material; however, since this is not a synthetic route, it has issues of reproducibility and disease transmission concerns. Plasma-polymer deposition provides a route to surface modification while maintaining the bulk material properties and structure; at the same time, the deposition also produces a thin (nanometers) layer of the desired surface chemistry [13–17]. Plasma surface modification can also take the form of an *etch*, where the original polymer surface chemistry is modified, often by an argon or oxygen plasma to introduce new chemical functionalities. These functionalities can be a graft, where an etched surface is exposed to a monomer that reacts with the surface, or a plasma-polymer coating.

Plasma-polymerized allylamine (ppAAm) has been used to prepare cell-supporting planer surfaces, with higher cell numbers being found compared to equivalent surfaces prepared using hexane (ppHex) [18–24]. Other plasma polymers have been formed using a range of monomers, including allyl alcohol, acrylic acid, acetone, and toluene [24, 25]. Coatings may readily be produced that follow the contour of the underlying surface, and are sterile as-prepared from the plasma environment. Plasma-derived coatings on 2D substrates have been used for the study of protein adsorption and cell attachment, although only recently have these been deposited within macroscopic porous materials coatings to provide 3D modification [26, 27].

A common problem with cultures in porous 3D scaffolds is that excessive colonization of the periphery occurs, caused by the attachment and proliferation of cells closest to the majority of the media. Plasma-polymer deposition has been shown to form a radial chemical gradient when a porous object is placed in the plasma, as a result of the restriction of diffusion of the depositing species to the inner surfaces [27, 28]. This effect has been used to produce a cell adhesive *core* and a *sheath* that is less cell adhesive using ppAAm and ppHex, respectively [27]. Here we describe the use of both ppAAm alone to enhance the attachment of 3T3 fibroblasts on a porous poly(D,L-lactic acid) ($P_{DL}LA$) scaffold produced by supercritical carbon dioxide processing, and the effects of an additional ppHex sheath coating. It should, however, be noted that since this is a coating method it can be applied to any material and any porosity, although it is likely that the deposition times will need to be varied to provide equivalent results on different sized objects with different types of open porosity. The present work was only conducted with fibroblasts, although research using stem cells is currently being undertaken.

We are unaware of any other methods used to produce surface chemical gradients in scaffolds in order to control cell distribution, although modification of scaffold material using plasma, protein adsorption, and a wide range of other adsorbates have been detailed but without taking advantage of patterning [29].

1.2 Experimental Design

The plasma-polymer coating method presented here is designed to achieve a uniform cell distribution in porous scaffolds. It is demonstrated with 3T3 fibroblasts on a porous $P_{DL}LA$ scaffold produced by super-critical carbon dioxide ($scCO_2$) processing; although, it is applicable with slight modification to other cell types on other porous materials. First, the use of the ppAAm coating as a modification to enhance cellular adhesion to the scaffold is tested. Second, scaffolds coated with ppAAm and an additional deposition of a ppHex *sheath* layer on the periphery are described in terms of their ability to support cell adhesion through the scaffold. Surface analysis was conducted by X-ray photoelectron spectroscopy (XPS) to characterize the plasma polymer distribution. As-prepared scaffolds were used as controls with XPS carried out after polymer deposition. The ability of 3T3 fibroblasts to ingress and adhere to the scaffold was assessed globally using microcomputed tomography with osmium tetroxide staining of the cells, which was sufficient to distinguish them from the scaffold background. Electron microscopy was used to locally assess cell morphology. An Alamar Blue assay was also used to assess metabolic activity on ppAAm-modified scaffolds as a comparison to that observed on the unmodified scaffolds. For this assay, 6 repeats were used. Control surface chemistries were produced as planer samples on glass cover slips coated with the plasma polymers under the same conditions as the scaffolds. Water contact angle measurements were conducted to assess the wettability of flat surfaces using deionized water, with an average of 5 repeats on each surface being taken. Normally the control samples were coated in the same plasma cycle as the other samples, taking care that substrates were not too close together, as shielding/shadowing problems would cause coating variation.

1.3 Materials

- Deionized water, ~18M ohm cm^{-2}
- Poly(D,L-lactic acid) mol weight 65 kDa (Purac)
- Allylamine (Sigma)
- Hexane (Sigma)
- Phosphate-buffered saline (Oxoid)—store at 4°C
- Penicillin 500 U mL^{-1} (Sigma)
- Streptomycin 0.5 mg mL^{-1} (Sigma)

- Amphotericin B 1.25 μg mL^{-1} (Sigma)
- Trypsin (Sigma)
- 3T3 Fibroblasts (ECACC)
- Alamar Blue (Biosource)
- Hanks balanced salt solution pH 7 (without phenol red) (InVitroGen)—store at 4°C
- Ethanol/water mixtures (by volume in deionized water): 0%, 25%, 50%, 75%, 90%, 95 %, 100 %
- Hexamethyldisilazane (Sigma)
- Glass cover slips 22 mm by 22 mm (TAAB)
- LIVE/DEAD Viability/Cytotoxicity Assay Kit (Molecular Probes, L3224)—store at <−20°C, protect from light.
- DABCO UV mountant (Vector)
- Paraformaldehyde (Sigma)
- 2% osmium tetroxide solution diluted before use with PBS to make a 1% solution

1.4 Methods

1.4.1 Scaffold preparation

Poly(D,L-lactic acid) ($P_{DL}LA$) was used in this study for the production of porous scaffolds. PTFE molds were used that fit neatly into a high-pressure autoclave [30] (although a similar high-pressure/temperature controlled vessel would be suitable), which was then pressurized with $scCO_2$ to liquefy the polymer. On release of the CO_2 as gas, foamed scaffolds were formed.

Place the powdered $P_{DL}LA$ in a PTFE container and liquefy the polymer in $scCO_2$ at 35°C and 17.32 MPa [31]. PTFE containers having a 10-mm diameter and 10-mm depth were used in this study. A schematic of the $scCO_2$ apparatus is shown in Figure 1.1.

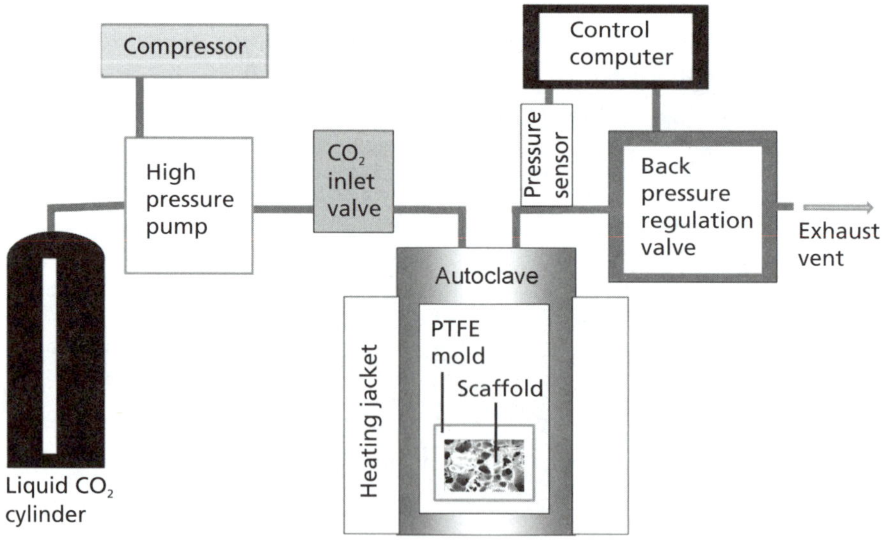

Figure 1.1 Schematic of the supercritical CO_2 apparatus for producing foamed polymer scaffolds.

Release the pressure over 30 minutes to form the scaffolds by the release of carbon dioxide [32].

A *skin* is normally formed around the edge of the scaffold due to the interaction with the mold walls as the gas is released. A thin layer of polymer remains, which contains much smaller pores and must be removed. Remove the outer skin of the scaffold using a blade to reveal the 85% porous material having pores in the range ~160–300 μm.

Wash the materials using deionized water (18M ohm cm^{-2}) by incubation for 24 hours on a roller mixer. This step allows any soluble impurities to be removed, which is encouraged by agitation.

Blow dry using nitrogen or air dry in sterile conditions.

1.4.2 Deposition of plasma polymers

A radio-frequency plasma apparatus constructed from a boro-silicate glass T-piece sealed with metal end plates was employed for the plasma-polymer deposition. An RF potential (13.56 MHz) was applied to copper electrodes external to the chamber, using manual impedance matching to stabilize the plasma. Monomer ingress is controlled using a series of values, adjusted to maintain a constant pressure within the chamber, which is monitored by an internal pressure sensor [33]. A quartz crystal microbalance is also fitted to monitor the mass of the polymer and the rate of deposition. As with most plasma-polymerization systems, this system was constructed in-house. A schematic is presented in Figure 1.2 [20].

Degas monomers by freezing and reducing pressure during the warm up. Repeat this several times if necessary.

1. Insert scaffolds into the plasma coating chamber, and label the face on the support that will be shielded during deposition.
2. Evacuate the chamber to 10^{-2} torr or lower for ~5 minutes.
3. In this study, deposition conditions were altered to assess the differences of plasma-grafted and plasma-deposited polymers at 3-W and 20-W input powers. All scaffolds were pretreated in oxygen plasma stabilized at 300 mtorr with an input power of 3W for 3 minutes.

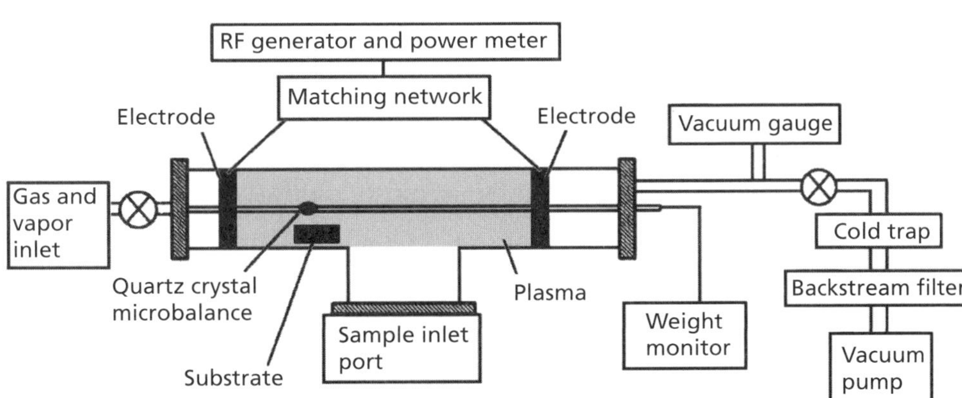

Figure 1.2 Schematic of the plasma coater.

4. Monomer vapor should then be flooded into the chamber with conditions differing dependant on the treatment:

   (a) For grafted polymers, the etched samples should then be exposed to allyamine vapor for a further 10 minutes.

   (b)For plasma-deposited polymers (ppAAm), stabilize the allylamine vapor in the chamber at 300 mtorr and ignite plasma at an input power of either 3W or 20W for 4 minutes.
5. If adding ppHex, stabilize the hexane vapor in the chamber at 300 mtorr and light plasma at an input power of 20W for 5 minutes. The deposition rate of ppHex is lower than that of ppAAm, allowing only the outermost pores to be coated. Note: Flat chemically modified surfaces were prepared as above by first depositing ppAAm, followed by the deposition of ppHex after partial masking of the surface.
6. Return to a 10^{-2} vacuum to remove any hazardous vapor before removing samples from the chamber. *Tip:* When using allylamine all inlets and o-rings should be cleaned prior to use, using suitable solvents such as acetone for metal parts and water for o-rings. Allylamine polymerizes easily and can leave residues in glassware and in vacuum lines. If starting conditions are not clean, the identity of the afforded surface coating will be unknown. This is particularly relevant when depositing different polymers in subsequent runs. The cleaning of the plasma chamber via oxygen plasma etch should be carried out between depositions to ensure reproducibility. Furthermore, degradation of the o-rings in needle valves is a common occurrence, leading to poor flow rate reproducibility. Regular inspection of these items is recommended so that they can be replaced before they fail. Samples are best left for at least 24 hours before use to minimize the effects of any surface residual reactive species (e.g., radicals) after plasma-polymer deposition.

1.4.3 Surface analysis

1.4.3.1 X-ray photoelectron spectroscopy

1. Quantitative surface analysis should be conducted using X-ray photoelectron spectroscopy (XPS) using monochromated Al Kα radiation to allow small spot analysis.
2. Mechanically section the scaffold at 2-mm below and parallel to the circular face.
3. Collect spectral data from areas across the sample at a 1-mm interval. *Tip:* The topography of the porous sample is likely to degrade the spectral quality unless the sample position is manually fine tuned at each analysis point.
4. Use the elemental nitrogen concentration to determine the relative amount of ppAAm at each point. On a flat surface a ppAAm coating thickness could be readily calculated; however, on the sectioned surface of the scaffold this is not possible [17].

1.4.3.2 Water contact angle

The measurement of water contact angles is a quick method to assess the surface modification using the wettability of the surface. Taking measurements at different positions allows analysis of the changing wettability across the surface. A KSV CAM200 instrument was used in this study.

1. Dispense a ~1-μL droplet of deionized water (18M ohm cm^{-2}) onto the sample surface, and immediately take an image as the droplet rests and the injection needle is removed.
2. The drop shape can be used along with tangents to the drop at the solid/liquid contact line to estimate the water contact angle through the droplet. A Young-Laplace function is fit to the drop profile and the angle measured between this and a straight line placed through the intersection of the drop and surface by the operator.
3. At least five repeating static contact angle measurements should be carried out to give an average value.

1.4.4 Cell culture on scaffolds

1. Prepare a solution of phosphate-buffered saline (PBS) with 1× and 5× antibiotic/antimycotic (500 U mL^{-1} penecillin, 0.5 mg mL^{-1} streptomycin, 1.25 mg mL^{-1} amphotericin B).
2. Prewet samples using PBS 5× antibiotic/antimycotic solution for 1 hour on a roller mixer.
3. Exchange the solution for a 1× antibiotic/antimycotic solution and incubate samples for 24 hours on a roller mixer.
4. Place scaffolds in a 24-well unmodified plate (Nunc).
5. Prepare cell culture media: 10% fetal calf serum, 1% glutamine in DMEM at 37°C.
6. Remove cells from the passage culture. Here we investigated the culture of 3T3 fibroblasts derived from an albino Swiss mouse embryo, although similar preparations can be carried out using other cell types.
   (a) Remove the media and wash cells with PBS.
   (b) Add 1-ml 0.5% trypsin in PBS and incubate at 37°C for 5 minutes. Note: The trypsin concentration should be adjusted according to cell type.
   (c) Remove cells in the solution and add them directly into 5-ml cell culture media.
   (d) Centrifuge at ~36 RCF – 200 RCF for 5 minutes.
   (e) Resuspend cell pellet in media.
7. Seed scaffolds with 3T3 fibroblasts to a density of 2×10^6 cells per scaffold.
8. Incubate for an appropriate time at 37°C, 5% CO_2. In this study 24–25-hour cultures were used for the assessment of metabolic activity and cell viability, with 7-day cultures allowing observation of cell colonies over a longer period.

1.4.5 Alamar Blue assay

1. Prepare Alamar Blue working solution 10% in Hanks Buffered Saline Solution (HBSS). HBSS without a phenol red indicator should be used.
2. Remove scaffolds from cell culture media and wash three times in HBSS to remove any phenol red, unbound cells, and proteins from the media.
3. Incubate scaffolds in assay solution for 1 hour with gentle agitation.
4. Take 100-μL aliquots of the assay solution from each scaffold and place in a 96 well plate.

5. Measure fluorescence at an excitation wavelength of 560 nm and emission at 590 nm using a fluorescence plate reader.

1.4.6 Cell viability assay on scaffolds

An assay using fluorescent probes can be conducted using a fluorescent microscope, although more detailed imaging can be obtained using a confocal system, especially when 3D structures are under investigation. Cell viability can be assessed after seeding onto the scaffolds using a two-color fluorescence cell viability assay.

1. Culture cells for an appropriate time. In this study, cell viability was assessed after 25 hours.
2. Following protocol for the live/dead viability/cytotoxicity assay kit (Molecular Probes), scaffolds should be removed from the culture media and washed three times in PBS to remove or dilute the serum in the media.
3. Warm the live/dead viability assay to room temperature.
4. Add 20 μL of the 2-mM ethidium homodimer-1 stock solution to 10-mL phenol red free HBSS, and vortex to mix.
5. Add 5 μL of the 4-mM calcein AM stock solution and vortex again to mix thoroughly to make the live/dead assay working solution.
6. Add working solution prewarmed to 37°C to each scaffold to ensure all cells are covered with the solution.
7. Incubate for 40 minutes at room temperature under sterile conditions. This step should be carried out in a covered vessel to minimize evaporation.
8. Wash the scaffolds in PBS via pipette, being careful not to remove any cells through high shear stress.
9. Using DABCO UV mountant, fix the scaffold.
10. When dry, cut into sections to reveal the interior of the scaffold cross section.

1.4.7 Scanning electron microscopy

1. Remove the scaffolds from the cell culture and wash three times in PBS.
2. Prepare 4% paraformaldehyde in PBS and incubate over the scaffolds overnight at 4°C.
3. Wash in PBS.
4. If conducting microcomputer tomography, also incubate scaffolds for a further 2 hours in 1% osmium tetroxide solution prepared in deionized water.
5. Wash with deionized water.
6. Dehydrate scaffolds through a series of ethanol concentrations (25%, 50%, 70%, 90%, 95%, and 100%).
7. Submerge samples in hexamethyldisilazane (HMDS) for 2 minutes before air drying in a fume hood. Note: HMDS is volatile and toxic and should only be used in a ventilated fume hood.
8. Sputter coat samples with ~10–20 nm of gold.
9. SEM images should be taken at ~10 kV to minimize the risk of sample degradation.

1.4.8 Microcomputed tomography of scaffolds

A 3D reconstruction of cell distribution can be achieved using a high-resolution micro-CT system. A μCT 40, Scanco Medical system was used in this work.

1. Set scanner voltage to 55 kV and current at 145 mA, scanning samples at a 8-µm voxel resolution with an integration time of 300 ms.
2. Image reconstruction can be afforded by taking ~20 slices from the center of the scaffold, analyzing for osmium tetroxide stained cells.
3. Radio dense areas can be compared to give an indication of cell distribution.
4. Cell areas calculated from each slice allow an average to be calculated.

1.5 Data Acquisition, Anticipated Results, and Interpretation

The use of plasma polymers to chemically modify materials allows varied functional groups to be investigated. By overlaying one polymer over another and gradually changing the coverage, it is possible to obtain a gradient change in surface chemistry [17]. Here this is particularly useful as the surface presents amine and other nitrogen-containing functionalities [19]; the change in surface chemistry promotes cell attachment and an overlaid hydrocarbon surface is used to hinder cell adhesion in specific regions. This is first carried out on a planar model plasma-polymer modified surface to readily confirm that the desired cell response is achieved, and then on the porous scaffold [17]. To counteract the greater probability of cell adhesion during culture at the periphery of the scaffold, a gradual increase of the cell adhesive nature of the scaffold surface towards the core of the scaffold is achieved using a ppAAm-ppHex gradient. Investigation of the surface chemistry is therefore paramount to study the effects of this plasma polymer deposition technique. X-ray photoelectron spectroscopy and water contact angle measurements were made to assess the surface, with a cell culture being carried out to observe the effects of the plasma polymer coating on cell distribution, attachment, and viability on the modified scaffolds.

1.5.1 Surface analysis

1.5.1.1 XPS

X-ray photoelectron spectroscopy (XPS) allows elemental analysis of the surface to be conducted. In this study, XPS was carried out on a Kratos Axis Ultra instrument using monochromated Al Kα radiation, a magnetic immersion lens, and charge compensating electron flood. Average readings were conducted over areas measuring 0.3 × 0.7 mm using an analysis time of approximately 20 minutes. Elemental and functional quantification was obtained using CASA software (developed by Neal Fairly, United Kingdom). Synthetic peak shapes of the Gaussian/Laurenzian ratio between 50 to 70 were used. A linear background was applied to the core levels. Empirically determined sensitivity factors, supplied by the instrument manufacturers, have been used to quantify the elemental compositions. For XPS, the accuracy of the elemental quantification may be as low as 15% due to uncertainties in the sensitivity factors and background shape; however, the

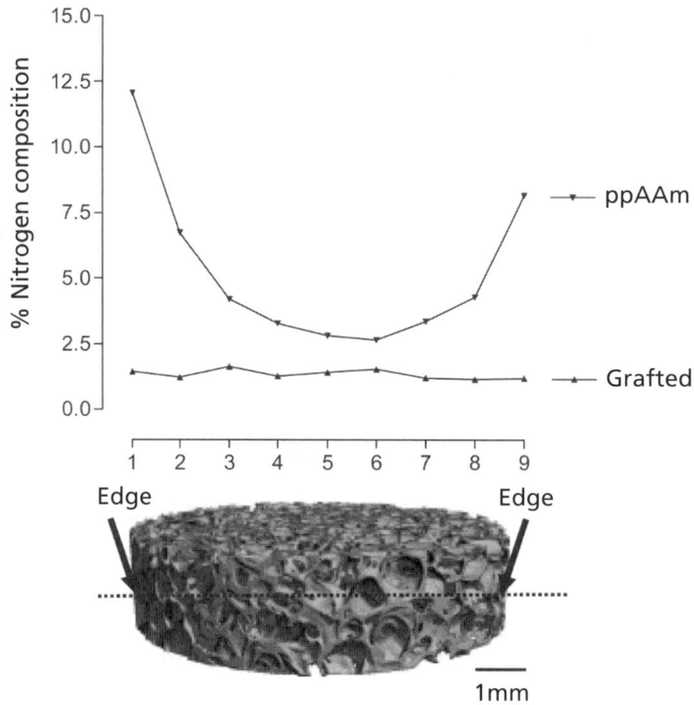

Figure 1.3 Surface nitrogen concentration as determined by XPS. Measurements were conducted at set intervals across the internal diameter of grafted and ppAAm-deposited scaffolds (20W input power) as depicted by the dotted line in the computed tomography image. A background level of 0.39 % nitrogen was recorded using unmodified $P_{DL}LA$ scaffolds as the control. (Image reprinted with permission from Wiley-VCH, copyright 2005.)

precision is significantly higher as indicated by the error bars estimated using a Monte Carlo analysis of the data.

After chemical modification, the scaffolds were mechanically sectioned and XPS analyses acquired in a straight line at 1-mm intervals from edge to edge passing through the center. Consideration of the nitrogen concentration revealed that the grafted allylamine coating was consistent across the cross-section of the sample, whereas ppAAm treatment resulted in a coating of variable thickness. High nitrogen concentrations were detected for the ppAAm-treated scaffold at the exterior, which fell to lower concentrations towards the center of the sample, yet were still significantly greater than the uncoated control analysis, seen in Figure 1.3. The exact position of the analysis relative to the edge results in the variable maximum nitrogen concentration on the two sides of the section. A true measure of the nitrogen concentration should be achieved by analyzing the exterior surface of the other half of the section. In this study, the ppAAm deposited on the outside using 20-W input power was found using this method to give rise to 13.7 %. Subsequently, a thin ppHex coating was deposited for 5 minutes as described in Section 1.4.2. Analysis of this section revealed that deposition of ppHex on the ppAAm surface modified the profile of the surface nitrogen, indicated by a decrease in nitrogen concentration at the outer analysis point commensurate with an overlayer of ppHex. The change in the profile is consistent with the analysis of the top surface, although the absolute compositions are not directly comparable because the section analysis contains cut $P_{DL}LA$ that could not have been coated. The combination of these two analyses confirms that the sequential deposition resulted in ppHex localized at the peripheral regions of the scaffold. This provides a route to modify the radial nitrogen functionality distribution from one decreasing from the outer surface to one that was lower at the outer surface compared to the adjacent inner region.

1.5.1.2 Water contact angle

Wettability of surfaces gives an indication of the terminal surface chemistry and is particularly useful when comparing a change in chemistry (e.g., from hydrophilic amine to hydrophobic alkane). On flat surfaces, an average contact angle using at least five droplets gives a good estimation of the true value. Anomalies can occur due to surface scratches or contamination (either chemically or by dust), and it is important not to make a measurement on the same sample spot more than once. The difference observed in the water contact angles of ppHex ($87° \pm 2.7°$) and ppAAm ($38° \pm 2.1°$) will influence protein adsorption and/or their conformation once adsorbed; therefore, it is anticipated that cells are driven to preferentially adhere to the more hydrophilic ppAAm surface. This was observed on flat substrates as demonstrated in Figure 1.4.

1.5.2 Investigation of cell culture on modified scaffolds

1.5.2.1 Alamar Blue assay

An Alamar Blue assay is used for the investigation of cellular metabolic activity. Here the assay was carried out after a 24-hour culture to observe the responses of cells after being seeded onto ppAAm scaffolds. The Alamar Blue dye changed from blue to red by mitochondrial enzymes. An average of six repeats were carried out for each scaffold with a one-way analysis of variance followed by a Tukey-Kramer post-hoc test being carried out to determine the significant differences in metabolic activity (significance >95%).

The ppAAm scaffolds were found to show a higher metabolic activity compared to untreated $P_{DL}LA$ scaffolds (Figure 1.5). Plasma-deposited polymers showed higher activity compared to grafted polymers although higher input powers showed little increase.

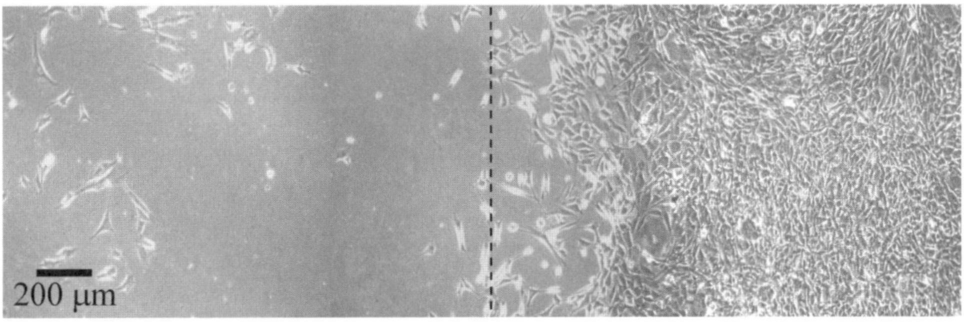

Figure 1.4 Phase contrast image of 3T3 fibroblasts cultured for 7 days on a glass surface coated with ppHex on the left and ppAAm on the right. (Image reprinted with permission from Wiley-VCH, copyright 2006.)

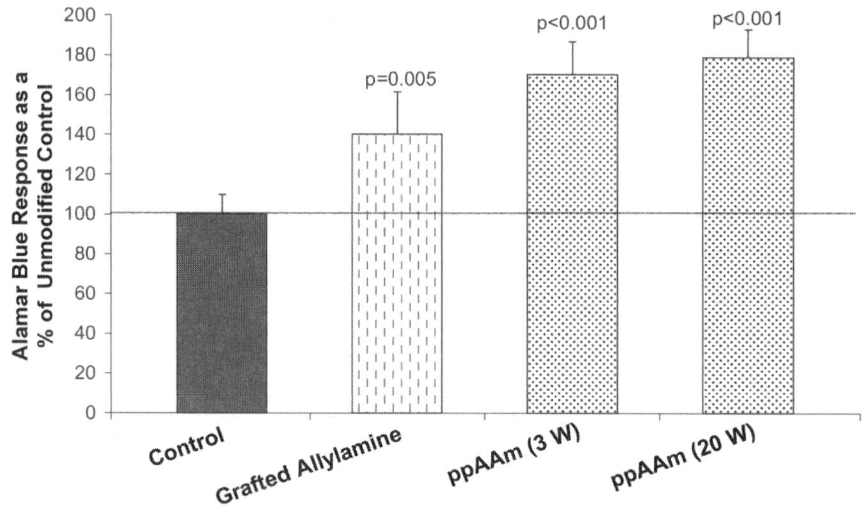

Figure 1.5 Alamar Blue activity of the modified/unmodified scaffolds. Statistical significance (p) is determined by the analysis of variance (ANOVA) using the Tukey-Kramer multiple comparison post-test. (Image reprinted with permission from Wiley-VCH, copyright 2005.)

1.5.2.2 Cell viability assay

A live/dead stain assessed using confocal microscopy can indicate the viability of cultured cells. Segments of the modified scaffolds were cut after 25 hours in the culture and stained (Figure 1.6). The green fluorescence indicates the presence of live cells with no dead cells apparent. Both ppAAm only and ppAAm/ppHex-modified scaffolds were analyzed, showing similar responses on all modified surfaces after this time in culture.

1.5.2.3 Scanning electron microscopy

Scanning electron microscopy (SEM) is a useful tool for the investigation of topography, both of the scaffold material itself and of the cultured cells. Fixation of the cells is necessary to lock in their morphology. The spreading of cells often indicates a good response to a substrate, although the exact morphology will be largely dependent on the cell type. Here the fibroblasts were found to cluster together on untreated $P_{DL}LA$, indicating that they preferred to adhere to each other over the surface. The rounded nature of these cells further suggests that the surface chemistry was not conducive for cell attachment. Grafted allylamine surfaces presented a mixture of rounded and stellate-flattened cells indicating the surface modification improved cell adhesion. The cells on ppAAm-coated scaffolds were well spread, indicating an affinity for the surface. Cell density and morphologies on modified scaffolds is shown in Figure 1.7.

1.5.2.4 Microcomputed tomography

The distribution of cells through the scaffold can be determined using X-ray microcomputed tomography (μCT) using osmium tetroxide to label the cells to provide sufficient X-ray absorption contrast to distinguish them from the $P_{DL}LA$. Figure 1.8 shows reconstructed μCT sections though the center of Figure 1.8(a, i) $P_{DL}LA$, Figure

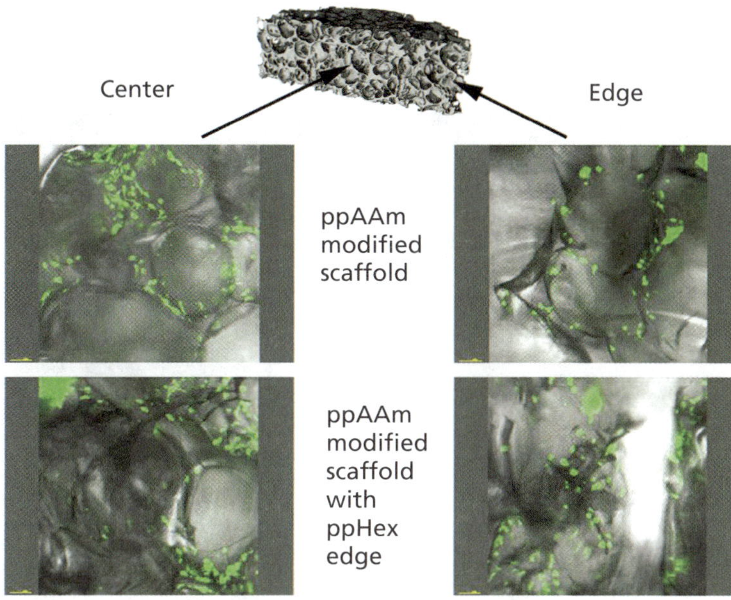

Figure 1.6 Confocal images of scaffolds showing cell viability after 25 hours using live/dead assay. Green represents live cells with no visible red areas denoting dead cells.

1.8(a, ii) P_{DL}LA coated with ppAAm, and Figure 1.8(a, iii) P_{DL}LA coated with ppAAm followed by ppHex on the outer edge of the scaffold, along with a graph showing comparative cell area data for the three surfaces [Figure 1.8(b)]. The cells are indicated in red, showing a high density restricted to outermost pores of the unmodified scaffold. The inhomogeneity of this cell colony would be likely to lead to tissue formation only around the periphery of the scaffold. After ppAAm modification (data shown for a 20-W deposition), a marked increase in cellular penetration into the scaffold was observed. One method to quantify the cell distribution is to assess the cell number in slices through the central region of the scaffold. Here 20 slices were taken with a separation of 8 μm. An outer edge region was imposed to allow a comparison of cell numbers attaching to the outer edge and those penetrating into the core of the scaffold; a circle having a radius of 3.54 mm was chosen to dissect the sample into two parts having equal volumes. Caution should be taken when imposing such regional markers, the positioning of such may give rise to dramatic changes in cell distribution, especially if using different sample shapes and volumes.

From the μCT reconstructed images, an increase in cell density penetrating the core of the scaffold is clear after ppAAm modification, although a higher concentration of cells in the outer region can be seen when the data is presented in a graphical form [Figure 1.8(b)]. The addition of a ppHex coating shows a marked effect on the distribution of cells. A slight reduction of cells was observed at the edges, but most importantly a greater cell density was observed in the core of the scaffold, providing a fairly homogenous distribution. A major point of interest is the high density of cells at the upper half of the scaffold. This is probably a result of the favorable possibility of cells settling on the top of the scaffold.

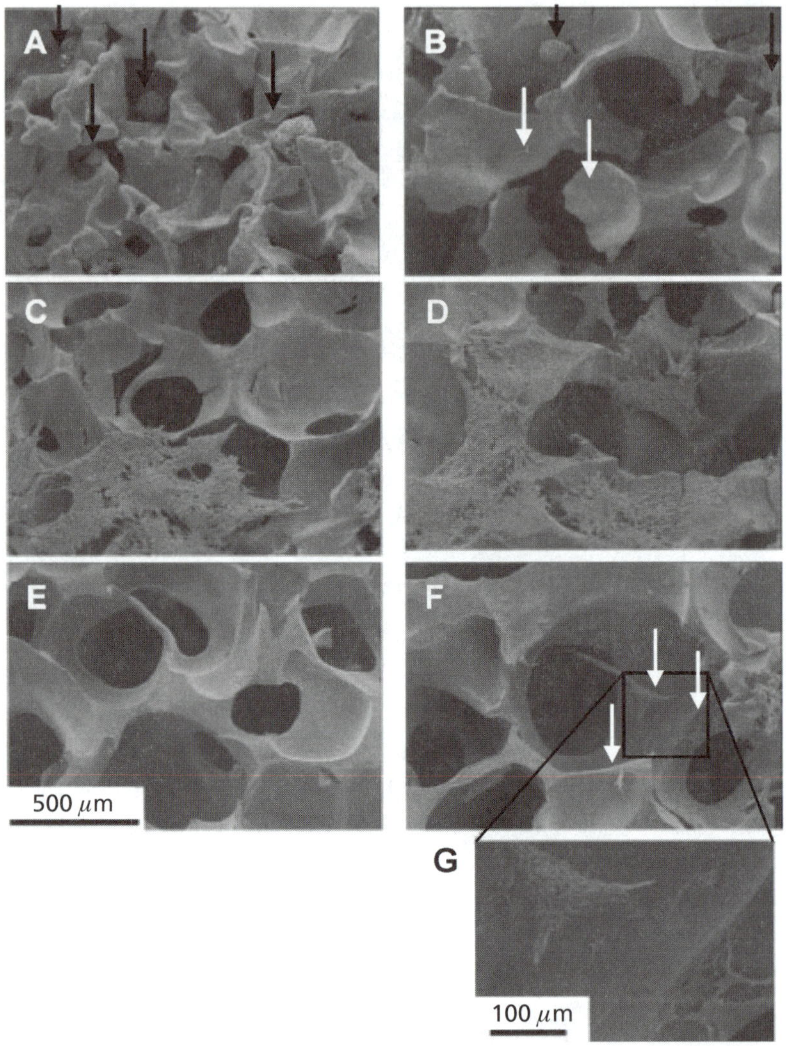

Figure 1.7 SEM images of 3T3 fibroblasts cultured for 24 hours on (a) unmodified $P_{DL}LA$, (b) allylamine grafted $P_{DL}LA$, ppAAm modified $P_{DL}LA$ at (c) 3-W and (d) 20-W input power. Images (a–d) are from the outer edges of the scaffold and (e, f) are representative of the unmodified/grafted (e) and plasma-polymerized 3W (f) inner surfaces. All images are of the same magnification. Images (e, f) were taken approximately in the center of the scaffold. White arrows denote cells that have assumed characteristic fibroblast morphology and black arrows denote cells that have not. Image (g) shows a higher magnified region of (f), highlighting cell adhesion on the modified scaffold. (Image reprinted with permission from Wiley-VCH, copyright 2005.)

1.6 Discussion and Commentary

We have illustrated that chemical surface modification can be performed using plasma polymerization to form a nanometer thin, conformal coating while retaining the bulk properties of the substrate. This technique is very versatile, allowing coatings to be produced on substrates of any shape and size using monomers chosen for the cell type required [e.g., if ppAAm does not encourage cell adhesion, plasma polymerized acrylic acid (pAAc) usually does] [34]. Here we present a method successfully using plasma poly-

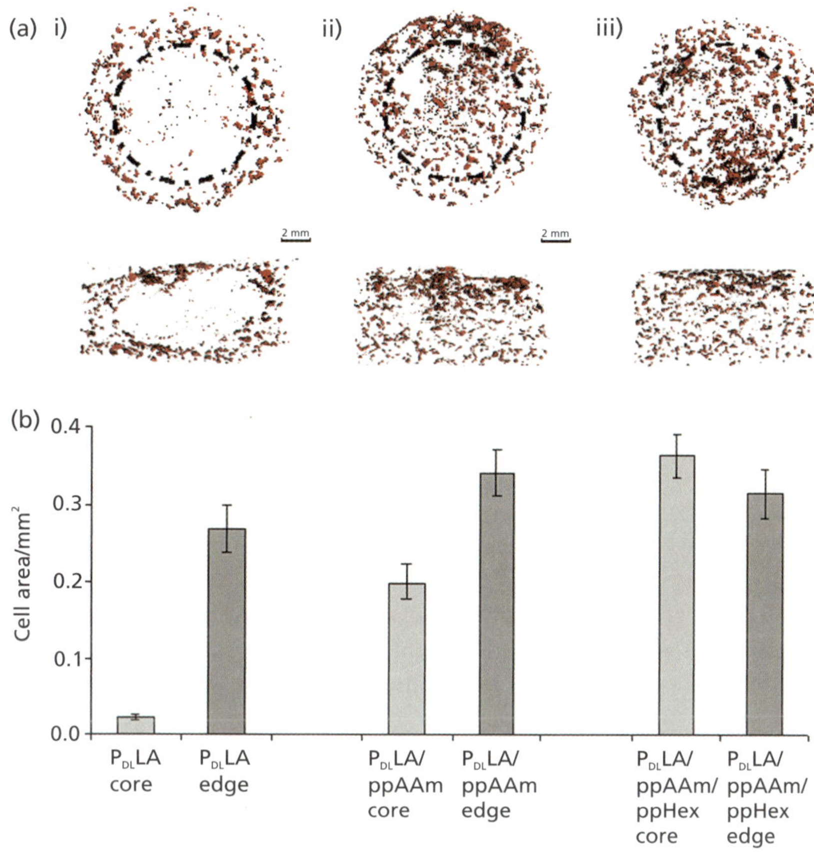

Figure 1.8 (a) Reconstructed images of 3T3 fibroblast density on scaffolds using microcomputed tomography: (i) $P_{DL}LA$, (ii) $P_{DL}LA$/ppAAm (20W), and (iii) $P_{DL}LA$/ppAAm (20W)/ppHex. The lower images show a cross-section of 2 mm cut through the center of the scaffold. (b) The cumulative cell area within a 0.01 mm central slice of the scaffold, within and outside a central region denoted by the black dotted lines in (a).

mer deposition to chemically modify the interior of porous scaffolds promoting cell attachment. Furthermore, problems associated with inhomogenous cell distributions caused by preferential colonization of the outer edges of the scaffold have been overcome by the addition of a plasma-polymerized hexane coating on the outermost scaffold regions. We demonstrate the efficiency of this method to produce modified $P_{DL}LA$ scaffolds populated by an evenly distributed culture of 3T3 fibroblasts, showing excellent viability and increased overall metabolic activity (indicating an increase in cell number) compared to those on untreated $P_{DL}LA$ scaffolds.

In this chapter we present the methodology of plasma-polymer deposition, including a protocol to assess variation in plasma-coating conditions if applied to other scaffold types. Allylamine grafting via pre-etching the substrate in oxygen was shown to increase metabolic activity compared to untreated $P_{DL}LA$ scaffolds; however, depositing a ppAAm gave rise to a further increase, as indicated by the Alamar Blue assay (Figure 1.5). Previous reports have suggested that functionalization using amine groups promotes preferential adsorption of cell-adhesive proteins such as vironectin and fibronectin, and therefore gives rise to more receptive surfaces for cell adhesion [35].

Elemental analysis of the grafted and plasma polymerized coating at different input powers showed increased nitrogen content indicating the presence of surface nitrogen groups (Figure 1.3).

Grafted polymers showed only a modest increase in surface nitrogen, although this was uniform through the thickness, and it was enough to elicit an increase in cell attachment and activity. Fibroblast morphology on allylamine-grafted surfaces was found to be spread and more characteristically stellate-shaped as would be seen on tissue culture plastic, rather than rounded with cells forming clusters on unmodified $P_{DL}LA$. This response was, however, localized at the outer edges of the scaffold and did not promote cell adhesion in the core of the scaffold.

Plasma-deposited polymers were found to have a higher nitrogen surface concentration than the grafted surfaces. Nitrogen levels were higher at the edges and dropped towards the center to levels still approximately twice that found on grafted polymers. 3T3 fibroblasts were found to adhere in high numbers although again formed higher densities at the edges of the scaffolds, with fewer becoming established at the core. The live/dead assay indicated that surface modifications allowed cell culture with excellent viability, along with the Alamar Blue assay, which demonstrated increased metabolic activity on all amine functionalized surfaces. Higher input power during plasma coating also gave rise to a slight increase in metabolic activity, suggesting that surfaces prepared at 20W are more suited to cell culture applications. This is possibly because these materials are more cross-linked and may contribute to longer-term stability of the functionalization during culture conditions.

The addition of a ppHex coating on the outer edges of the 20-W ppAAm-coated scaffolds allowed a greater ingress of cells into the scaffold, giving rise to an almost homogeneous distribution except for the upper section. This was probably due to shielding of the bottom scaffold face during cell culture, which is likely to be circumvented by suspending the scaffold in the culture media.

In this chapter, we have covered aspects of plasma coating methodology onto planer and porous 3D scaffolds, demonstrating the use of ppAAm and ppHex as useful surface chemical modifications to guide cell attachment and enhance activity over 3T3 fibroblasts cultured directly on unmodified $P_{DL}LA$. Surface analysis methods have been reported to follow the effects of coating conditions to ensure optimized cell culture. This method can be extended to use different monomers to incorporate differing functionalities onto substrates of almost any size and shape, although coating conditions may have to be adjusted to suit the application using procedures detailed within this article. To assess the responses of different cell types to chemistry, it may be useful to observe cell growth on plasma polymer–modified planer surfaces prior to experimentation on 3D scaffolds.

Troubleshooting Table: Maximum of 8 Critical Step Items

Problem	Potential Explanation	Potential Solutions
Plasma polymer deposition not achieved.	Plasma in chamber not optimized in area of sample.	Manual impedance matching requires modification while observing the location of the plasma glow and reflected power.
Scaffold shows physical change after plasma polymerization.	Plasma conditions too harsh resulting in too great an energy transfer into the polymer. Scaffolds should also be thoroughly dehydrated prior to modification.	Reduce incident RF power and treatment time.
WCA for ppHex too low or ppAAm to high.	Contamination during/after coating.	Make sure glassware, monomers, and vacuum lines are clean. Degas monomers thoroughly immediately before use. (Prepolymerized allylamine will give a much more intense pink plasma, which may indicate a fresh monomer is required or vacuum lines need cleaning.)
Cells do not attach well to the inner surfaces of the scaffold.	ppAAm coating not completely entering the scaffold, or ppHex layer too thick.	This may result from the use of larger samples than reported here. Use of longer deposition times for ppAAm will ensure better distribution of coating into scaffold and/or shorter deposition times for ppHex.
Cells do not adhere to the planar surface intended to promote adhesion.	Cell type requires a different surface chemistry to encourage adhesion.	Use another plasma polymer, first trying one with an opposite surface charge (e.g., if ppAAm does not work, try plasma polymerized acrylic acid).
Cell location using X-ray μCT is indistinct.	Check voxel size (cells protrude only 5 microns). Contamination by radiodense material (i.e., with PBS or inclusion of radio dense materials, or osmium tetroxide–absorbing materials in the culture media).	Check scan parameters. Verify scan information with the live/dead stain or histology. Beam can be hardened by the addition of a metal filter to reduce the scaffold signature.

1.7 Application Notes

Plasma polymerization can be used to form chemical coatings on all surfaces, and has been widely used on planer substrates. In this chapter, we explain the versatility of the method and the application of allylamine coatings for enhanced cell culture of fibroblasts, which was chosen as a model to illustrate the method. The main advance reported here is the extension of this technique to the chemical modification of porous 3D scaffolds for tissue engineering applications. We give information on how to assess the effects of coating conditions on cell culture, comparing grafting and plasma polymerization at two different input powers. The addition of a second coating of plasma polymerized hexane on the outer edges of the scaffold allows a greater ingress of cells into the core by restricting initial adhesion on the periphery. The uniform cell distribution achieved is an important prerequisite to viable tissue formation.

The method described can be applied to a variety of materials where the bulk properties are already optimized. This may be particularly important for the study of cells with surfaces having defined elastic properties, for instance. In our study, $P_{DL}LA$ was used as a scaffold material due to its biodegradability, whereas others may use copolymers or blends of $P_{DL}LA$/poly(glycolic acid) for their specific material properties. Although the chemical modification does not affect the bulk properties, there may be a reduction in the dissolution of degradable materials due to the coating acting as a barrier at the interface. Variation of the coating conditions allows fine tuning for optimization. Our report demonstrates such an optimization procedure, showing that excellent 3T3 fibroblast attachment and viability can be achieved within the inner core of porous scaffolds using ppAAm.

1.8 Summary Points

1. We have shown how plasma-polymerized allylamine chemical modification can enhance 3T3 fibroblast adhesion while it is reduced by plasma-polymerized hexane. Glass cover slip samples were used to readily assess the cell type response and this was then applied in porous scaffolds.
2. Grafted and plasma polymerized allylamine surface coatings were compared in terms of cell viability using the Alamar Blue assay, revealing an improved total cell metabolic activity on both, compared to the unmodified $P_{DL}LA$. ppAAm had the highest metabolic activity. XPS results showed that ppAAm had higher surface concentrations of amino groups corresponding to higher cellular activity.
3. On flat surfaces, plasma-polymerized hexane was shown to reduce cell attachment, in comparison to neighboring ppAAm regions. The application of ppHex on the outer edge of scaffolds drastically improved cell distribution throughout the scaffold, which was observed using microcomputed tomography for osmium tetroxide–stained cells.
4. Adequate surface characterization is necessary to ensure the desired surface chemistry is obtained. Water contact angle measurements are useful for comparing surfaces or examining changes in surface chemistry, although it was necessary to carry out a detailed analysis of chemical composition for this new process using XPS.

Acknowledgments

The authors acknowledge financial support from the Medical Research Council (Grant reference number: G0701849).

References

[1] Mandal, B. B., and S. C. Kundu, "Osteogenic and Adipogenic Differentiation of Rat Bone Marrow Cells on Non-Mulberry and Mulberry Silk Gland Fibroin 3D Scaffolds," *Biomaterials*, Vol. 30, 2009, pp. 5019–5030.

[2] Obradovic, B., et al., "Towards Functional Cartilage Equivalents: Bioreactor Cultivation of Cell-Polymer Constructs," *Contemporary Studies in Advanced Materials and Processes*, Vol. 413, 2003, pp. 251–256.

[3] Lin, C. H., et al., "A Scaffold-Bioreactor System for a Tissue-Engineered Trachea," *Biomaterials*, Vol. 30, 2009, pp. 4117–4126.

[4] Levenberg, S., et al., "Engineering Vascularized Skeletal Muscle Tissue," *Nat. Biotechnol.*, Vol. 23, 2005, pp. 879–884.

[5] Lee, J. Y., J. W. Lee, and C. E. Schmidt, "Neuroactive Conducting Scaffolds: Nerve Growth Factor Conjugation on Active Ester-Functionalized Polypyrrole," *Journal of the Royal Society Interface*, Vol. 6, 2009, pp. 801–810.

[6] Zhang, H. N., C. Y. Lin, and S. J. Hollister, "The Interaction Between Bone Marrow Stromal Cells and RGD-Modified Three-Dimensional Porous Polycaprolactone Scaffolds," *Biomaterials*, Vol. 30, 2009, pp. 4063–4069.

[7] Koenig, A. L., V. Gambillara, and D. W. Grainger, "Correlating Fibronectin Adsorption with Endothelial Cell Adhesion and Signaling on Polymer Substrates," *J. Biomed. Mater. Res. Part A*, Vol. 64A, 2003, pp. 20–37.

[8] Scotchford, C. A., et al., "Protein Adsorption and Human Osteoblast-Like Cell Attachment and Growth on Alkylthiol on Gold Self-Assembled Monolayers," *J. Biomed. Mater. Res.*, Vol. 59, 2002, pp. 84–99.

[9] Tidwell, C. D., et al., "Endothelial Cell Growth and Protein Adsorption on Terminally Functionalized, Self-Assembled Monolayers of Alkanethiolates on Gold," *Langmuir*, Vol. 13, 1997, pp. 3404–3413.

[10] Cooper, E., et al., "Rates of Attachment of Fibroblasts to Self-Assembled Monolayers Formed by the Adsorption of Alkylthiols onto Gold Surfaces," *J. Mater. Chem.*, Vol. 7, 1997, pp. 435–441.

[11] Scotchford, C. A., et al., "Growth of Human Osteoblast-Like Cells on Alkanethiol on Gold Self-Assembled Monolayers: The Effect of Surface Chemistry," *J. Biomed. Mater. Res.*, Vol. 41, 1998, pp. 431–442.

[12] Keselowsky, B. G., D. M. Collard, and A. J. Garcia, "Surface Chemistry Modulates Fibronectin Conformation and Directs Integrin Binding and Specificity to Control Cell Adhesion," *J. Biomed. Mater. Res. Part A*, Vol. 66A, 2003, pp. 247–259.

[13] France, R. M., et al., "Attachment of Human Keratinocytes to Plasma Co-Polymers of Acrylic Acid Octa-1,7-Diene and Allyl Amine Octa-1,7-Diene," *J. Mater. Chem.*, Vol. 8, 1998, pp. 37–42.

[14] Daw, R., et al., "A Comparative Study of Cell Attachment to Self Assembled Monolayers and Plasma Polymers," *J. Mater. Chem.*, Vol. 8, 1998, pp. 2583–2584.

[15] Daw, R., R. D. Short, and I. M. Brook, "Effect of Functional Group Concentration of Cellular Attachment," *J. Dent. Res.*, Vol. 77, 1998, p. 1263.

[16] France, R. M., et al., "Plasma Copolymerization of Allyl Alcohol 1,7-Octadiene: Surface Characterization and Attachment of Human Keratinocytes," *Chem. Mater.*, Vol. 10, 1998, pp. 1176–1183.

[17] Zelzer, M., et al., "Investigation of Cell-Surface Interactions Using Chemical Gradients Formed from Plasma Polymers," *Biomaterials*, Vol. 29, 2008, pp. 172–184.

[18] Mitchell, S. A., N. Emmison, and A. G. Shard, "Spatial Control of Cell Attachment Using Plasma Micropatterned Polymers," *Surf. Interface Anal.*, Vol. 33, 2002, pp. 742–747.

[19] Shard, A. G., et al., "A NEXAFS Examination of Unsaturation in Plasma Polymers of Allylamine and Propylamine," *J. Phys. Chem. B*, Vol. 108, 2004, pp. 12472–12480.

[20] Dehili, C., et al., "Comparison of Primary Rat Hepatocyte Attachment to Collagen and Plasma-Polymerised Allylamine on Glass," *Plasma Processes and Polymers*, Vol. 3, 2006, pp. 474–484.

[21] Alexander, M. R., et al., "Plasma Polymer Chemical Gradients for Evaluation of Surface Reactivity: Epoxide Reaction with Carboxylic Acid Surface Groups," *J. Mater. Chem.*, Vol. 14, 2004, pp. 408–412.

[22] Bible, E., et al., "The Support of Neural Stem Cells Transplanted into Stroke-Induced Brain Cavities by PGLA Particles," *Biomaterials*, Vol. 30, 2009, pp. 2985–2994.

[23] Yang, J., et al., "A High-Throughput Assay of Cell-Surface Interactions Using Topographical and Chemical Gradients," *Advanced Materials*, Vol. 21, 2009, pp. 300–304.

[24] d' Agostino, R., *Plasma Deposition, Treatment, and Etching of Polymers: The Treatment and Etching of Polymers*, New York: Academic Press, 1990.

[25] Yasuda, H., *Plasma Polymerization*, New York: Academic Press, 1985.

[26] Barry, J. J. A., et al., "Using a Core-Sheath Distribution of Surface Chemistry Through 3D Tissue Engineering Scaffolds to Control Cell Ingress," *Advanced Materials*, Vol. 18, 2006, pp. 1406–1410.

[27] Barry, J. J. A., et al., "Using Plasma Deposits to Promote Cell Population of the Porous Interior of Three-Dimensional Poly(D,L-Lactic Acid) Tissue-Engineering Scaffolds," *Adv. Funct. Mater.*, Vol. 15, 2005, pp. 1134–1140.

[28] Zelzer, M., et al., "Influence of the Plasma Sheath on Plasma Polymer Deposition in Advance of a Mask and Down Pores," *The Journal of Physical Chemistry B*, Vol. 113, 2009, pp. 8487–8494.

[29] Stevens, M. M., and J. H. George, "Exploring and Engineering the Cell Surface Interface," *Science*, Vol. 310, 2005, pp. 1135–1138.

[30] Davies, O. R., et al., "Applications of Supercritical co2 in the Fabrication of Polymer Systems for Drug Delivery and Tissue Engineering," *Adv. Drug Del. Rev.*, Vol. 60, 2008, pp. 373–387.

[31] Pini, R., et al., "Sorption and Swelling Of Poly(D,L-Lactic Acid) and Poly(Lactic-Co-Glycolic Acid) in Supercritical CO_2: An Experimental and Modeling Study," *Journal of Polymer Science Part B-Polymer Physics*, Vol. 46, 2008, pp. 483–496.

[32] Mather, M.L., et al., "Image-Based Characterization of Foamed Polymeric Tissue Scaffolds," *Biomedical Materials*, Vol. 3, 2008.

[33] Bible, E., et al., "Attachment of Stem Cells to Scaffold Particles for Intracerebral Transplantation," *Nature Protocols*, Vol. 4, 2009, pp. 1440–1453.

[34] Haddow, D. B., et al., "Comparison of Proliferation and Growth of Human Keratinocytes on Plasma Copolymers of Acrylic Acid/1,7-Octadiene and Self-Assembled Monolayers," *J. Biomed. Mater. Res.*, Vol. 47, 1999, pp. 379–387.

[35] Yang, J., et al., "Fabrication and Surface Modification of Macroporous Poly(L-Lactic Acid) and Poly(L-Lactic-Co-Glycolic Acid) (70/30) Cell Scaffolds for Human Skin Fibroblast Cell Culture," *J. Biomed. Mater. Res.*, Vol. 62, 2002, pp. 438–446.

CHAPTER

2

Three-Dimensional Cultures in Soft Self-Assembling Nanofibers

Núria Marí-Buyé,[1] Maria Teresa Fernández Muiños,[1] and Carlos E. Semino[1,2,3]

[1]Tissue Engineering Laboratory, Department of Bioengineering, Institut Quimíc de Sarrià, Universidad Ramon LLull, Via Augusta 390, Barcelona, Spain, [2]Translationalcentrum fur Regenerative Medizine (TRM), Universität Leipzig, Johannisallee 30, Leipzig 04103, Germany, [3]Center for Biomedical Engineering, Biological Engineering Division, NE47-383, Massachusetts Institute of Technology, 500 Technology Sq., Cambridge, MA, United States, Corresponding author: Carlos E. Semino, address: Tissue Engineering Laboratory, Department of Bioengineering, Institut Quimíc de Sarrià, Universidad Ramon LLull, Via Augusta 390, Barcelona 08017, Spain, semino@mit.edu, phone +34 932 672 000, fax +34 932 056 266.

Abstract

Here we describe a technique for culturing cells in self-assembling nanofiber scaffolds, an environment that closely mimics the structural context of cells in vivo. This material provides a truly three-dimensional matrix for cells, which allows migration, organization, proliferation, differentiation and, thus, development of their cellular function. Furthermore, self-assembling peptide nanofibers may be easily designed to contain biologically active motifs, for instance, ligands of the extracellular matrix, which would enhance cell behavior for specific applications. We have already described the good performance of this system for different studies and cell types, such as mouse embryonic stem cells differentiation, mouse embryonic fibroblast self-organization, maintenance of hepatocyte function, endothelial cells adhesion, and capillary morphogenesis.

Key terms
differentiation
nanobiomaterials
stem cell
3D scaffolds

2.1 Introduction

Cell culture, maintenance, and differentiation studies in the last decades have been mainly focused on exploring experimental conditions using two-dimensional (2D) cultures, which strictly do not represent the in vivo situation. Although these systems have helped to understand the main cellular molecular mechanisms that govern basic cell processes, it is known that cell-cell and cell-matrix interactions in three-dimensional (3D) systems are crucial to integrate the extensive signaling pathways, the biophysics, and the biomechanics that regulate the development, homeostasis, and regeneration of tissues. For this reason, three-dimensional systems based in the use of natural or synthetic scaffolds may substantially provide to the cells a new integrative level, a new order of complexity, which is an environment where cells can grow, interact, create cellular networks, extend process, migrate, and so forth. This is why, 3D culture systems could give the minimal structural and mechanical input to cells for them to access the necessary environment instruction, and therefore engage in proper proliferation and differentiation as well as morphogenesis, a key factor in the development of functional tissues.

Protein components of connective tissue extracellular matrix, such as collagens, laminins, and fibronectins, have been identified extensibility [1–4]. Interestingly, because of their capacity to form 3D scaffolds and hydrogels, these molecules have been used as natural biomaterials to culture cells in an environment more similar to the extracellular milieu. The most used are collagen type I and complex basement membrane components (Matrigel), which is a mix of collagen type IV, laminin 1, fibronectin, and others. These molecules naturally self-assemble forming a molecular network that ends in spontaneous scaffolds, with a nanometric porous size and mechanical and structural properties of soft tissues—ideal properties for 3D culture.

Molecular self-assembly is the spontaneous organization of chemical entities under thermodynamic equilibrium conditions into structurally stable macromolecules. The driving force of the process is controlled by weak noncovalent interactions such as hydrogen bonds, ionic bonds, electrostatic interactions, van der Waals interactions, and so forth. In recent years, scientists have identified the key parts of molecules—mainly proteins—responsible for the self-assembling process in order to develop new biomaterials [5]. Interestingly, polypeptides with alternating hydrophilic and hydrophobic residues form water-soluble β-sheet structures by self-assembling in the presence of salts [6–9]. One of these peptides, Lysβ-21, corresponding to residues 41–61 of the egg white lysozyme, presents β-sheet configuration and forms gels in water as deduced by IR spectrum and phase diagram data [10]. By molecular design, a family of self-assembling peptides can be obtained. Some of these new peptides are termed DN1, RAD16-I, and KLD12; they are soluble in water and by changing the ionic strength and/or the pH of the solution, with salts of buffers, they form soft hydrogels. In particular, the molecular self-assembling process that ends in the development of a nanofiber network is illustrated with the peptide RAD16-I (Figure 2.1). Self-assembling peptides of this class are good candidates to culture cells because their structural (nanoscale network) and biomechanical properties are similar to natural extracellular matrices [11].

The main advantage of self-assembling peptides over their natural counterparts (proteins) is that they are stable at room temperature for long period of time, which makes them very convenient for storage and distribution purposes. When desired, they can be easily turned into gels by increasing the ionic strength (i.e., in physiological solutions) or adjusting the pH to neutrality (Figure 2.1). Also, cells can be easily encapsulated into

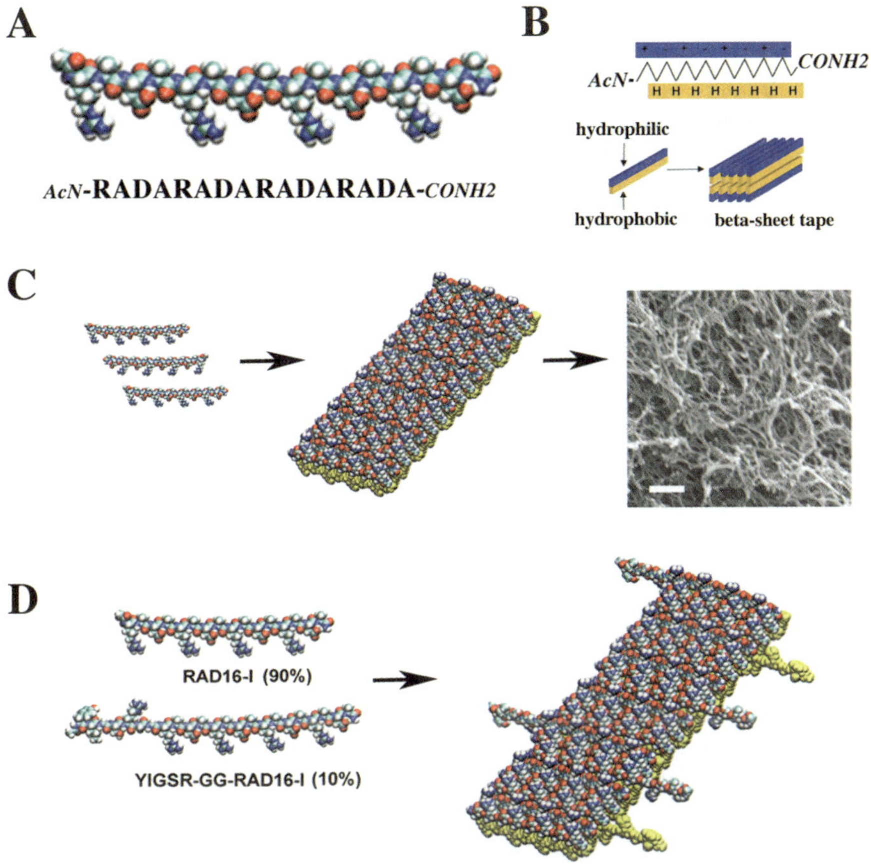

Figure 2.1 Peptide RAD16-I self-assembles into a nanofiber network. An example of a class of self-assembling peptide scaffold of nanometric fibers with injectable properties. The scaffold is biocompatible, biodegradable, and will allow cell seeding. (a) The material per se has not instructive capacity for cells, only structural features (nanofiber network). (b) A molecular model of the nanofiber developed by the self-assembling of RAD16-I molecules. *Note:* The nanofiber is formed by a double tape of assembled RAD16-I molecules in antiparallel b-sheet configuration (top tape in color blue color} and bottom tape in yellow). (c) A RAD16-I nanofiber network by SEM. The white bar represents 200 nm. (d) The peptide RAD16-I can be easily functionalized by solid-phase synthesis by extending at the N-termini. Peptides RAD16-I and its functionalized derivated peptide YIGSR-GG-RAD16-I (AcN-YIGSR-GG- RADARADARADARADA-CONH$_2$) with their respective blending proportions (left). Molecular model of the nanofiber tape obtained after blending peptide RAD16-I (90%) with peptide YIGSR-GG-RAD16-I (10%). *Note:* The minimum-binding peptide domain for the 67-kDa laminin receptor YIGSR—the motif is extending at the sides of the nanofiber tape for proper cellular receptor recognition at the nanoscale level (right).

the nanofiber network in a truly 3D environment. Hence, this class of biomaterial scaffold has often been used to promote in vitro maintenance, growth, and differentiation of a variety of cell types including chondrocytes, hepatocytes, endothelial cells, osteoblasts, neuronal cells, as well as embryonic and somatic stem cells [12–22]. Moreover, a series of in vivo studies has been performed to study implanted cell integration and biosafety as well as protocols to promote or enhance bone, cardiac, and neural tissue regeneration. In the next sections the detailed description of the most relevant cases in vitro and in vivo will be performed.

2.2 Experimental Design

This chapter describes two protocols for the 3D culture of cells using self-assembling peptides as scaffolds. In the encapsulation method, cells are homogeneously mixed with a peptide solution (Figure 2.2, steps 1.1 and 1.2), which is subsequently induced to self-assemble, embedding the cells in a truly 3D environment (Figure 2.2, step 1.3). In the sandwich method cells are disposed as a monolayer in between two gel layers. First the self-assembling of the lower layer is induced, followed by cell attachment, and later the addition and gelation of the upper peptide layer (Figure 2.2, steps 2.1–2.5). One key factor for the success of these cultures is the adjustment of the concentration of the gel for each different study, since it is well known that matrix viscoelasticity affects cellular behavior. As routine controls, the same conditions may be run in two dimensions. It is recommended to culture cells in other 3D matrices, such as collagen type I, which would have better control conditions.

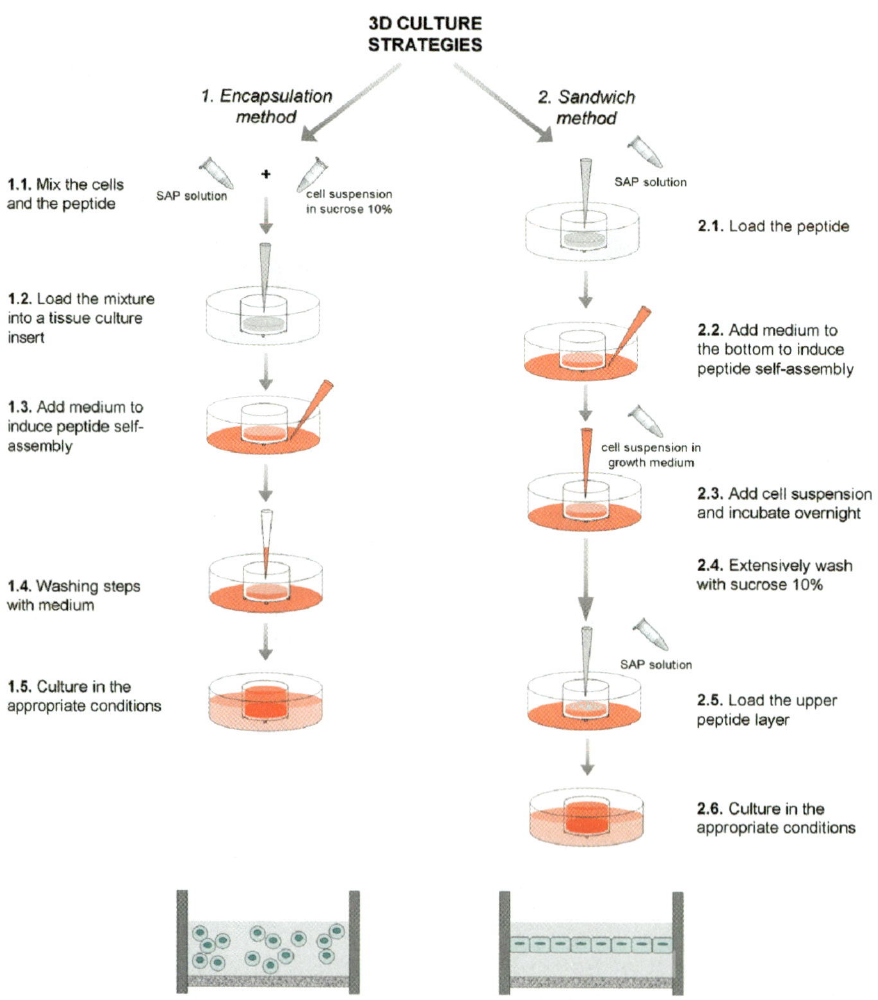

Figure 2.2 Schematic representation of the protocol for 3D cultures in self-assembling peptides. Two strategies are shown: the encapsulation method, where cells are randomly dispersed within the gel, and the sandwich method, where cells are disposed in a monolayer in between two hydrogel layers. SAP stands for self-assembling peptide.

2.3 Materials

2.3.1 Reagents

- RAD16-I peptide solution (PuraMatrix, BD Biosciences)
- Sucrose (tissue culture grade, Sigma)
- Water (tissue culture grade, PAA)
- 0.05%/0.02% Trypsin-EDTA (Invitrogen)
- Cell culture inserts (0.4-μm pore, 12-mm diameter, Millipore)
- Cell growth medium (the appropriate for each cell type)
- *p*-formaldehyde (Sigma)
- Phosphate saline buffer (PBS, tissue culture grade, PAA)
- Isopentane (Sigma)
- Cryomolds (VWR)
- Tissue-Tek O.C.T. (VWR)
- Liquid nitrogen
- 5-bromo-2-deoxyuridine (BrdU, Sigma)
- Anti-BrdU mouse monoclonal antibody IgG1 FITC-conjugated (BD Pharmingen)
- Hydrochloric acid
- Blocking buffer: 20% fetal bovine serum, 0.1% Triton X-100 and 1% dimethyl sulfoxide in PBS
- Live/Dead Viability/Cytotoxicity Kit (Invitrogen)
- RIPA buffer (Sigma)
- Complete protease inhibitor cocktail tablets (Roche)
- PhosSTOP phosphatase inhibitor cocktail tablets (Roche)
- BCA Protein Assay (Pierce)
- 4′, 6-Diamidino-2-phenylindole dihydrochloride (DAPI, Sigma)
- DAB substrate (Roche)
- PCR DIG probe synthesis kit (Roche Diagnostics)
- Silver nitrate (Sigma)
- TRIzol (Invitrogen)
- RNA lysis buffer (RNeasy Mini kit, Quiagen)
- Proteinase K (Roche)
- 1,9-dimethyl dimethylene blue (DMMB, Sigma-Aldrich)
- Sodium chloride (Sigma-Aldrich)
- Glycine (Sigma-Aldrich)
- Ethylenediaminotetracetic acid (EDTA, Sigma-Aldrich)
- Tris base (Sigma-Aldrich)
- Shark cartilage (Sigma-Aldrich)
- Hoescht 33258 solution (Invitrogen)
- DNA (Sigma-Aldrich)
- SuperFrost Plus Slides (VWR)

- TNE buffer: 10-mM Tris base, 1-mM EDTA, 200-mM NaCl, and adjust pH to 7.4 with concentrated HCl

2.3.2 Equipment

- Cryostat (Leica)
- Fluorescence microscope with long distance objective (Nikon)
- Spectrophotometer (Perkin Elmer)
- Fluorimeter (Perkin Elmer)

2.4 Methods

2.4.1 Self-assembling peptide preparation

Prepare a solution of the commercial peptide RAD16-I (BD PuraMatrix, 1% (w/v) in water) at the desired final concentration in 10% (w/v) sucrose. For the encapsulation method, the prepared solution must be two-fold more concentrated than the final gel. Typically, final concentrations are used in the range 0.15–0.5% (w/v).

If modified peptides are used, mix them with the RAD16-I up to a ratio 95:5 (prototypic: modified). Higher amounts of modified peptides may changes the rheological properties of the final material, so that the experiments would not be comparable. These are synthesized by extension of the RAD16-I sequence at the amino terminal. In order to keep the active sequence free, two glycines are added as spacers between the main chain and the new sequence (X), as exemplified by the following expression: $AcN\text{-}X\text{-}GG\text{-}(RADA)_4\text{-}CONH_2$.

Thoroughly mix the components by placing the solution tube into an ultrasonic bath for 20 minutes. The resulting solution may be stored at +4°C for several months.

2.4.2 Cell encapsulation into the self-assembling peptide

1 Prepare a suspension of the cells in culture medium.
2. Centrifuge cells for 5 minutes at the usual centrifuge force for each cell type.
3. Remove the supernatant and suspend the cells in 3–5 ml of 10% (w/v) sucrose and count the cells.
4. Place the tissue culture inserts (one per encapsulation) into a 6-well plate.
5. Centrifuge cells again.
6. Remove the supernatant and suspend the cells in 10% (w/v) sucrose to get the desired final concentration (usually between $2{\cdot}10^6$–$4{\cdot}10^6$ cells/ml, which corresponds to $1.6{\cdot}10^5$–$3.2{\cdot}10^5$ cells per encapsulation). Sucrose solution at 10% (w/v) is an isotonic and nonionic medium. Hence, it allows maintaining cells while avoiding peptide gelation during the mixing process.
7. Sonicate the peptide for approximately 5 minutes. Although this step may enhance the encapsulation process, do not prolong sonication much more, because the material may become temporarily stiffer.

8. Take the necessary volume of the cell suspension for the desired number of encapsulations (40 μL of cell suspension per encapsulation) plus approximately 10% of extra volume. Place it into a standard microcentrifuge tube.
9. Mix the cell suspension with an equal volume of the already prepared RAD16-I solution to obtain the final suspension of cells in the desired peptide concentration in 10% (w/v) sucrose. Mix by pipetting approximately 10 times and avoid bubble formation. This step must be performed carefully but quickly at the same time, because cells are in quite hostile conditions due to the peptide low pH (around 3.5) until the medium starts buffering the suspension.
10. Load 80 μL of the suspension to each insert and add 0.5 ml to the bottom of the insert in order to wet the membrane. At this moment, the media diffuses into the gel so that the ions induce the spontaneous self-assembling of the peptide.
11. Let the peptide gel for approximately 20 minutes in the flow cabinet. The manipulation of the gels when they are not properly formed yet may break the construct.
12. Add 40 μL of medium in the inner wall of the insert and let it slide slowly to the gel. Place the plate in the incubator and wait 20 minutes more. This step and the consecutive medium additions will favor the leaching of the sucrose.
13. Add 60 μL of medium slowly into the insert by allowing it to flow down the wall. Aspirate the medium in the wells, rich in sucrose, and add 0.5 ml of the fresh medium. Place the plate in the incubator and wait 10 minutes.
14. Add 60 μL more into the insert in the same way. Place the plate in the incubator and wait 10 minutes.
15. Repeat step 14.
16. Aspirate the medium in the well. Add 2.5 ml of the fresh medium into the well and an additional 200 μL into the insert.
17. Place the plate in the incubator (37°C, 5% CO_2, humidified atmosphere).
18. Change the medium every day by removing 0.5 ml from the well and adding 0.5 ml of the fresh medium into the insert.

2.4.3 Sandwich method

1. Prepare a suspension of the cells in a culture medium.
2. Place the tissue culture inserts (one per sandwich) in a 12-well plate. Prepare as many as needed.
3. Load 40 μl of the RAD16-I peptide solution 0.5% (w/v) into the bottom of a tissue culture insert to obtain a 0.5-mm-thick hydrogel. Depending on the desired thickness the volume of the loaded solution may be changed.
4. Add 0.5 ml of the culture medium below the tissue culture insert to initiate self-assembling (as detailed in Section 2.4.2.10) and let the process take place for 20 minutes.
5. Carefully add 200 μl of medium on the top of the formed gel by allowing it to flow down the wall. Equilibrate the cultures for 30 minutes in the incubator at 37°C and 5% CO_2.

6. Add the volume of cell suspension necessary to get the desired final density (cells/cm^2) over the gel. A density of 65,000 cells/cm^2 has successfully been used for hepatocytes.
7. Add 650 μL in the well and let the cells attach to the gel overnight in the incubator.
8. The next day, wash unattached cells by rinsing them three times with a solution of 10% (w/v) sucrose. This step is important to eliminate the medium and avoid gelation of the peptide solution when it is subsequently loaded over the cells.
9. Load 40 μL of the peptide solution 0.5% (w/v) on top of the cell monolayer to entrap them in a sandwich-like culture, and wait 30 minutes. The medium in the well will diffuse up to the new peptide layer and induce gelation.
10. Equilibrate by carefully adding 20 μL of medium on top of the gel and waiting for 20 minutes.
11. Repeat step 10.
12. Add 50 μL of medium into the tissue culture insert.
13. Maintain the 3D cultures in a humidified incubator equilibrated with 5% CO_2 at 37°C.
14. Change the medium every day by replacing the 650 μL in the well with fresh medium, which will diffuse up to the culture without disturbing the upper hydrogel layer.

2.4.4 Cell isolation and culture of isolated cells

Some postculture analysis techniques, such as cell counting, kinetic studies, or even immunofluorescence, require cell isolation from the 3D constructs.

1. Wash the cultures with PBS (without calcium and magnesium).
2. Treat 3D cultures with 0.05%/0.02% trypsin/EDTA in the same insert and use the micropipette to mechanically disrupt the peptide scaffold by several up and down aspirations until about 50% of the clusters are extracted as determined by phase contrast microscopy.
3. Add the serum-containing medium to inhibit trypsin.
4. Place the suspension in a regular tissue culture flask and incubate overnight in humidified atmosphere with 5% CO_2 at 37°C.

2.4.5 Cryosections of the 3D cultures

Obtaining slices of the 3D cultures in self-assembling peptides is usually a very tough step, especially when the constructs are very soft and fragile. In these cases, the chances of breaking the structures when manipulating are high and, thus, it is recommended to assay them whole-mount. Even when the constructs are stiffer, take into account that the mechanical properties are not as good as for tissues.

1. Wash the cultures with PBS and fix them with 2% *p*-formaldehyde for 2 hours.
2. Rinse with PBS.
3. Incubate the 3D cultures in 30% sucrose at 4°C for 2 hours.
4. Transfer the construct to a cryomold containing the O.C.T. medium.
5. Freeze the embedded culture using an isopentane bath immersed in liquid nitrogen. Use a tip or spatula to maintain the desired orientation of the sample.

6. Take off the OCT-embedded construct from the mold. The frozen structures may be stored at –80°C.
7. Use a cryostat to make the sections of the cell mass and place them on charged glass slides (SuperFrost Plus Slides). Slices between 10–20 μm are usually performed.

2.4.6 Cell proliferation study using 5-bromodeoxyuridine (BrdU) uptake analysis

Cell proliferation into the constructs may be assessed with BrdU (5-bromo-2-deoxyuridine), which is an analog of thymidine that can be incorporated into the newly synthesized DNA of replicating cells (S-phase stage). Cellular nuclei with BrdU can be detected using a monoclonal antibody against this molecule.

1. Add BrdU to the culture medium at a concentration of 10 μM and use it to incubate the 3D culture overnight.
2. Fix cells with 2% *p*-formaldehyde in PBS (pH 7.4) at room temperature for 2 hours.
3. Treat cells with 2N HCl in PBS for 30 minutes at 37°C to achieve the denaturation of DNA and allow the subsequent binding of the antibody.
4. Wash the samples with PBS several times until neutral pH is reached.
5. Treat samples with blocking buffer for 2 hours.
6. Incubate samples with an anti-BrdU monoclonal antibody FITC-conjugated for 2 hours.
7. Extensively wash with blocking buffer to eliminate the unbound antibody.
8. Analyze samples under fluorescence microscopy.

2.4.7 Cell viability

Cell viability may be assessed by fluorescence with a live/dead viability/cytotoxicity assay. On one hand, calcein AM substrate is cleaved by estearases in live cells, which produces a green fluorescence in the cytoplasm. On the other hand, ethidium homodimer-1 (EthD-1) stains red fluorescence when associated to DNA, which is only observed in membrane-compromised cells.

1 Freshly prepare a solution of 2-μM calcein AM and 2-μM EthD-1 in PBS. Concentrations may be adjusted depending on the cell type. Vortex the solution and keep it in the dark.
2. Rinse the specimens with PBS and cover them with the aforementioned solution.
3. Incubate cells for 40 minutes in the dark.
4. Extensively rinse the constructs with PBS. Because of the tendency of these hydrogels to retain dye molecules, an extended washing step will often be the difference between a blurry or a great picture.
5. Visualize the samples under the fluorescence microscope.

2.4.8 Protein analysis

There are different techniques for the analysis of proteins like western blot or ELISA that may be used also for the 3D cultures. The details of these protocols are well known and are not the aim of this chapter. However, one common step in all of them is the extraction and quantification of total protein from the sample in order to obtain the protein solution and to normalize the results. In order to obtain reliable results, one must take into account that the protocol for protein extraction and quantification followed in 3D cultures slightly differs from the protocol used in 2D cultures.

1. Prepare lysis buffer with RIPA buffer and protease inhibitors. Add phosphatase inhibitors in case of phosphorilated proteins study.
2. Suspend 3D culture samples in the lysis buffer and mechanically disrupt the peptide scaffold.
3. Sonicate the cell suspension for 5 minutes to complete cell disruption and centrifuge at 14,000 rpm for 5 minutes in order to remove cell and scaffold debris.
4. Determine total protein levels at the supernatant fraction using a detergent-compatible protein quantification kit as BCA.
5. Maintain samples at –20°C until analyzed.

2.4.9 Sample staining

2.4.9.1 Immunostaining

The immunostaining technique is described here for whole-mount samples. However, if a lot of background from the hydrogel is usually observed, it would be recommended to work on slices.

1. Rinse the constructs with PBS and fix them with 1% (w/v) *p*-formaldehyde for 2 hours at room temperature.
2. Wash twice with PBS and incubate with blocking buffer for 4 hours at room temperature on an orbital shaker.
3. Prepare a solution of the primary antibody in the blocking buffer at the appropriate dilution (follow the company protocols). An antibody titration experiment may be performed before.
4. Incubate the constructs with this solution overnight at 4°C.
5. Remove the primary antibody and wash three times with blocking buffer.
6. Prepare a solution of a secondary antibody in the blocking buffer at the appropriate dilution (follow the company protocols).
7. Incubate the constructs with the secondary antibody (fluorescent or reporter enzyme-conjugated, such HRP or ALP) for 4 hours at room temperature.
8. Remove the secondary antibody and wash three times with the blocking buffer.
9. Prepare a solution of 10 mg/ml DAPI in methanol:water (50:50). This stock solution must be stored at –20°C. Dilute this stock solution 1:10,000 in PBS to yield the working solution.
10. Cover the samples with DAPI nuclear dye for 5 minutes and rinse generously with the blocking buffer.
11. Observe the samples under microscopy, fluorescence, or bright field, depending on the type of secondary antibody.

2.4.9.2 In situ hybridization

RNA in situ hybridization is used to measure and localize mRNAs and other transcripts within tissue sections or whole mounts. In this type of 3D culture this technique can be performed over the whole 3D culture sample (whole mount) or over slices.

1. Fix the 3D culture samples with 2% (w/v) *p*-formaldehyde for 2 hours.
2. Make cryosections (as described in Section 2.4.5).
3. Perform the in situ hybridization with a complementary DNA DIG-labeled probe for the mRNA in study.
4. Follow the usual protocol for in situ hybridization for embryos, in case of whole mount, and for tissue sections, in case of slices.
5. Perform the inmunostaining (as previously described) for DIG using an anti-DIG primary antibody and a secondary antibody HRP-conjugated against the first one.
6. Add a DAB substrate to localize the mRNA in study in the slice or whole mount.

2.4.9.3 Toluidine blue

This staining is performed to study chondrogenic phenotype since toluidine blue dye forms complexes with anionic glycoconjugates such as proteoglycans (PG) and glycosaminoglycans (GAG), which are the main components of the chondrocyte extracellular matrix.

1. Wash 3D cultures with PBS and fix them with 2% (w/v) *p*-formaldehyde for 2 hours at room temperature.
2. Wash twice with 0.1% Triton X-100 in PBS.
3. Incubate with 0.05% toluidine blue in water for 20 minutes.
4. Wash several times with PBS.
5. Analyze samples under microscope.

2.4.9.4 Nile red

This staining is used to study the adipogenic phenotype since Nile red stains intracellular lipid droplets. This dye is strongly fluorescent only in the presence of a hydrophobic environment.

1. Wash 3D cultures with PBS and fix them with 2% (w/v) *p*-formaldehyde in PBS for 2 hours at room temperature.
2. Meanwhile, prepare a stock solution of 1 mg/ml Nile red in DMSO and dilute it 1:100 in PBS to obtain the working solution.
3. Incubate the 3D cultures with the aforementioned working solution for 5 minutes.
4. Wash three times with PBS.
5. Inspect the samples under fluorescence microscopy.

2.4.9.5 von Kossa

This staining is based on the substitution of calcium ions in carbonate and phosphates salts by silver cations, which subsequently reduce, producing black nodules in the calcium phosphate deposits. Therefore, this assay is used to detect mineralization in the cultures and, thus, state the osteogenic differentiation.

1. Wash the 3D cultures twice with PBS and fix the constructs with 1% (w/v) *p*-formaldehyde solution for 1 hour at room temperature.
2. Strictly rinse the fixed cultures with distilled water until *p*-formaldehyde and PBS are completely removed. Make sure to remove phosphate traces, otherwise they will precipitate with the following silver solution.
3. Incubate the samples with a solution of 5% (w/v) silver nitrate for 1 hour in the dark.
4. Wash the samples with abundant distilled water to remove the excess silver nitrate solution.
5. Place the sample under a strong light source for 10 minutes.
6. Inspect the samples at the microscope (reflection mode) to assess the presence of black nodules (mineralized cells).

2.4.10 sGAG quantification

2.4.10.1 Sample preparation

1. Prepare a solution of 250 ng/ml proteinase K in Tris-HCl.
2. Incubate the samples overnight with the aforementioned solution at 60°C.
3. Centrifuge at 14,000g and separate supernatant.

2.4.10.2 DMMB (1,9-dimethyl-dimethylene blue) assay for sGAG quantification

This assay is based on the ability of sulfated GAGs (mainly chondroitin-6-sulfate) to bind the cationic dye 1,9-dimethylmethylene blue (DMMB). This interaction produces a change in the absorption spectrum of DMMB that can be measured using the spectrophotometer.

1. Prepare the DMMB working solution: 0.16% DMMB, 0.24% NaCl, 0.30% glycine, and 10-mM HCl.
2. Prepare standards for chondroitin-6-sulfate from shark cartilage with concentrations between 0 and 100 μg/ml to get the calibration curve.
3. In a 96-well plate, incubate 20 μl of standards and sample supernatants, obtained as previously described, with 200 μl of DMMB working solution.
4. Read the absorbance at 520 nm in a spectrophotometer.
5. Use the obtained calibration curve to calculate the amount of chondroitin-6-sultafe in each sample.
6. Normalize the results with the total amount of DNA obtained with Hoescht dye for each sample as described later.

2.4.10.3 Hoescht assay for DNA quantification

This assay is based on the use of Hoechst 33258 dye, which is a fluorescent nucleic acid stain for quantitating double-stranded DNA (dsDNA).

1. Prepare the Hoescht working solution from the dilution 1:1,000 of a 10 mg/ml Hoescht stock solution with TNE buffer.

2. Prepare standards for DNA with concentrations between 0 and 10 ng/ml to get the calibration curve.
3. In a fluorescence 96-well plate, incubate 20 μl of standards and supernatants previously obtained from the sample preparation with 20 μl of Hoescht working solution.
4. Excite the samples at 352 nm and read the emission at 461 nm in a fluorimeter.
5. Use the obtained calibration curve to calculate the amount of DNA in each sample.

2.4.11 Lysis of 3D cultures for RNA extraction

In order to analyze gene expression in the 3D cultures, quantitative reverse transcription polymerase chain reaction (qRT-PCR) is very useful. The first step to perform this technique is the lysis of these cultures, which will be followed by the usual RNA extraction, cDNA synthesis, and the actual RT-PCR analysis.

1. Carefully remove the culture medium of the inserts and wells and wash the samples with PBS.
2. Add 0.5 ml of TRIzol or an alternative RNA lysis buffer into the insert.
3. Disrupt the sample by pipetting up and down with a micropipette and transfer it to a RNase- and DNase-free microcentrifuge tube. A pestle may be necessary to help in the disaggregation of some samples.
4. The homogenized samples may be stored at –80°C for at least 1 year or can sit at room temperature for several hours to proceed with the RNA extraction according to the manufacturer's instructions of the respective kits.

2.5 Data Acquisition, Anticipated Results, and Interpretation

In this section, we selected a number of examples that illustrate the versatility and the advantages of the self-assembling culture system. In this way, we have decided to present the most characteristic and quantitative data to help the reader proceed faster in the implementation of these techniques in his or her own experiments. Therefore, we show an example of an adult hepatocyte culture in a sandwich system as well as an adult hepatic stem cell and mouse embryonic fibroblast culture after encapsulation in self-assembling peptide scaffolds.

Maintenance of functional hepatocytes in vivo is a major challenge as these cells quickly lose their metabolic properties in culture. Recently, we have developed a bioengineered platform that replaces the use of the collagen type I (in the traditional culture sandwich technique) by self-assembling peptide hydrogel sandwich layers functionalized with biologically active motifs. In this synthetic sandwich system, adult hepatocytes showed similar parenchymal morphology, presence of functional bile canaliculi structures, CYP3A2 induction by dexamethasone, urea production, secretion of proteins such as apolipoprotein (class A1, E, J), a-1-microglobulin, a-1-macroglobulin, retinol binding protein, fibronectin, a-1-inhibitor III, and biotin-dependent carboxylases [20]. Therefore, we combined RAD16-I with modified self-assembling peptides containing the integrin-binding sequence RGD, the 67 KDa laminin receptor binding sequence YIGSR (YIG), or the heparin binding sequence present in collagen IV TAGSCLRKFSTM (TAG) in order to obtain a functionalized matrix scaffold. We analyzed several liver-specific functions in terms of gene expression by means of quantitative PCR, examined albumin, hepatocytes nuclear factor 4-alpha (HNF4-alpha), multi-drug-resistant protein 2 (MDR2), and tyrosine aminotrasferase (TAT). In addition, we prepared two sandwich dimensions with layers of 1 mm and 0.5 mm, respectively, in order to assess mass transfer phenomena due to the diffusion capacity of nutrients, toxins, and gases. As expected, gene expression analysis for the 0.5-mm sandwich layers indicates that, in general, peptide hydrogel and collagen cultures remained mainly in the same levels of expression (Figure 2.3). Expression values that fell between –1 and +1 were considered the same as fresh hepatocytes. In general, it was observed that albumin and HNF4-alpha had already reached the expression levels of freshly isolated hepatocytes. In the case of albumin, all the peptide hydrogel cultures were significantly different from collagen. For HNF4-alpha, significant differences were only observed for RAD16-I and YIG. In addition, MDR2 remained down-regulated in almost all conditions tested, except for YIG, which reached the relative levels of freshly isolated hepatocytes, and was significantly different than collagen [Figure 2.3(b)]. However, RAD16-I and TAG presented a slight but statistically significant up-regulation in MDR2 compared to collagen [Figure 2.3(b)]. Moreover, TAT in collagen cultures remained somehow down-regulated, but its expression in peptide hydrogel sandwich cultures was comparable to the positive control (freshly isolated hepatocytes), and significantly different than collagen cultures [Figure 2.3(b)] [20]. In addition, hepatocyte-specific functionality was evaluated and compared with the classical collagen sandwich system by assessing cell-specific albumin and urea secretion. In all culture systems, the albumin secretion gradually increased between 3 and 7 days of culture and remained stable thereafter [Figure 2.4(a)]. As shown by immunoblotting, albumin was expressed at a level that was similar in all hepatocyte cultures on day 7 [Figure 2.4(b, c)]. This indicates the versatility and reliability of the new sandwich method, indicating that it is possible to design and develop a cellular matrix analog to instruct cells in vitro to promote function maintenance.

Self-assembling peptides provide a microenvironment with particular properties that favor the culture of mature or primitive cell types with diverse possibilities: cell maintenance, proliferation, or differentiation [12, 16, 18]. In our group, several studies have been performed with mouse embryonic fibroblasts (MEFs), some of them based on differentiation in different mesodermal-derived tissues like bone, cartilage, or fat [21]. After culturing MEFs for several days and weeks in theses 3D encapsulations, we stained for calcium deposition (von Kossa), for glycosaminoglycan (GAG) synthesis (toluidine blue), and for cell-lipid accumulation (Nile red) to assess osteogenic, chondrogenic, and adipogenic commitment, respectively. Interestingly, MEFs encapsulated in self-assembling peptides showed a default chondrogenic commitment suggesting that during the culture cells underwent a process that recreates, in part, mesodermal induction, progressing into cartilage differentiation. In order to demonstrate the presence of cartilage in our cultures, we determined the presence of collagen type II and glycosaminoglycans (GAGs) in the 3D constructs. The synthesis of the key ECM component of cartilage, collagen type II, was assessed by a western blot of samples cultured during 15 days [Figure 2.5(a)]. Results showed that collagen type II is expressed only in the constructs, but not in control flask cultures, demonstrating the chondrogenic commitment of the cells in the 3D system. Moreover, we first observed that the samples stained positive with

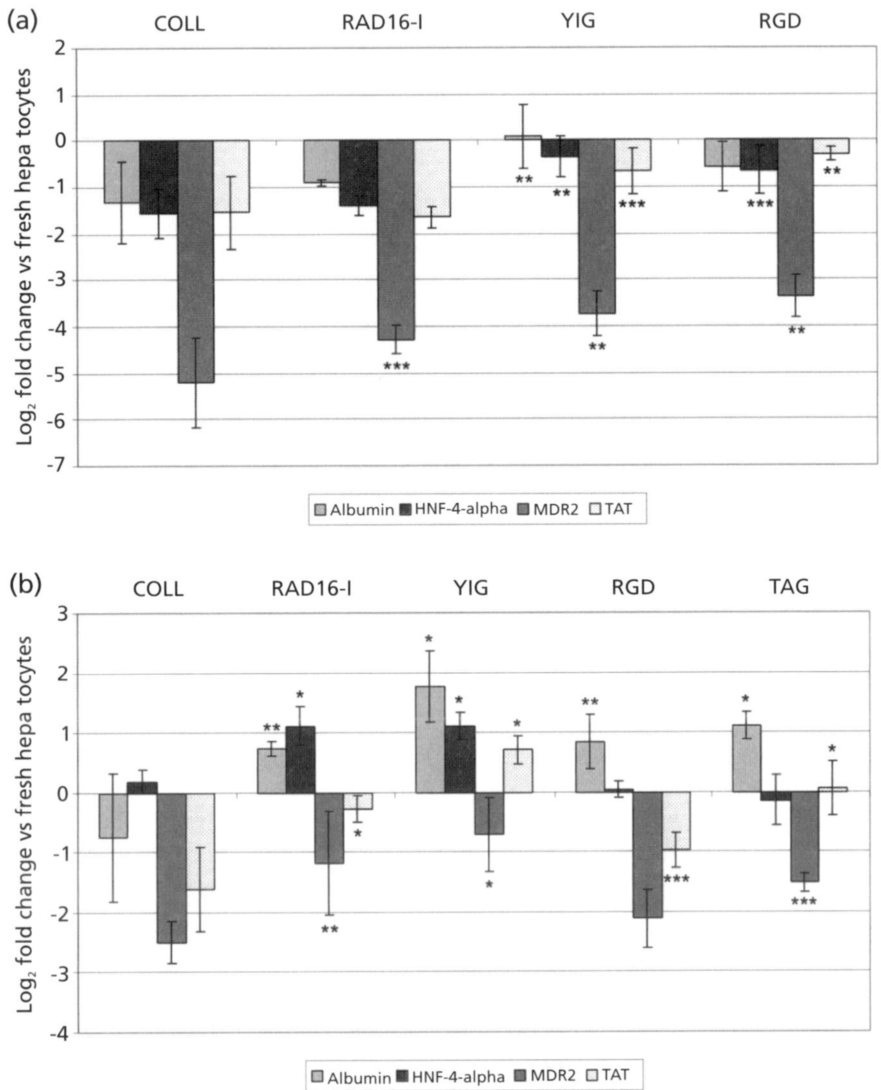

Figure 2.3 Quantitative PCR analysis of liver-specific genes in hepatic cultures in 1-mm and 0.5-mm matrices. The expression of liver-specific genes in the 1-mm and 500-μm hydrogel cultures were examined by means of qPCR and were expressed as a Log_2-fold change relative to freshly isolated hepatocytes in (a) 1 mm and (b) 0.5 mm hydrogel systems. Expression levels were normalized to 18s RNA levels, which were invariant per cell across the different culture systems. Data were obtained from four independent experiments, each of which was performed normalizing to the 18s corresponding to each hepatocyte isolation. Data are presented as mean ± SD (Fisher's PLSD statistical significance compared to collagen sandwich cultures * $p < 0.001$, ** $p < 0.01$, *** $p < 0.05$).

toluidine blue, which is a dye that indicates the presence of glycosylated proteoglycans (or GAGs). We therefore quantified the presence of GAGs in the 3D construct by a colorimetric method using chondroitin sulfate as controls [Figure 2.5(b)]. We observed a pronounced increment of GAGs during culture time, indicating the synthesis and accumulation of GAGs, and reconfirming the chondrogenic commitment of the samples. It is important to say that the method detects general glycosylated proteoglycans, which could be aggrecan, perlecan, and so forth.

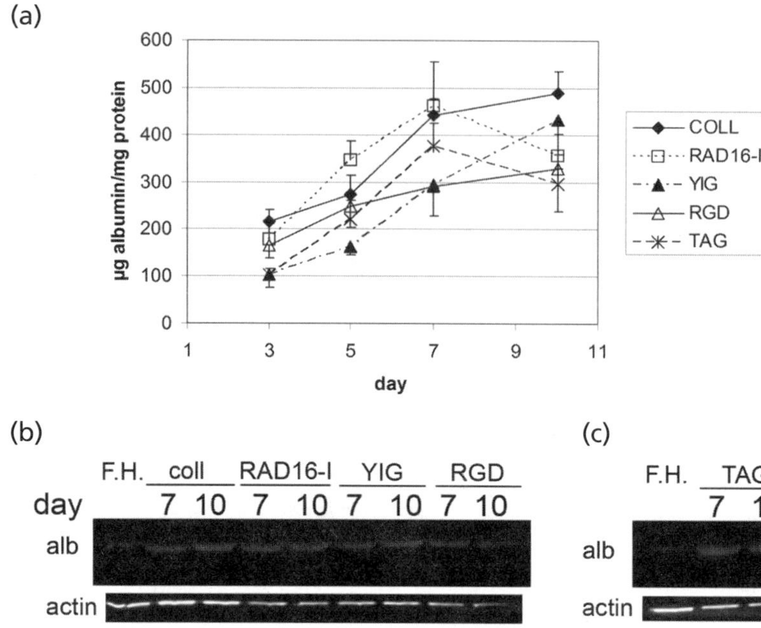

Figure 2.4 (a) Analysis of secreted rat albumin present in the media normalized by total protein present in the cellular lysate. Data are presented as mean ± SD from two different experiments. COLL: collagen. (b, c) Albumin western blot of the cellular lysate. F.H: Freshly isolated hepatocytes.

In another work, we investigated the ability of the self-assembling peptide scaffolds to foster tissue-like function by adult rat hepatocyte stem cell line Lig-8. In regular flask cultures (2D), Lig-8 cells divide actively, and express the markers for definitive endoderm HNF3β and hepatocyte lineage such as CK8, α-fetoprotein, and albumin; however, the cells lack the expression of mature hepatocyte markers. In 3D peptide scaffold, these cells present nonexponential cell kinetics and spheroidal morphology with mature hepatocyte phenotype. The differentiated progeny cells display an increased expression of albumin, binucleation, an up-regulation of transcription factor C/EBPα, and an expression of cytochrome P450's CYP1A1, CYP1A2, and CYP2E1, all characteristic of mature hepatocytes. Interestingly, CK8 and α-fetoprotein remained expressed, suggesting the development of cell cluster units (spheroids) containing a more complex cellular structure: adult stem cells and their differentiating progeny [13]. This demonstrates the ability of a designed biological material to provide a microenvironment in which adult stem cells regain their intrinsic ability to continuously produce differentiating progeny cells. This bioengineered system provides a physiological approach to stem cell differentiation for future biomedical and pharmaceutics applications [13]. Since direct immunofluorescence staining in the 3D constructs is difficult due to the presence of high background, we developed an alternative way involving isolation of the spheroids from the gels and their reculture on a flask. In this way, the spheroid colonies obtained (flat) can be easily compared with the regular Lig-8 colonies. Here, we present one example of an immunoflorescence staining using a liver developmental marker, C/EBPα, and a CCAAT enhanced-binding protein highly expressed in hepatocytes and other endodermal tissues, which was only expressed in 3D-derived spheroid colonies (Figure 2.6).

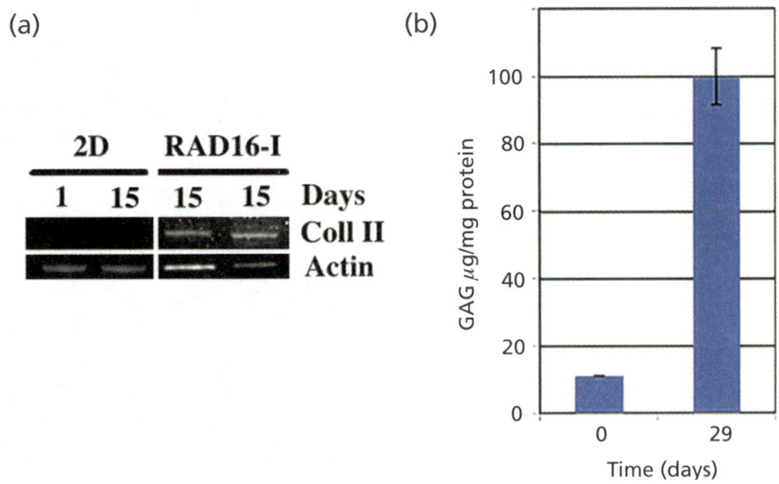

Figure 2.5 Collagen type II and glycosaminoglycans in the 3D-MEF-constructs. (a) Collagen type II was analyzed by a western blot in MEFs cultured in flask cultures (2D) after 1 and 15 days in culture, and in RAD16-I (3D) during 15 days in culture with a fibroblast medium (FM). (b) Glycosaminoglycans (GAGs) from 3D self-assembling peptide cultures of MEF at days 0 and 29 were quantified with DMMB (1,9-dimethyl-dimethyleneblue) using chondroitin sulfate as the standard.

2.6 Discussion and Commentary

We provided examples from results obtained in our laboratory using the main two systems that were developed to study cell behavior in three-dimensional cultures: the sandwich system and cell encapsulation. In the first, we basically adapted the use of the self-assembling peptides instead of collagen type I with a clear intention of developing a platform able to control matrix cell instruction or signaling (due to the use of a functionalized synthetic matrix), and layer dimensions. In this way, the hepatocyte cultures are an ideal system because they can be cultured in defined media. Then, our working hypothesis was that by controlling media composition, matrix signaling, and biophysics it was possible to adjust the parameters to obtain ideal culture conditions in which hepatocytes would maintain their functional adult phenotype for longer periods of time. This is exactly what we observed by changing the gel geometry and the different peptide motifs anchored to the self-assembling scaffold, since different signaling caused defined responses and, thus, we were able to keep adult rat hepatocytes properties for a long time [20]. The platform can be easily translated to other cell types that require culture conditions similar to the hepatocytes, such as pancreatic, epithelial intestine, or renal cells, which require a high demand of gas exchange as well as nutrients and toxins diffusion in 3D systems. These cell types required something very important to function—a polarization effect. This could be easily provided, for instance, by changing the matrix composition from top to bottom, or just by creating asymmetrical environmental conditions using different media composition in each side of the sandwich or the different biomechanical properties of each layer. The system could be adapted and customized for each case, providing a versatile platform. Eventually, it could be adapted for 96 multiwell plates for toxicology and pharmacology applications, with the eventual use of automatization for high throughput screenings (HTS).

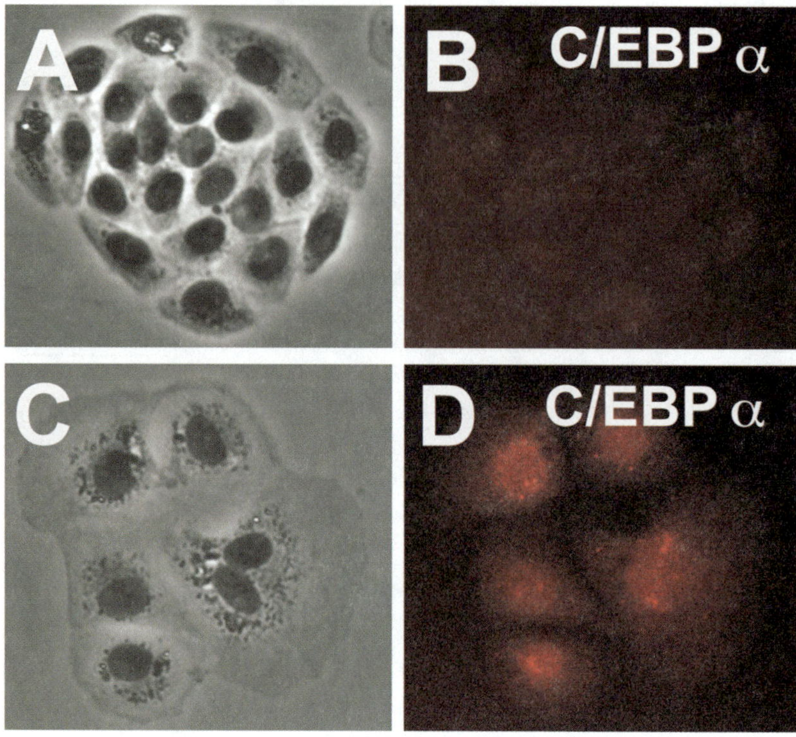

Figure 2.6 Hepatocyte differentiation by 3D culture peptide scaffold. Lig-8 hepatic stem cells were cultured in an adherent culture or in a RAD16-I peptide scaffold. Spheroids were isolated and analyzed approximately 16 hours after transfer to the adherent culture. (a) Adherent cell colony (phase contrast); (b) respective in situ immunofluorescence for adherent colonies with anti-C/EBPα; (c) isolated peptide scaffold spheroids (phase contrast; note binucleated cells); (d) respective in situ immunofluorescence for isolated peptide scaffold spheroids with anti-C/EBPα.

Then, we described the use of an encapsulation method, which creates truly three-dimensional environments for cells that do not require a polarized environment. In this way, mouse embryonic fibroblasts (MEFs) or adult hepatic stem cells are ideal candidates to study cell growth and differentiation. We cultured MEFs in this synthetic matrix and we observed that the cells initially developed a rich cell network that contracted the gels forming a highly elastic tissue-like structure. When we analyzed this spontaneous process we realized that the obtained tissue-like structures showed cartilage properties. Biomechanically, the constructs presented a viscoelastic component similar to soft cartilage confirmed by the presence of GAGs and collagen type II, two important components in the extracellular matrix of cartilage. We therefore realized that the synthetic neutral gel, in terms of intrinsic signaling, provide to the MEFs a biomechanical and structural environment similar to early embryonic tissues, but missing the chemical signaling from the matrix; this could explain the fact that the cells "dedifferentiated" to an early mesodermal progenitor to direct a default chondrogenic commitment in an autonomous way [21]. In this way, other cells, such as fibroblastic-like cells, from other species, including human, could be "environmentally reprogrammed" in order to obtain primitive cells from their lineage and to be used for regenerative purposes [23].

Finally, we described the capacity of these self-assembling peptide cultures to induce autonomous hepatic commitment to adult liver stem cells. This cell line, Lig-8, presents properties of adult stem cells including active cell division and the expression of the definitive endoderm marker HNF3β, and hepatocyte lineage markers such as CK8, α-fetoprotein, and albumin. After culturing Lig-8 cells in self-assembling peptide, those acquired properties of mature hepatic cells, including an increased expression of albumin, binucleation, the up-regulation of transcription factor C/EBPα, and the expression of cytochrome P450's CYP1A1, CYP1A2, and CYP2E1 [13]. This clearly indicates that these cells present the potential to become hepatocyte-like cells but they require a special microenvironment, a truly 3D environment to develop spheroid clusters where cells undergo a transition from stem cells to mature hepatocytes, as it is in vivo. The system provides an intrinsic property required for the cells to spontaneously differentiate—the microenvironment.

In this way, the platform we present here could provide an adequate 3D culture system to different cell types, depending on the requirement of cell polarization (sandwich technique) or cell network formation (encapsulation technique) in order to differentiate into particular tissues. Most importantly, independently, if the cells are of embryonic or adult origin, or if stem cells are present or not, cells in these systems would have better conditions to produce functional tissues that can be used for future reparative and regenerative medicine, pharmacology, or toxicology platforms [24].

2.7 Troubleshooting

Some common problems happen when classical methods developed for cell culture in two dimensions (2D) are adapted to 3D cultures. During the performance of these methods, the following issues may arise.

Troubleshooting Table

Problem	Explanation	Potential Solutions
High cell death	Cells are suspended in peptide solution at low pH for too long during encapsulation (step 1.1 and 1.2, Figure 2.2).	Work quickly between cell-peptide solution preparation and gel induction by medium addition (from step 1.1 to 1.3, Figure 2.2).
Gel breaking	Abrupt movement or premature washing before gel formation.	Strictly follow the necessary waiting time for gel formation.
Gel floating	Entrapped bubbles in the gel.	Gently mix cells and peptide solution, avoiding bubble formation.
Unattached upper peptide layer	Presence of residual medium at the time of loading the upper layer, causing premature gelation.	Increase the number of washings with 10% sucrose solution.
Fluorescence background	The self-assembling peptide cultures are not well blocked. Hydrogel tends to retain many small molecules, such as dyes.	Increase the time and concentration of serum and blocking time. Increase the number and duration of washing steps.
Constructs break when assayed	Hydrogels are soft and fragile.	Reinforce the gel by the addition of a few drops of 2% (w/v) agarose.

2.8 Application Notes

We have provided some examples of the 3D-culture platform developed by our group and others [10–22]. The main objective in this new technique is the clear gain of function obtained by the fact that cells are in an environment more similar to an in vivo situation. This clear advantage creates at the same time a challenge, because cells require more parameters to be controlled as the system increases its complexity. It is important to consider and to remember that a 3D system will be required to control biophysical parameters, such as the diffusion constant, the stiffness of the matrix, and the need for assisting or supporting systems such as medium flow to reduce problems associated to the mass transfer phenomena. In other words, the 3D culture systems belong to an interdisciplinary platform, where not only the material development is important, but also mechanics, biophysics, and biology play and important role. In this way, complex systems such as cell networks in the 3D milieu can only access the next level of integrity or emergent state where they become a real functional tissue. This is by far the most important consequence of growing and differentiating cells in 3D, as compared to 2D systems where the level of integrity and function is very poor. The fact that synthetic scaffolds can reproduce conditions in vitro similar to their natural counterparts (extracellular matrix proteins) indicates that we can rationally study the effect of each new component added to the matrix (growth factor, polysaccharide, or signalling peptide). In addition, the big advantage of the synthetic materials over the natural scaffolds in based in their potential predictive toxicology (acute and chronic toxicity test, pharmacodynamics, and genotoxicity). The biomaterial synthesis process can be highly controlled as well as safety applied out of shelf. For future translational applications, biomaterials will play an important role, such as vehicles for cell, growth factor, and drug delivery, tissue matrix replacement during wound healing, and medical devices. It is our hope that the study, design, and development of this class of biomaterials will, combined with other platforms, promote the development of new therapeutic approaches for reparative and regenerative medicine, cancer, and biopharmaceutics.

2.9 Summary Points

1. We have developed two platforms for culturing cells in a 3D system: an encapsulation and a sandwich method.
2. The encapsulation method is compatible for culturing cells that normally required a truly 3D environment because they form cellular networks, such as fibroblasts, mesenchymal stem cells, hematopoietic stem cells, and so forth.
3. The sandwich method is ideal for cells and stem cells that will require the presence of a polarized environment, such as the presence of a basement membrane, or organ-derived cells, such as from the liver, pancreas, or kidney.
4. Cell encapsulation, as well as the sandwich method, is compatible for several quantitative methodologies to assess, for instance, specific molecular markers, produced metabolites, or enzymatic activities.
5. The main gain in the use of a 3D method (encapsulation or sandwich), is that the cells have access to a next level of organization where intrinsic properties and functions of complexity will arise, obtaining better and reliable tissue constructs.

Acknowledgments

Núria Marí-Buyé acknowledges financial support from DURSI (Generalitat de Catalunya) and the European Social Foundation (2006FI 00447). Maria Teresa Fernández Muiños gratefully acknowledges her fellowship from Fundació Obra Social "La Caixa." The research carried on by the author was supported in part by the Institut Quimíc de Sarrià, Universidad Ramon LLull, and the Grant Award Marató TV3 to Carlos E. Semino.

References

[1] Charonis, A. S., et al., "Binding of Laminin to Type IV Collagen: A Morphological Study," *J. Cell Biol.*, Vol. 100, 1985, pp. 1848–1853.

[2] Beck, H., I. Hunter, and J. Engel, "Structure and Function of Laminin: Anatomy of a Multidomain Glycoprotein," *FASEB J.*, Vol. 4, 1990, pp. 148–160.

[3] Engel, J., "Laminins and Other Strange Proteins," *Biochemistry*, Vol. 31, 1992, pp. 10643–10651.

[4] Yurchenco, P. D., and J. J. O'Rear, "Basement Membrane Assembly," *Methods and Enzymol.*, Vol. 145, 1994, pp. 489–518.

[5] Ball, P., "Polymers Made to Measure," *Nature*, Vol. 367, 1994, pp. 323–324.

[6] Piggion, E., et al., "Conformational Studies on Polypeptides. The Effect of Sodium Perchlorate on the Conformation of Poly-L-Lysine and of Random Copolymers of L-Lysine and L-Phenylalanine in Aqueous Solution," *Biopolymers*, Vol. 11, 1972, pp. 633–643.

[7] Rippon, W. B., H. H. Chen, and A. G. Walton, "Spectroscopic Characterization of Poly(Glu-Ala)," *J. Mol. Biol.*, Vol. 75, 1973, pp. 369–375.

[8] Seipke, G., H. A. Arfmann, and K. G. Wagner, "Synthesis and Properties of Alternating Poly(Lys-Phe) and Comparison with the Random Copolymer Poly(Lys 51, Phe 49)," *Biopolymers*, Vol. 13, 1974, pp. 1621–1633.

[9] Brack, A., and L. E. Orgel, "Beta Structures of Alternating Polypeptides and Their Possible Prebiotic Significance," *Nature*, Vol. 256, 1975, pp. 383–387.

[10] Aggeli, A., et al., "Responsive Gels Formed by the Spontaneous Self-Assembly of Peptide into Polymeric b-Sheet Tapes," *Nature*, Vol. 386, 1997, pp. 259–262.

[11] Semino, C. E., "Can We Build Artificial Stem Cell Compartments?" *J. Biomed. Biotech.*, Vol. 3, 2003, pp. 164–169.

[12] Kisiday, J., et al., "Self-Assembling Peptide Hydrogel Fosters Chondrocyte Extracellular Matrix Production and Cell Division: Implications for Cartilage Tissue Repair," *Proc. Natl. Acad. Sci. USA*, Vol. 99, 2002, pp. 9996–10001.

[13] Semino, C. E., et al., "Functional Differentiation of Hepatocyte-Like Spheroid Structures from Putative Liver Progenitor Cells in Three-Dimensional Peptide Scaffolds," *Differentiation*, Vol. 71, 2003, pp. 262–270.

[14] Narmoneva, D. A., et al., "Endothelial Cells Promote Cardiac Myocyte Survival and Spatial Reorganization: Implications for Cardiac Regeneration," *Circulation*, Vol. 110, 2004, pp. 962–968.

[15] Semino, C. E., et al., "Entrapment of Migrating Hippocampal Neural Cells in Three-Dimensional Peptide Nanofiber Scaffold," *Tissue Eng.*, Vol. 10, 2004, pp. 643–655.

[16] Bokhari, M. A., et al., "The Enhancement of Osteoblast Growth and Differentiation In Vitro on a Peptide Hydrogel-PolyHIPE Polymer Hybrid Material," *Biomaterials*, Vol. 25, 2005, pp. 5198–5208.

[17] Genové, E., et al., "The Effect of Functionalized Self-Assembling Peptide Scaffolds on Human Aortic Endothelial Cell Function," *Biomaterials*, Vol. 26, 2005, pp. 3341–3351.

[18] Garreta, E., et al., "Osteogenic Differentiation of Mouse Embryonic Stem Cells and Mouse Embryonic Fibroblasts in a Three-Dimensional Self-Assembling Peptide Scaffold," *Tissue Eng.*, Vol. 12, 2006, pp. 2215–2228.

[19] Sieminski, A. L., et al., "Primary Sequence of Ionic Self-Assembling Peptide Gels Affects Endothelial Cell Adhesion and Capillary Morphogenesis," *J. Biomed. Mater. Res. A*, Vol. 87A, 2008, 494–504.

[20] Genové, E., et al., "A Synthetic Functionalized Self-Assembling Peptide Hydrogel Enhance Maintenance of Hepatocyte Activity In Vitro," *Journal of Cellular and Molecular Medicine*, 2010.

[21] Quintana, L., et al., "Early Tissue Patterning Recreated by Mouse Embryonic Fibroblasts in a Three-Dimensional Environment," *Tissue Eng. Part A*. Vol. 1, 2009, pp. 45–54.

[22] Hernández Vera, R., et al., "Interstitial Fluid Flow Intensity Modulates Endothelial Sprouting in Restricted Src-Activated Cell Clusters During Capillary Morphogenesis," *Tissue Eng. Part A*, Vol. 15, No. 1, 2009, pp. 175–185.

[23] Quintana, L., N. I. zur Nieden, and C. E. Semino, "Morphogenetic and Regulatory Mechanisms During Developmental Chondrogenesis: New Paradigms for Cartilage Tissue Engineering," *Tissue Eng. Part B Rev.*, Vol. 15, No. 1, 2009, pp. 29–41.

[24] Semino, C. E., "Self-Assembling Peptides: From Bioinspired Materials to Bone Regeneration," *Journal of Dental Research*, Vol. 87, No. 7, 2008, pp. 606–616.

CHAPTER

3

3D Fibrin Matrices as Scaffold for Depot and Release of Bioactive Molecules

Heike Hall

Cells and BioMaterials, Department of Materials, ETH Zurich, Switzerland, Corresponding author: Heike Hall, address: ETH Zurich, Department of Materials, HCI E415, Cells and BioMaterials, Wolfgang-Pauli-Strasse 10, CH-8093 Zurich, Switzerland, phone: +41 44 633 69 75, fax: +41 44 632 10 73, e-mail: heike.hall@mat.ethz.ch

Abstract

This chapter describes how to produce, use, and analyze 3D fibrin hydrogel matrices as versatile tools for tissue engineering and regenerative medicine. Rationally designed 3D fibrin hydrogel matrices provide adhesion sequences and, in addition, are able to store and release bioactive molecules that induce cell type-specific responses, thus providing favorable growth and differentiation conditions for different cell types including progenitor and stem cells. The 3D fibrin matrices can be used as in vitro 3D culture systems that allow cell infiltration and thereby release entrapped or covalently immobilized bioactive molecules. When applied in vivo, ideally the speed of tissue regeneration correlates with the removal of 3D fibrin hydrogel matrices, thus mimicking a natural healing process. In our group we used 3D fibrin hydrogel matrices to analyze stimulatory factors that induce angiogenesis and nerve regeneration in vitro and matrix-released gene transfer to stimulate endogenous wound healing in vitro as well as in vivo.

Key terms
bioactive molecules
depot
extracellular matrix
fibrin matrices
release system

3.1 Introduction

Hydrogel matrices are highly swollen 3D cross-linked structures produced by the reaction of one or more monomers or by association bonds such as hydrogen bonds and strong van der Waals interactions between the chains [1]. They are freely permeable for small molecules such as gas, water, and nutrients, and because of their fibrous structure they can simulate to a certain extent the natural extracellular matrix (ECM). Hydrogel matrices are usually composed of soluble precursor solutions that can be applied at the site of action and are induced to polymerize under physiological conditions (37°C and pH 7.4). These matrices provide a versatile platform for molecular interactions with target cells or tissues since they can be composed of native or synthetic monomers that provide a 3D scaffold for cellular growth and differentiation. In addition, hydrogel matrices are used as depots for growth factors or drugs released by hydrolytic degradation of the matrices or on specific cellular demand [2–5] (reviewed in [6–8]).

Fibrin(ogen) is a natural scaffold material that is used extensively for medical applications and as matrices for tissue engineering. Although fibrin(ogen) is derived from human blood, it is food and drug administration (FDA)-approved because of its very favorable wound-healing inductive capacities. In the healthy body, fibrinogen circulates as an inactive precursor in the blood stream and is recruited to the site of injured vasculature where it becomes activated through proteolytic cleavage. Fibrin leaks out into the surrounding tissue and forms fibrin clots by initial physical association followed by covalent cross-linking through the concerted activity of thrombin and factor XIIIa [9–14]. The fibrin clot is a complex network, composed of fibrils with different diameters and strengths. The composition and mechanical properties depend largely on the molecular details at the site of fibrin clot formation [14–17]. Fibrin clots provide a natural wound healing matrix that is, also in the native situation, remodeled through cellular activities to form the tissue-specific mature ECM. Cells such as fibroblasts and endothelial cells secrete proteolytic enzymes (usually plasmin and matrix metalloproteinases, MMPs) that become activated at the cell surface close to the leading edge of the migrating cell and degrade the matrix very locally, allowing cell migration into the fibrin clot [8, 18–22]. Several groups controlled the release of growth factors from fibrin hydrogels by using different fibrin concentrations, various crosslink densities, and precipitation of growth factors by heparin-binding peptides or polymer microspheres [23–26]. Moreover, 3D fibrin matrices can be used as scaffold and release system by covalently introducing bifunctional peptides or directly cell type-specific adhesion sequences, growth factors, or condensed plasmid DNA by the activity of transglutaminase factor XIIIa. In order to do so, a factor XIII recognition sequence (e.g., NQEQVSPL) needs to be placed at the N-terminus of the peptides/proteins to be incorporated [27–35]. This feature of 3D fibrin matrices transforms the natural wound healing material into a highly versatile tool to analyze cell growth and differentiation under quasi-controlled 3D experimental conditions. Furthermore the simplicity in production enables a large variety of biomedical applications.

The 3D fibrin matrices described here use factor XIIIa, the natural crosslink enzyme, to simultaneously crosslink fibrinogen precursors to form a fibrin network with covalently incorporated bioactive molecules. As factor XIIIa incorporates the bioactive molecules at fibrin crosslink sites, the mechanical properties of the modified hydrogel matrices decrease with increasing concentrations of incorporated bioactive molecules [36]. Moreover, the fibrin fiber structure changes through incorporation of large concentrations of bioactive molecules [36]. The conclusion is that mechanical properties and fiber structures of modified 3D fibrin hydrogels result from the equilibrium between crosslink density and the amount of incorporated bioactive molecules. Therefore, 3D fibrin matrices allow the design of different fiber structures depending on the amount of incorporated bioactive molecules, thus providing very different conditions for infiltrating cells.

For experimental use of such modified 3D fibrin matrices, one must consider that by changing the 3D fibrin matrix on the molecular level through altering the mechanical properties and/or the fiber structure by incorporation of bioactive molecules, the degradation time of such a matrix might decrease. This feature is especially important when 3D fibrin matrices are used as in vitro systems where different cell types secrete varying amounts of degrading enzymes (plasmin and MMPs) thus scaffold stability and release functions need to be carefully balanced. When using 3D fibrin matrices for in vivo experiments, the removal of the 3D scaffold depends on the native degradation mechanisms, which lead to the release of bioactive molecules at the speed of the regenerating tissue.

3.2 Experimental Design

The 3D fibrin matrices can be used to test the controlled release and role of bioactive molecules in vitro and in vivo. As native tissues are composed of hierarchical 3D structures, 3D tissue culture systems are highly desirable and provide many advantages over 2D surfaces that are commonly used in cell culture. Here we provide 3D fibrin matrices as a tool to study the efficiency of biologically active molecules under standardized conditions that allow good availability combined with ease in production and maintenance. An analysis of cellular responses within 3D fibrin matrices can be performed using conventional techniques such as biochemical methods and fluorescence or confocal microscopy. Moreover, multiple assays can be performed in parallel thus allowing proper statistics. Several applications are possible including the search for proangiogenic factors whose activity can be assessed by the formation and length of vascular tubes formed in vitro [29–31, 33, 34], factors that favor nerve regeneration as determined by the growth of neurites and in vitro myelination by Schwann cells [28, 37, 38] and proliferation or differentiation of stem cells can be determined [8, 39, 40]. Prior to the actual experiment several questions need to be addressed:

- Which bioactive substance will be tested?
- How can one incorporate the bioactive molecules into the 3D fibrin matrix?
- Which cell type(s) will be used during the experiments?
- Do these cells secrete MMPs and/or plasmin to degrade the 3D fibrin matrix?
- Selection of experimental setup: placement of cells on, into, between two layers of the 3D fibrin matrix?
- How to analyze the biological response?

3.3 Materials

3.3.1 Chemicals

- Human fibrinogen (Fluka or Sigma)
- PBS (Sigma P3813)
- TBS (10 mM Tris/HCl, pH 7.4, 150 mM NaCl)
- $CaCl_2$
- Double-distilled water
- Thrombin (Sigma T6884)
- Factor XIII (e.g., Fibrogammin P 1250, CLS Behring GmbH, Marburg, Germany)
- Collagen type I (stock solution 3.41 mg/ml, BD Bioscience)
- Fluorescein diacetate (AppliChem)
- Dimethyl-sulfoxid (DMSO, Sigma)
- WST-1 proliferation assay (Roche)
- Hoechst nuclear stain-33342 (Invitrogen/Molecular Probes)
- Aprotinin (Sigma)
- GM6001 (also named Ilomastat, Chemicon)
- 0.25% Trypsin (Gibco BRL)

3.3.2 Equipment/Infrastructure

- Tissue culture plates 24 or 48 wells (NUNC corning)
- Eppendorf pipettes 1,000, 200, 20 μl
- Fluorescence microscope equipped with a camera and fluorescence filters (DAPI, FITC, TRITC) (e.g., Zeiss Axiovert 200)
- Confocal laser scanning microscope (e.g., Leica SP5)
- Dialysis tubes (e.g., Spectra/Por)
- Sterile pore filters (5 μm, 0.2-μm pore size)
- Spectrophotometer that allows UV detection
- Quartz cuvettes for spectrophotometer
- Sterile working environment for tissue culture
- Incubators for tissue culture (37°C, 5% CO_2)
- Horizontal shaker for microtiter plates
- Fluorescence and absorbance plate reader (e.g., Tecan infinite M200)

3.4 Methods

3.4.1 Preparation of 3D fibrin matrices

3.4.1.1 Fibrinogen solution

Time required: 2 days

1. Store human fibrinogen at –20°C.

2. Prewarm fibrinogen for 15 minutes at room temperature.
3. Dissolve 50-mg fibrinogen in 3-ml double distilled water in 30-mm diameter Petri dishes for 1–2 hours at room temperature
4. Inject dissolved fibrinogen into a dialysis tube.
5. Dialyze for 24h at room temperature in a 4 l TBS buffer (10 mM Tris/HCl pH 7.5, 150 mM NaCl). Stir constantly and replace the TBS buffer once.
6. Filter sterilized dialyzed fibrinogen solution by sequentially using a 5-μm followed by 0.2-μm pore size filter.
7. Determine the protein content at 280 nm in a spectrophotometer.
8. Calculate the fibrinogen concentration using the Lambert-Beers law, according to the following equation:

$$c_{fib}\left[\frac{mg}{ml}\right] = \frac{M_{fib}[g/mol]A_{280}b}{d[cm]\varepsilon_{280}(fib)}$$

   c_{fib} = the fibrinogen concentration
   M_{fib} = molecular weight of fibrinogen (341,000 g/mol)
   A_{280} = absorbance intensity at 280 nm
   d = thickness of the quartz curvette (often 1 cm)
   $\varepsilon_{280}(fib)$ = extinction coefficient at 280 nm (528,550 L mol^{-1} cm^{-1})
   b = dilution factor (valid for the equation between 10 and 100)
9. Prepare aliquots of appropriate size and store at −20°C until use.

3.4.1.2 Formation of 3D fibrin matrices

Time required: 1–2 hours, depending on the number of samples. Wear gloves as you work with human fibrinogen that might potentially be hazardous for your health.

See the schematic in Figure 3.1(a) and also Table 3.1.

1. Prepare the following stock solutions:
   - Fibrinogen: > 8 mg/ml, store at –20°C until use
   - Thrombin: 0.1 U/ml, store at –20°C until use
   - Factor XIII: 20 U/ml, store at –20°C until use
   - $CaCl_2$: 125 mM in double distilled water, store at 4°C
   - TBS (10 mM Tris/HCl pH 7.5, 150 mM NaCl), store at 4°C

   All solutions need to be sterile.
2. Determine the final amount of the 3D fibrin matrix that you need per well, per animal (not per experiment). (Example: 100 μl of 3D fibrin matrix per well of a 48-well plate, 250 μl per well of a 24-well plate.)
3. Prepare one Eppendorf tube per 3D fibrin matrix to be produced.
4. Prepare a fibrinogen master mix solution for each Eppendorf tube containing: fibrinogen, $CaCl_2$, factor XIII, and TBS.
5. Start the polymerization by addition of thrombin.
6. Mix well and transfer immediately into final container.
7. Let the 3D fibrin matrix polymerize for 10 minutes at room temperature.
8. Add buffer, tissue culture medium, or other solution to prevent drying.
9. Perform planned assay.

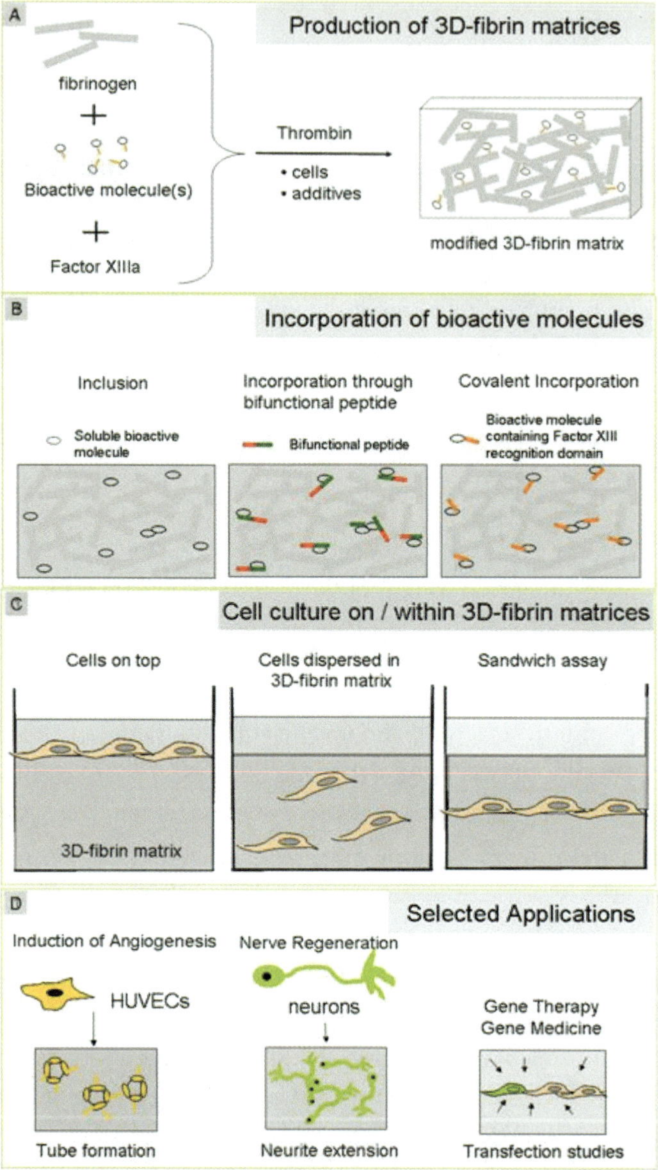

Figure 3.1 (a) Schematic representations of 3D fibrin matrix formation, (b) different possibilities to incorporate bioactive molecules, (c) in vitro cell cultivation on top and within 3D fibrin matrices, and (d) some selected applications.

Table 3.1 Pipetting Scheme for 200 μl of 2 mg/ml 3D Fibrin Matrix

Substance	Concentration of Stock Solution	Used Volume	Final Concentration
Fibrinogen	8 mg/ml	50 μl	2 mg/ml
Thrombin	0.1 U/ml	2.5 μl	1.25 mU/ml
Factor XIII	200 U/ml	2.5 μl	500 mU/ml
$CaCl_2$	125 mM	1.3 μl	0.8 mM
TBS		143.7 μl	

3.4.2 Introduction of bioactive molecules

Time required:

- Inclusion of bioactive molecules: 1–2 hours as for the preparation of 3D fibrin matrices.
- Insertion of bifunctional peptides: weeks (design, purchase of peptides).
- Insertion of bioactive proteins that contain an N-terminal factor XIII recognition sequence (NQEQVSPL): Weeks – month (PCR-design, cloning and expression, and characterization of the protein).

Three possible ways are commonly used to introduce bioactive molecules into 3D fibrin matrices. The decision needs to be made according to the chemical nature, availability, and purpose of the bioactive molecule to be delivered and further analyzed [see schematic Figure 3.1(b)]. This chapter only provides a short overview on the currently used procedures and might help in choosing one procedure over another. The included references provide more information on the actual procedures, as a detailed description would go beyond the scope of this chapter.

1. Inclusion of soluble bioactive molecules:
   - Simplest and easiest method [23–26].
   - Depends only on biophysical characteristics, such as solubility of the bioactive molecule within the fibrinogen master mix solution.
   - Release is completely driven by diffusion and depends on the concentration gradient towards the culture medium.

2. Insertion of bioactive molecules through a bifunctional peptide that contains the N-terminal factor XIII recognition sequence (NQEQVSPL), and a binding site for the bioactive molecule (such as a DNA or heparin-binding sequence).
   - The peptide needs to be synthesized or purchased.
   - An example for a bifunctional peptide used to bind/complex plasmid DNA combined with the factor XIII recognition sequence [35, 41]:
     factor XIII-recognition DNA-binding
     NQEQVSPL-$(G)_3$-CH$(K)_6$-HC
   - An example for a bifunctional peptide comprising the factor XIII recognition sequence and a heparin-binding site [28].
     factor XIII-recognition Heparin-binding
     dLNQEQVSPK(bA)FAKLAARLYRKA
   - Method is relatively complicated as it involves several components whose relative concentrations towards each other need to be carefully adjusted.
   - No covalent attachment of the bioactive molecule, therefore relatively fast release.
   - Release depends on concentration gradient and ionic strength of culture conditions.

3. Insertion of bioactive proteins that contain an N-terminal factor XIII recognition sequence (NQEQVSPL).
   - Most time-consuming method, as it requires modification of a protein by recombinant DNA technology to introduce N-terminal NQEQVSPL.
   - Examples: Introduction of N-terminal NQEQVSPL into vascular endothelial growth factor $(VEGF)_{121}$, nerve growth factor (NGF), or a specific $\alpha v\beta 3$ integrin binding domain (L1Ig6) using PCR technology [29, 37, 42].

3.4.3 Cell Culture

Time required:

- Determination of optimal fibrin concentration: 2 days–1 week for one experiment.
- Test for plasmin or matrix metalloproteinase (MMP) activity: 2 days–1 week for one experiment.
- Determine the optimal culture conditions: 2 days–1 week for one experiment.

3.4.3.1 Determination of optimal fibrin concentration

To avoid early matrix degradation in vitro and in vivo, the concentration of fibrin for each experimental setup needs to be optimized.

1. Produce 3D fibrin matrices with different concentrations (e.g. 2, 3, 4, and 8 mg/ml) in 24- or 48-well plates (adapt pipetting scheme from Table 3.1).
2. Let polymerize for 10 minutes at room temperature but avoid drying the surface (e.g., place into a humid chamber).
3. Place desired cell type at 80% confluence on top of 3D fibrin matrices.
4. Add the corresponding tissue culture medium.
5. Place the cultures at 37°C and 5% CO_2.
6. Monitor cell growth and matrix degradation daily by phase-contrast microscopy.
7. Change the medium every other day.
8. Take images at designated time points and determine when the 3D fibrin matrix begins to dissolve.

3.4.3.2 Test for plasmin or matrix metalloproteinase (MMP) activity

Plasmin and MMPs are proteolytic enzymes that are secreted from different cell types in different amounts. Plasmin and MMPs both contribute to degradation of 3D fibrin matrices and might, when extensively secreted, interfere with the experiment. Therefore inhibition experiments in the presence of a plasmin inhibitor (aprotinin) or a MMP inhibitor (GM6001) or in the presence of both might be necessary.

1. Perform the same experiment as described above in the presence of:
   - Plasmin inhibitor aprotinin (e.g., 50 and 5 μg/ml [38]);
   - MMP inhibitor GM6001 (e.g., 6, 12.5, or 60 μM [36]);
   - Both inhibitors.
2. Add the inhibitors into the tissue culture medium.
3. Analyze cell attachment and growth as well as matrix degradation as described above.

3.4.3.3 Determine the optimal culture conditions

See the schematic in Figure 3.1(c).

1. Cells cultured *on top* of a 3D fibrin matrix.
   - Produce 3D fibrin matrix with fibrin concentration as determined in 1.
   - Test different cell densities (e.g., 50–80%) confluence and monitor cell attachment, cell viability, and cell proliferation for several days.

2. Cells placed directly *into* the 3D fibrin matrix.
   - Certain cell types such as fibroblasts can be cultivated when dispersed directly into the fibrinogen precursor mix solution. The advantage of this is that the cells are surrounded by the 3D matrix and form 3D adhesion structures.
   - Produce 3D fibrin matrix with fibrin concentration as determined in 1.
   - Introduce different cell numbers directly into the fibrinogen precursor master mix solution and reduce the amount of TBS accordingly (use the pipetting scheme of Table 3.2).
   - Monitor cell attachment, cell viability and cell proliferation for several days.
3. Cells placed *between* two layers of fibrin: Sandwich assay. Cell types that do not grow when dispersed directly within the 3D fibrin matrix but still need direct contact to the matrix from all sides can be cultivated between two hydrogel sandwiches. The first 3D fibrin matrix is produced, cells are seeded on top and are allowed to attach and spread. Then they are covered by a second 3D fibrin matrix. Often cell types do not like fibrin matrices as a substrate for cell adhesion; therefore, blending the 3D fibrin matrix with collagen type I to provide different cell attachment sites is recommended.

3.4.4 Data acquisition, important controls, and staining procedures

Time required:

- Release of bioactive molecules from 3D fibrin matrices: ~ 1 week.
- Determine biological response of bioactive molecule in 3D fibrin matrix: variable.

3.4.4.1 Release of bioactive molecules from 3D fibrin matrices

1. Include/incorporate bioactive molecules into 3D fibrin matrices.
2. Rinse solidified matrices once with 250-μl PBS for 48 well plates and with 500 μl for 24-well plates to remove the unbound molecules from the surface of the matrices.
3. Overlay the matrices with 500- or 250-μl PBS, respectively, and place at 37°C, 5% CO_2 while gently shaking on a horizontal shaker.
4. Remove PBS supernatant every 24 hours and replace with fresh PBS.

Table 3.2 Pipetting Scheme for 100 μl of 8 mg/ml 3D Fibrin Matrix for Cell Culture Experiments

Substance	Concentration of Stock Solution	Used Volume	Final Concentration
Fibrinogen	25 mg/ml	32 μl	8 mg/ml
Thrombin	0.1 U/ml	1.25 μl	1.25 mU/ml
Factor XIII	200 U/ml	1.25 μl	500 mU/ml
$CaCl_2$	125 mM	1.3 μl	1.6 mM
Optional: collagen type I	1 mg/ml	1 μl	10 μg/ml
Optional: additives	1 mg/ml	2.0 or 0.2 μl	50 or 5 μg/ml
Aprotinin, GM6001, cells	2.5 mM	0.24, 0.6, and 2.4 μl	6, 12.5, or 60 μM (e.g., 20,000/ml)
TBS		64.2 μl (reduce volume according to the additives)	

5. Repeat this procedure daily and collect all the supernatants and store at 4°C for further analysis.
6. After the last removal of supernatants, digest the 3D fibrin matrices with 0.025% trypsin for 60 minutes at 37°C.
7. Collect the solubilized fibrin matrix to determine the concentration of the remaining bioactive molecules.
8. Repeat the release experiments three times in duplicate.
9. Calculate the cumulative release of the bioactive molecule over time.
10. Compare the differences between the mean values by two-tailed ANOVA and accept statistical significance for $p < 0.05$. Statistics can be performed by using a statistic software (e.g., Origin 7.5).

3.4.4.2 Determine biological response of bioactive molecules in 3D fibrin matrices

Perform actual experiments within 3D fibrin matrices: for example, tube formation of endothelial cells [30, 31, 33, 34, 42], differentiation of progenitor or stem cells [39], nerve regeneration [37, 38], or transfection of cells with therapeutically relevant plasmid DNA [43, 44] [see Figure 3.1(d)].

3.4.4.3 Important controls

Determine the biological activity of matrix-released bioactive molecules

- Compare biological activity of matrix-released bioactive molecules with freshly produced/prepared bioactive molecules.

Fluorescein diacetate staining to determine cell viability

Fluorescein diacetate (FDA), a nonfluorescent fatty acid ester of fluorescein, enters living cells; in these cells, it may be rapidly hydrolysed by esterases to produce fluorescein, which can be used as a marker for cell viability.

1. Prepare stock solution of FDA (5 mg/ml in DMSO).
2. Remove tissue culture medium.
3. Rinse cells twice with TBS.
4. Stain cells with FDA (final concentration: 5 μg/ml dissolved in TBS) for 1–2 minutes at room temperature.
5. Remove staining solution and wash cells twice with TBS.
6. Analyze cells immediately by fluorescence microscopy (FITC filter).
7. Determine the number of living cells by taking 2 photos/well.
8. Count living (green) and total cell number (blue, as determined by Hoechst nuclear stain; see following method) for each condition by either manual counting or by using Image J image processing.
9. Perform three independent experiments and calculate mean values +/− standard deviation.
10. Compare the differences between the mean values by two-tailed ANOVA and accept the statistical significance for $p < 0.05$. Statistics can be performed by using Origin 7.5.

Hoechst nuclear stain to determine the absolute cell number

1. Prepare Hoechst stain solution: 1 μl from stock solution into 2-ml TBS.
2. Remove the tissue culture medium.
3. Rinse once with TBS (avoid drying of the cells).
4. Add staining solution to cells for 1–5 minutes.
5. Remove the Hoechst stain.
6. Rinse once with TBS and add the cell culture medium.
7. Analyze with the fluorescence microscope (DAPI filter).
8. Determine the cell number for each condition using either manual counting or Image J image processing in at least three experiments carried out in duplicate.
9. Determine mean values +/– standard deviation.
10. Compare the differences between the mean values by two-tailed ANOVA and accept statistical significance for $p < 0.05$. Statistics can be performed by using Origin 7.5.
11. Use the data to normalize the cell viability and/or cell proliferation.

WST-1 cell proliferation assay The proliferation substrate does not harm the cells and can therefore be repeatedly used with one single culture. The advantage is that the number of cultures is reduced and an individual culture can be analyzed at different time points.

1. Thaw WST-1 reagent and vortex carefully such that no precipitates are visible.
2. Remove the cell culture medium and add fresh medium.
3. Add one-tenth of the volume of the culture medium of WST-1 reagent to the culture dish.
4. Incubate the cells for 1–3 hours at 37°C, 5 % CO_2.
5. Transfer cell culture medium into Eppendorf tubes.
6. Feed cells with the fresh cell culture medium and place back into the incubator (37°C and 5% CO_2) for further cultivation.
7. Measure absorbance at 450 nm.
8. In parallel, determine the cell number (by Hoechst nuclear stain) for each condition in at least three experiments carried out in duplicate.
9. Calculate mean values +/– standard deviation.
10. Correlate cellular activity (WST-1 assay) with the absolute cell number (determined by Hoechst nuclear stain) to obtain cellular activity/cell.
11. Compare the differences between the mean values by two-tailed ANOVA and accept statistical significance for $p < 0.05$. Statistics can be performed by using Origin 7.5.

3.5 Data Analysis, Anticipated Results, and Interpretation

A broad spectrum of cellular readouts can be obtained by using the 3D fibrin matrix system. Information on efficiencies of different bioactive molecules released with time can be obtained in a quantitative manner. As in vitro culture conditions are more defined than in vivo experiments this 3D culture system allows the easy correlation of the investigated biological effect/response, with cell viability and cell proliferation being important parameters that validate the entire test system. After analyzing the cell number by

Hoechst nuclear stain, all obtained values can be normalized to the individual cell. This gives an ideal tool to determine the biological activity per cell.

In addition, cell morphology can be visualized by confocal microscopy using FDA staining in addition to Hoechst nuclear stain. Both techniques allow 3D reconstruction of the cell population growing within two layers of the 3D fibrin matrix or entirely dispersed within the matrix by using a relevant software package such as Imaris 6.2 (Bitplane, Switzerland, http://www.bitplane.com/). These microscopy data combined with quantitative evaluation of the analyzed biological effect/response allow interesting conclusions on cellular functions and behavior that might be more relevant than data obtained in conventional 2D tissue culture assays.

3.6 Discussion and Commentary

3D tissue culture systems are one way to overcome the limited relevance of conventional tissue culture studies for in vivo applications. Here we combine such improved techniques with the release of bioactive molecules to provide both a 3D scaffold and a sustained release system for bioactive molecule(s). As bioactive molecules need to be released, several options are discussed to include or to incorporate them into 3D fibrin matrices. In addition several ways of cell culturing on top and within such a 3D fibrin matrix are described. Most important is that many samples can be performed in parallel such that statistical analysis will be possible. This feature provides an advantage to relevant in vivo studies that are often only performable in small numbers, and large individual variations between test animals complicate the analysis. For in vitro and in vivo use of 3D fibrin matrices, a careful balance needs to be established between the amount of incorporated molecules to be released and the mechanical stability of the 3D matrix. A further complication might be that different cell types secrete varying amounts of proteolytic enzymes that accelerate matrix degradation. Therefore, 3D fibrin matrices are preferentially used for short term applications between 1–7 days in vitro and 1–14 days in vivo. These time frames correspond roughly with the natural residing time of a fibrin clot that is remodeled throughout the healing process of a wound. Experiments to be performed using 3D fibrin matrices might include the determination of the efficiency of matrix-released growth factors or release of condensed plasmid DNA to stimulate the formation of new blood vessels and therefore improve wound healing [33–35, 41, 42]. In order to do so, human umbilical vein endothelial cells (HUVECs) were cultured within the matrices and process extensions were analyzed [see schematic in Figure 3.1(d)]. Additionally, we used such matrices to compare neurite extensions when PC12 neurons were cultivated on top or dispersed within the 3D fibrin matrices. Such experiments allowed assessment of degradation mechanisms used by neurons to remodel their extracellular matrix [see schematic in Figure 3.1(d)] [38]. Other groups have used 3D fibrin matrices to culture and differentiate mesenchymal stem cells for further analysis [8, 39, 40].

When comparing 3D fibrin matrices with other natural hydrogel matrices such as collagen type I, 3D fibrin matrices do not contract with time in culture as described for collagen type I matrices [45–47]. Moreover, 3D fibrin matrices can be blended with relevant extracellular matrix molecules that then provide the necessary cell attachment sites for optimal cell growth and differentiation (e.g., [30]). Here, inhibitions studies can be performed to analyze the involvement of different integrins binding to their respective extracellular matrix receptors. Therefore we think that 3D fibrin matrices provide a versatile tool for tissue engineering and allow quantitative cell function analysis in vitro as well as implantation in vivo providing a combined scaffold and release system.

Troubleshooting Table

Problem	Explanation	Potential Solution
Fibrin matrices do not polymerize.	Mixing of precursor solutions is not sufficient.	Mix all components very carefully prior to adding factor XIII and thrombin.
	Thrombin is inactive.	Use a freshly prepared aliquot of thrombin.
	Thrombin concentration is too low.	Test different concentrations of thrombin.
	Factor XIII is not active.	Use a fresh aliquot of factor XIII and test different concentrations.
Fibrin matrices polymerize too fast.	Thrombin and factor XIII act to fast.	Precool all solutions on ice.
	Some recombinant proteins contain traces of thrombin as thrombin is often used to remove the His-tag during the purification process.	Prepare fibrin matrices on ice. Work fast. Reduce thrombin concentration.
Cells die within the fibrin matrix.	Concentration of fibrinogen precursor is too high or too low.	Make a concentration series of different fibrinogen precursor solutions and test the optimal concentration for this specific cell type.
Cells do not adhere and stay round within the fibrin matrix.	Cells cannot interact with fibrin matrices as a substrate.	Use a fibrin matrix and place cells on top: Do cells adhere?
		If cells do not adhere add (e.g., 10 μg/ml collagen) type I to the fibrinogen precursor solution.
Cells degrade the 3D fibrin matrix to fast.	Cells secrete high amounts of MMPs and/or plasmin.	Add proteolytic inhibitors (aprotinin for plasmin; GM6009 for MMPs).
		Use higher concentrations of initial fibrin matrix.

3.7 Application Notes

The here introduced 3D culture system tries to bridge the gap between conventional 2D tissue culture systems and in vivo situations. As tissue function is very much dependent on 3D architecture, 3D fibrin hydrogel matrices might be a good compromise to analyze biological activity under controlled in vitro conditions but with increased complexity as compared to conventional tissue culturing. This chapter provides only a selection of possible ways to produce relevant assay systems as well as an extract of analysis tools that can be performed with standard methodology. Many more relevant tests that allow examination of coculture systems, production of mixed hydrogel matrices consisting of different monomers, and the development of a simpler, more versatile release system might be desirable in future experiments.

3.8 Summary Points

1. We have developed a 3D fibrin matrix system that can be modified to store and release bioactive molecules in a controlled manner that induces cell-type specific responses. This 3D matrix system simulates the native ECM to a certain extent and provides a versatile tool to analyze various biological questions under

quasi-controlled in vitro conditions. As many samples can be processed in parallel, statistical data can be obtained and compared to each other.

2. The 3D fibrin matrices have turned out to be very versatile because of their natural origin and their compatibility with in vitro and in vivo use. They are easy to handle and to modify. Experimentation requires no special equipment besides a tissue culture facility and access to conventional fluorescence and/or confocal microscopy.
3. Detailed protocols are provided for fibrinogen dissolution, 3D fibrin matrix production, and performance of release studies for bioactive molecules.
4. Protocols are introduced for three possible ways to cultivate cells on top, dispersed in, and between sandwiches of 3D fibrin matrices. Furthermore, strategies to optimize culture conditions for different cell types are provided.
5. An extensive section is dedicated to necessary controls that validate the system and allow quantification of cellular responses to individual cells.

Acknowledgments

This work was supported by the Gebert Rüf-Foundation GRS-053/05 and ETH Zurich. Tessa Lühmann and Markus Rimann are acknowledged for their critical reading and commenting on the manuscript.

References

[1] Peppas, N. A., "Time- and Position-Dependent Drug Delivery in Controlled-Release Systems," *J. Pharm. Sci.*, Vol. 76, No. 3, 1987, p. 267.

[2] Tarvainen, T., et al., "Drug Release from Poly(Acrylic Acid) Grafted Poly(Vinylidene Fluoride) Membrane Bags in the Gastrointestinal Tract in the Rat and Dog," *J. Control Release*, Vol. 66, No. 1, 2000, pp. 19–26.

[3] Zarif, L., "Elongated Supramolecular Assemblies in Drug Delivery," *J. Control Release*, Vol. 81, No. 1–2, 2002, pp. 7–23.

[4] Misra, G. P., and R. A. Siegel, "New Mode of Drug Delivery: Long Term Autonomous Rhythmic Hormone Release Across a Hydrogel Membrane," *J. Control Release*, Vol. 81, No. 1–2, 2002, pp. 1–6.

[5] Drury, J. L., and D. J. Mooney, "Hydrogels for Tissue Engineering: Scaffold Design Variables and Applications," *Biomaterials*, Vol. 24, No. 24, 2003, pp. 4337–4351.

[6] Lutholf, M. P., and J. A. Hubbell, "Synthetic Biomaterials as Instructive Extracellular Microenvironments for Morphogenesis in Tissue Engineering," *Nat. Biotechnol.*, Vol. 23, 2005, pp. 47–53.

[7] Ahmed, T. A., E. V. Dare, and M. Hincke, "Fibrin: A Versatile Scaffold for Tissue Engineering Applications," *Tissue Eng. Part B Rev.*, Vol. 14, No. 2, 2008, pp. 199–215.

[8] Breen, A., T. O'Brien, and A. Pandit, "Fibrin as a Delivery System for Therapeutic Drugs and Biomolecules," *Tissue Eng. Part B Rev.*, February 27, 2009.

[9] Weisel, J. W., et al., "A Model for Fibrinogen: Domains and Sequence," *Science*, Vol. 230, 1985, pp. 1388–1391.

[10] Ariens, R. A. S., et al., "Role of Factor XIII in Fibrin Clot Formation and Effects of Genetic Polymorphisms," *Blood*, Vol. 100, 2002, pp. 743–754.

[11] Lorand, L., and R. M. Graham, "Transglutaminases: Crosslinking Enzymes with Pleiotropic Functions," *Nat. Rev. Mol. Cell. Biol.*, Vol. 4, No. 2, 2003, pp. 140–156.

[12] Blombäck, B., and N. Bark, "Fibrinopeptides and Fibrin Gel Structure," *Biophys. Chem.*, Vol. 112, 2004, pp. 147–151.

[13] Mosesson, M. W., "Fibrinogen and Fibrin Structure and Functions," *J. Thromb. Haemost.*, Vol. 3, No. 8, 2005, pp. 1894–1904.

[14] Weisel, J.W., "Structure of Fibrin: Impact on Clot Stability," *Journal of Thrombosis and Haemostasis*, Vol. 5, 2007, pp. 116–124.

[15] Ryan, E., et al., "Influence of a Natural and a Synthetic Inhibitor of Factor XIII on Fibrin Clot Rheology," *Biophys. J.*, Vol. 77, 1999, pp. 2827–2836.

[16] Ryan, E., et al., "Structural Origins of Fibrin Rheology," *Biophys. J.*, Vol. 77, 1999, pp. 2813–2826.

[17] Rocco, M., et al., "Early Events in the Polymerization of Fibrin," *Ann. N.Y. Acad. Sci.*, Vol. 936, 2001, pp. 167–184.

[18] Pepper, M. S., et al., "Angiogensis: A Paradigm for Balanced Extracellular Proteolysis During Cell Migration and Morphogenesis," *Enzyme Protein*, Vol. 49, 1996, pp. 138–162.

[19] Pintucci, G., et al., "Angiogenesis and the Fibrinolytic System," *Semin. Thromb. Hemost.*, Vol. 22, No. 6, 1996, pp. 517–524.

[20] Hiraoka, N., et al., "Matrix Metalloproteinases Regulate Neovascularization by Acting as Pericellular Fibrolysins," *Cell*, Vol. 95, 1998, pp. 365–377.

[21] Hiller, O., et al., "Matrix Metalloproteinases Collagenase-3, and Membrane Type 1-Matrix Metalloproteinase Impair Clotting by Degradation of Fibrinogen and Factor XII," *J. Biol. Chem.*, Vol. 275, 2000, pp. 33008–33013.

[22] Hotary, K. B., et al., "Marix Metalloproteinases (MMPs) Regulate Fibrin-Invasive Activity Via MT1-MMP-Dependent and -Independent Processes," *J. Exp. Med.*, Vol. 195, 2002, pp. 295–308.

[23] Kipshidze, N., et al., "Endoluminal Reconstruction of the Arterial Wall with Endothelial Cell/Glue Matrix Reduces Restenosis in an Atherosclerotic Rabbit," *J. Am. Coll. Cardiol.*, Vol. 36, No. 4, 2000, pp. 1396–1403.

[24] Royce, S. M., M. Askari, and K. G. Marra, "Incorporation of Polymer Microspheres Within Fibrin Scaffolds for the Controlled Delivery of FGF-1," *J. Biomater. Sci. Polymer. Edn.*, 2004, Vol. 15, pp. 1327–1336.

[25] Jeon, O., et al., "Control of Basic Fibroblast Growth Factor Release from Fibrin Gel with Heparin and Concentrations of Fibrinogen and Thrombin," *J. Contr. Rel.*, Vol. 105, 2005, pp. 249–259.

[26] Jeon, O., et al., "Long-Term and Zero Order Release of Basic Fibroblast Growth Factor from Heparin-Conjugated Poly(L-Lactide-Co-Glycolide) Nanospheres and Fibrin Gel," *Biomaterials*, Vol. 27, 2006, pp. 1598–1607.

[27] Schense, J. C., and J. A. Hubbell, "Cross-Linking Exogenous Bifunctional Peptides into Fibrin Gels with Factor XIIIa," *Bioconjug. Chem.*, Vol. 10, No. 1, 1999, pp. 75–81.

[28] Sakiyama, S. E., J. C. Schense, and J. A. Hubbell, "Incorporation of Heparin-Binding Peptides into Fibrin Gels Enhances Neurite Extension: An Example of Designer Matrices in Tissue Engineering," *FASEB. J.*, Vol. 13, 1999, pp. 214–224.

[29] Hall, H., T. Baechi, and J. A. Hubbell, "Molecular Properties of Fibrin-Based Hydrogels for Angiogensis In Vitro," *Microvasc. Res.*, Vol. 62, 2001, pp. 315–326.

[30] Hall, H., et al., "Heterophilic Interactions Between Cell Adhesion Molecule L1 and Alphavbeta3-Integrin Induce HUVEC Process Extension In Vitro and Angiogenesis In Vivo," *Angiogenesis*, Vol. 7, No. 3, 2004, pp. 213–223.

[31] Hall, H., and J. A. Hubbell, "Matrix-Bound Sixth Ig-Like Domain of Cell Adhesion Molecule L1 Acts as an Angiogenic Factor by Ligating Alphavbeta3-Integrin and Activating VEGF-R2," *Microvasc. Res.*, Vol. 68, No. 3, 2004, pp. 169–178.

[32] Zisch, A. H., M. P. Lutolf, and J. A. Hubbell, "Biopolymeric Delivery Matrices for Angiogenic Growth Factors," *Cardiovasc. Pathol.*, Vol. 12, No. 6, 2003, pp. 295–310.

[33] Ehrbar, M., et al., "Endothelial Cell Proliferation and Progenitor Maturation by Fibrin-Bound VEGF Variants with Differential Susceptibilities to Local Cellular Activity," *J. Control Release*, Vol. 101, No. 1–3, 2005, pp. 93–109.

[34] Ehrbar, M., et al., "The Role of Actively Released Fibrin-Conjugated VEGF for VEGF Receptor 2 Gene Activation and the Enhancement of Angiogenesis," *Biomaterials*, Vol. 29, No. 11, 2008, pp. 1720–1729.

[35] Trentin, D., et al., "Peptide-Matrix-Mediated Gene Transfer of an Oxygen-Insensitive Hypoxia-Inducible Factor-1alpha Variant for Local Induction of Angiogenesis," *Proc. Natl. Acad. Sci. USA*, Vol. 103, No. 8, 2006, pp. 2506–2511.

[36] Urech, L., et al., "Mechanical Properties, Proteolytic Degrdability and Biological Modifications Affect Angiogenic Process Extension into Native and Modified Fibrin Matrices In Vivo," *Biomaterials*, Vol. 26, 2005, pp. 1369–1379.

[37] Sakiyama-Elbert, S. E., A. Panitsch, and J. A. Hubbell, "Development of Growth Factor Fusion Proteins for Cell Triggered Drug Delivery," *FASEB Journal*, March 20, 2001.

[38] Pittier, R., et al., "Neurite Extension and In Vitro Myelination Within Three-Dimensional Modified Fibrin Matrices," *J. Neurobiol.*, Vol. 63, No. 1, 2005, pp. 1–14.

[39] Willerth, S. M., A. Rader, and S. E. Sakiyama-Elbert, "The Effect of Controlled Growth Factor Delivery on Embryonic Stem Cell Differentiation Inside Fibrin Scaffolds," *Stem Cell Res.*, Vol. 3, 2008, pp. 205–218.

[40] Neuss, S., et al., "Secretion of Fibrinolytic Enzymes Facilitates Human Mesenchymal Stem Cell Invasion into Fibrin Clots," *Cells Tissues Organs*, April 24, 2009.

[41] Trentin, D., J. Hubbell, and H. Hall, "Non-Viral Gene Delivery for Local and Controlled DNA Release," *J. Control Release*, Vol. 102, No. 1, 2005, pp. 263–275.

[42] Zisch, A. H., et al., "Covalently Conjugated VEGF—Fibrin Matrices for Endothelialization," *J. Control Release*, Vol. 72, No. 1–3, 2001, pp. 101–113.

[43] Luhmann, T., et al., "Cellular Uptake and Intracellular Pathways of PLL-g-PEG-DNA Nanoparticles," *Bioconjug. Chem.*, Vol. 19, No. 9, 2008, pp. 1907–1916.

[44] Rimann, M., et al., "Characterization of PLL-g-PEG-DNA Nanoparticles for the Delivery of Therapeutic DNA," *Bioconjug. Chem.*, Vol. 19, No. 2, 2008, pp. 548–557.

[45] Angele, P., et al., "Influence of Different Collagen Species on Physico-Chemical Properties of Crosslinked Collagen Matrices," *Biomaterials*, Vol. 25, 2004, pp. 2831–2841.

[46] Bilic, G., et al., "Human Preterm Amnion Cells Cultured in 3-Dimensional Collagen I and Fibrin Matrices for Tissue Engineering Purposes," *American Journal of Obstetrics and Gynecology*, Vol. 193, 2005, pp. 1724–1732.

[47] Madhan, B., et al., "Stabilization of Collagen Using Plant Polyphenol: Role of Catechin," *International Journal of Biological Macromolecules*, Vol. 37, 2005, pp. 47–53.

Selected Bibliography

Imaris 6.2, Bitplane, Switzerland, http://www.bitplane.com/Image J Image Processing, http://rsbweb.nih.gov/ij.

CHAPTER

4

Designer Self-Assembling Peptide Scaffolds for 3D Tissue Cell Cultures

Fabrizio Gelain, Xiumei Wang, Akihiro Horii, Angus Hucknall, Sotirios Koutsopoulos, and Shuguang Zhang

Center for Biomedical Engineering NE47-379, Center for Bits & Atoms, Massachusetts Institute of Technology, Cambridge, MA, Corresponding author: Shuguang Zhang, address: Center for Biomedical Engineering NE47-379, Center for Bits & Atoms, Massachusetts Institute of Technology, 77 Massachusetts Avenue, Cambridge, MA 02139, United States, phone: 1-617-258-7514, fax: 1-617-258-5239, e-mail: Shuguang@mit.edu

Abstract

Biomedical researchers have become increasingly aware of the limitations of conventional 2D tissue cell cultures. They are now testing 3D cell culture systems, something between a Petri dish and a mouse. The important implications of 3D tissue cell cultures for basic cell biology, tumor biology, high-content drug screening, regenerative medicine, and beyond are far-reaching. It has become more apparent that 3D cell cultures offer a more realistic microenvironment for the cells in the nanofiber scaffolds where the cells can be observed and manipulated. A class of designer self-assembling peptide nanofiber scaffolds provides an ideal 3D culture system. The time has come to address the 3D questions because quantitative biology requires in vitro culture systems that more authentically represent the cellular microenvironment in a living organism. In doing so, in vitro experimentation can become truly more predictive of in vivo systems. This chapter describes methods to work on designer self-assembling peptide nanofiber scaffolds for 3D tissue cell cultures.

Key terms
3D cell culture
designer self-assembling peptides
hydrogel
matrix
nanofibers
scaffold
unidirectional cell migration

4.1 Introduction

Advancement of biology often requires development of new materials, methods, and tools. The introduction of the Petri dish over 100 years ago provided an indispensable tool for culturing cells in vitro, thus permitted detailed dissection of seemingly intractable biology and physiology systems into manageable units and well-defined studies. This simple dish has had a profound impact on our understanding of complex biology, especially cell biology and neurobiology. However, the Petri dish culture system, including multiwell plates, glass cover slips, and so fourth, is less than ideal for several reasons:

- It is a two-dimensional (2D) system, which is in sharp contrast to the 3D environment of natural tissues in animals and plants.
- The Petri dish surface without a coating is rigid and inert, again in sharp contrast to the in vivo environment where cells intimately interact with the extracellular matrix and with each other.
- The tissue cell monolayers cultured on coated 2D surface, such as poly-L-lysine, collagen gels, fibronectin, laminin, and Matrigel as well as other synthetic materials containing segments of adhesion motifs, have only part of the cell surface attached to the materials and interact neighboring cells. The remaining parts are often directly exposed to the culture media, unlike the tissue environment where every cell intimately interacts with neighboring cells and/or the extracellular matrix.
- Biomolecular diffusion in 2D cultures is drastically different from those in 3D culture systems. In 2D culture systems, cytokines, chemokines, and growth factors quickly diffuse in the media across the culture dish. This is again in sharp contrast to the in vivo environment where chemical and biological gradient diffusion systems play a vital role in signal transduction, cell-cell communications, and development.
- Cells cultured on a 2D Petri dish are not readily transportable; that is, it is nearly impossible to move cells from one environment to another without incurring changes in the cell-material and cell-cell interactions. For example, cell collections using trypsinization or mechanical scrap using rubber policeman have adverse effects on cell-environment interactions. In contrast, cells cultured on 3D substrates are more readily transportable without significantly harming cell-material and cell-cell interactions, thus providing a realistic way to study cell biology.

We believe that the development of new biological materials, particularly those biologically inspired nanoscale scaffolds mimicking the in vivo environment and serve as permissive substrates for cell growth, differentiation, and biological function is key. These materials will be useful not only in furthering our understanding of cell biology, but also for advancing biotechnology, tissue engineering, regenerative biology, and medicine.

The ideal biological scaffold should meet several criteria. The building blocks should be derived from biological sources; basic units should be amenable to design and modification to achieve specific needs; exhibit a controlled rate of material biodegradation; exhibit no cytotoxicity; promote cell-substrate interactions; elicit no or little immune responses and inflammation; afford economically scaleable material production, purification and processing; be readily transportable; be chemically compatible with aqueous solutions and physiological conditions; and integrate with other body tissues.

4.1.1 Discovery and development of self-assembling peptide scaffolds

Shuguang Zhang serendipitously discovered the self-assembling peptides while sequencing a yeast protein *Zuotin* in 1990. It took him more than a year to understand how the seemingly soluble short peptides underwent self-assembly to form naked-eye visible materials. He and his colleagues filed a U.S. patent application in 1992 (issued in 1997) and published the yeast protein [1] where the first self-assembling peptide was identified.

We therefore have extensive experience in this class of biological materials made from the designer self-assembling peptides [2–4]. These self-assembling peptides consist of greater than 99% water (w/v). They form a hydrogel when exposed to physiological media or salt solution [2–7]. The constituents of the scaffold are amphiphilic peptides that have alternating repeating units of positively charged lysine or arginine and negatively charged aspartic acid and glutamic acid. The unmodified scaffolds consist of alternating amino acids that contain 50% charged residues [2–4]. These peptides are characterized by their periodic repeats of alternating ionic hydrophilic and hydrophobic amino acids. Thus, they have tendency to form beta sheets that have distinct polar and nonpolar sides [2–4].

The first self-assembling peptide, EAK16-II, a 16 amino acid peptide, was found in a segment in a yeast protein, zuotin, which was originally characterized by binding to left-handed Z-DNA. A number of additional self-assembling peptides including RAD16-I and RAD16-II, in which arginine and aspartic acid residues substitute lysine and glutamic acids have been designed and characterized for salt-facilitated scaffold formation [2–7]. Stable macroscopic matrix structures have been self-organized through the self-assembly of aqueous peptide solutions introduced into physiological salt-containing solutions. Several peptide scaffolds have been shown to support cell attachment of a variety of mammalian primary and tissue culture cells [2–7].

4.1.2 The nanofiber structure of the peptide scaffold

The peptide scaffolds consist of individual interwoven nanofibers. The individual fibers are approximately ~10–20 nanometers in diameter. The fiber density correlates with the concentration of peptide solution that is used to produce the materials. Generic observation with scanning electron microscope revealed a nanofiber network and pore (diameters ranging from 50 to 200 nm) ensemble similar to those found with biologically derived substrates like Matrigel [5]. The mechanical properties of the scaffold and their self-assembly process have also been investigated. Rheology was used as a method for comparison of the relative mechanical stiffness of the assembled peptides. The storage moduli (G′) were measured at low frequencies. This information is useful in describing the type of mechanical environment that seeded cells are presented with and can serve as a macroscopic measure of the extent of interactions formed between assembled peptides The 1% w/v self-assembling peptides like RADA16 (G′ = 1630Pa), were generally found to exhibit reduced storage moduli when compared to Matrigel (G′ = 5408 Pa). Upon increasing the peptide concentration, the storage moduli can be significantly augmented to meet the requirements of the specific research application (cartilage regeneration, stem cell differentiation, and so forth).

4.1.3 A generic biological scaffold

The self-assembling peptide scaffold belongs to a class of biologically inspired materials. The self-assembly event creating the peptide scaffold takes place under physiological conditions. They float in aqueous solution and are readily transportable to different environments. Nanostructures formed by RADA16-I self-assembling peptide are depicted in Figure 4.1; a molecular interpretation of reassembly of RADA16-I is described in Figure 4.2. These new biological materials have become increasingly important not only in studying 3D spatial behaviors of cells, but also in developing approaches for a wide range of innovative medical technologies. One example is in the use of the peptide scaffolds to support neurite growth and differentiation. We reported that peptide scaffolds from RADA16-I and RAD16-II are a permissible substrate for primary neurons isolated from the cerebellum and hippocampus of newborn rats and mice to form extensive neurite outgrowth and active synapses on the peptide surface [3].

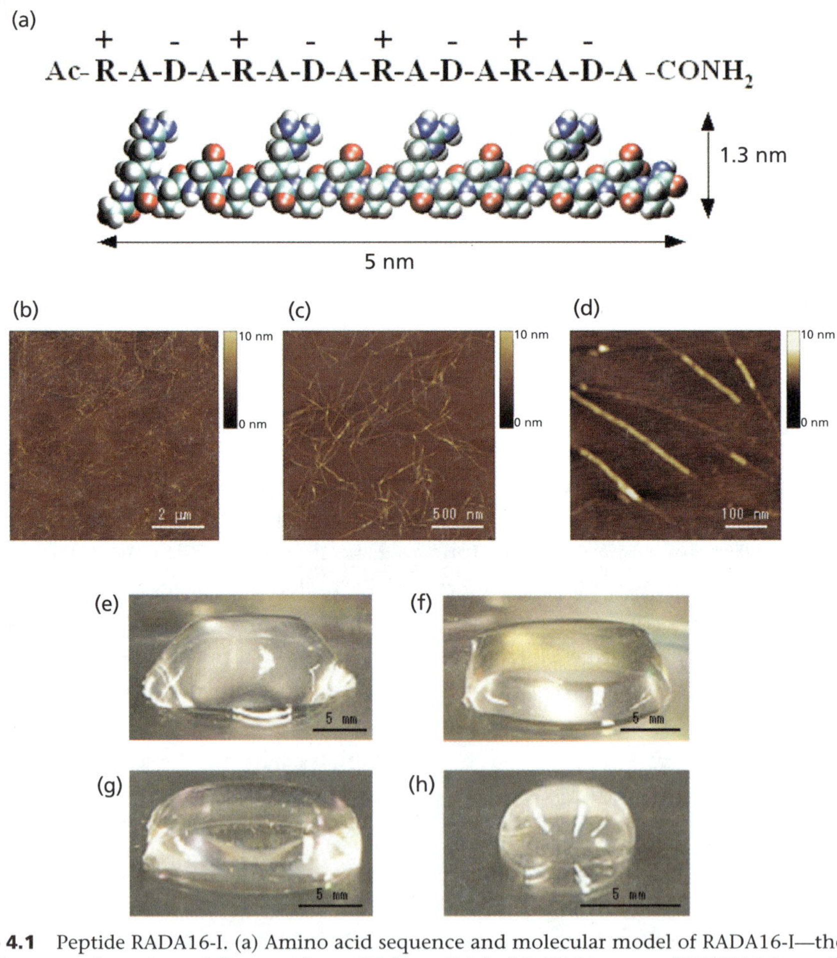

Figure 4.1 Peptide RADA16-I. (a) Amino acid sequence and molecular model of RADA16-I—the dimensions are ~5-nm long, 1.3-nm wide, and 0.8-nm thick; (b) AFM images of RADA16-I nanofiber scaffold, 8 μm × 8 μm; (c) 2 μm × 2 μm; (d) 0.5 μm × 0.5 μm. Note the different height of the nanofiber, ~2–5 nm, in (d) suggesting either a single or a double layer structure. Photographs of RADA16-I hydrogel at various conditions: (e) 0.5 wt% (pH 7.5); (f) 0.1 wt% (pH 7.5); and (g) 0.1 wt% (pH 7.5, PBS) before sonication. (h) Reassembled RADA16-I hydrogel after 4 time sonications, respectively. (Image courtesy of Hidenori Yokoi.)

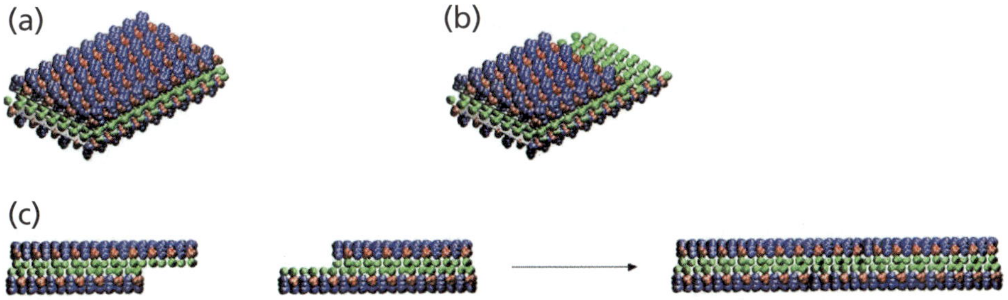

Figure 4.2 A proposed reassembly molecular model of self-assembling RADA16-I peptides. When the peptides form stable β-sheets in water, they form intermolecular hydrogen bonds along the peptide backbones. The β-sheets have two distinctive sides, one hydrophobic with an array of alanines and the other with negatively charged aspartic acids and positively charged arginines see Figure 4.2(a)]. These peptides form antiparallel β-sheet structures. The alanines form overlap packed hydrophobic interactions in water, a structure that is found in silk fibroin from silkworm and spiders. On the charged sides, both positive and negative charges are packed together through intermolecular ionic interactions in a checkerboard-like manner. These nanofiber fragments can form various assemblies similar to restriction-digested DNA fragments with (a) blunt ends and (b) semiprotruding ends. (c) These fragments with protruding and blunt ends could reassemble readily through hydrophobic interactions and hydrogen bonds. (Image courtesy of Hidenori Yokoi.)

4.1.4 Peptide scaffold fosters chondrocyte extracellular matrix production

In choosing a scaffold for cartilage repair, it is important to identify a material that can maintain high rates of proliferation of chondrocytes and high rates of chondrocyte synthesis of specific ECM macromolecules including type II collagen and glycosaminoglycans (GAGs) until they evolve into steady state tissue maintenance. We first used a RADA16 scaffold but it did not give the optimal results because it is a rather weak hydrogel. We then designed the KLD12 (n-KLDLKLDLKLDL-c) peptide scaffold, reasoning that since leucine is more hydrophobic than alanine, the leucines would likely pack more tightly in the nanofibers in aqueous conditions and thus provide a higher mechanical strength of the scaffold [4].

We used the self-assembling peptide KLD12 scaffold for cartilage repair and developed a method to encapsulate chondrocytes within the peptide scaffold. During 4 weeks of culture in vitro, chondrocytes seeded within the peptide scaffold developed a cartilage-like ECM rich in proteoglycans and type II collagen, indicative of a stable chondrocyte phenotype. Time-dependent accumulation of this ECM was paralleled by increases in material stiffness, indicative of the deposition of mechanically functional tissue. The content of viable differentiated chondrocytes within the peptide scaffold increased at a rate that was 4-fold higher than that in parallel chondrocyte-seeded agarose culture, a reference chondrocytes culture system. These results demonstrate the potential of self-assembling peptide scaffolds for the synthesis and accumulation of a true cartilage-like ECM in a 3D cell culture for cartilage tissue repair. The peptide KLD12 used in this study represents a designed self-assembling peptide made through molecular engineering that can be modified to suit specific cell and tissue application interests [4].

These results suggest that different cell types have different requirements for the scaffolds. We therefore systematically tailor-make peptide scaffolds for a variety of cell types.

4.1.5 Designer peptides appended with active motifs

A number of functional peptide motifs have been identified from extracellular matrix proteins. Some of the most important motifs are from collagens and laminins. Others comprise tissue-specific proteins including osteopontin, osteocalcin, osteonectin, nidogen, and netrins.

These functional motifs have been directly coupled on to the self-assembling peptide RADA16 and other self-assembling peptides, so as to obtain functional peptides linked to the C-termini of self-assembling cores. This method can directly introduce biological functions into the peptide scaffolds. After self-assembly of the nanofibers, these motifs are part of the local microenvironment. Many bioactive motifs have been selected to create a microenvironment niche to foster specific cell cultures. Since these functional motifs are modular, we can tailor-make and mix them in a combinatorial manner to achieve the optimal benefit or recreate an in vivo–like microenvironment.

It must be emphasized that the peptide nanofiber 3D scaffolds only need to create a temporary or initial scaffolding microenvironment to foster cell attachment, proliferation, migration, or differentiation. Cells may produce their own extracellular matrix proteins during that initial period. These peptide scaffolds will then be naturally degraded and the degradation product, amino acids, can be reused by cells.

Thus we developed a novel class of designer self-assembling peptides appended with a broad set of biological active motifs. A schematic representation is depicted in Figure 4.3. Blue lines represent generic self-assembling peptides (sapeptide); red, green, purple, yellow, and brown lines represent various functional peptide motifs. The functional motifs are on the C-termini since peptide synthesis starts from the C-termini to avoid imperfect coupling deletion during synthesis (~99% coupling per step). Self-assembling peptides sharing the same self-assembling backbone and showing different functional motifs can also be mixed together within the same scaffolds (Figure 4.4). It is generally known that when longer peptides are made, deletion may occur due to the coupling efficiency of the synthetic peptide chemistry. In order to preserve the fidelity of the func-

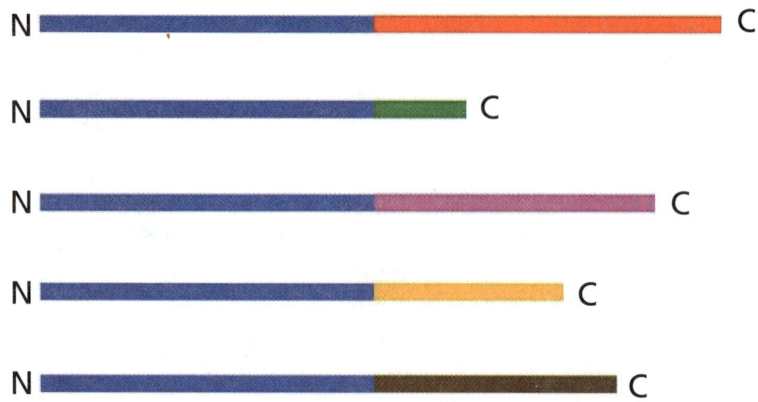

Figure 4.3 Direct extension of the functional motifs from the self-assembling peptides. The blue lines represent the sapeptide; the red, green purple, yellow, and brown lines represent various functional peptide motifs. The functional motifs are on the C-termini since peptide synthesis starts from C-termini to avoid functional motif deletion during synthesis. Since the self-assembling core has repeated motifs, any one amino acid deletion does not significantly alter its self-assembly.

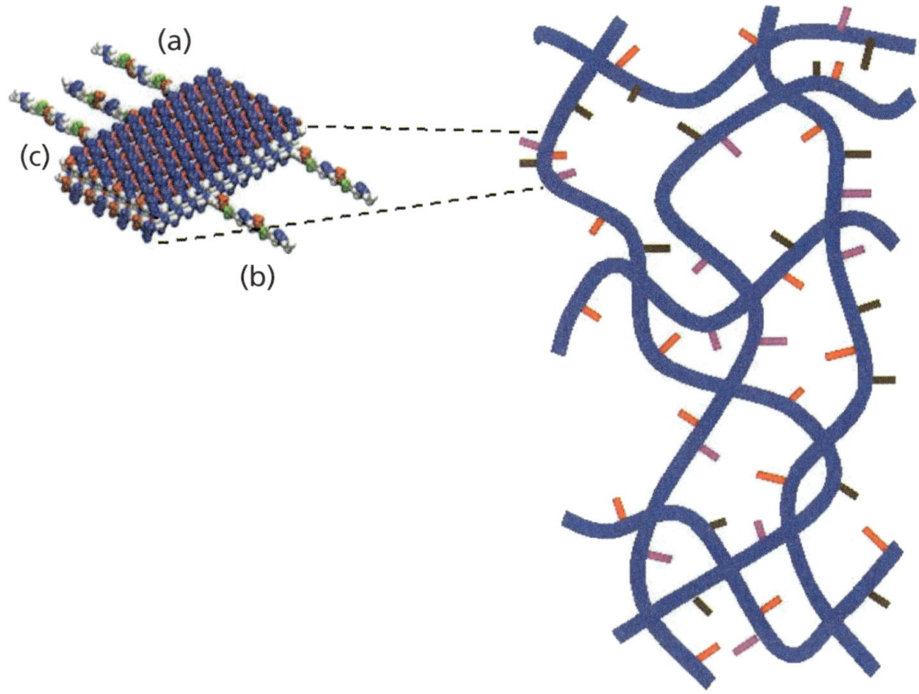

Figure 4.4 Schematic representation of a self-assembling peptide scaffold modified with various functional motifs. The density of these motifs can be easily adjusted simply by mixing different functionalized peptides in various ratios, 1:1, 1:2, 1:4, 1:10, 1:100, 1:1,000 or more depending on cell responsiveness. Either mono or multiple functional peptide motifs, labeled as A, B, and C, can be mixed at the same time.

tional peptide, they are designed to be on the C-termini in order to prevent residue alterations during chemically solid phase peptide synthesis, which has ~98% for coupling efficiency. The sequence of the sapeptide has repeating units; one deletion does not significantly alter its ability to undergo self-assembly.

A spacer comprising of two glycines is usually placed between the self-assembling sequence and the functional motif in order to provide a "joint" with sufficient degrees of freedom necessary for a correct exposure of the functional motifs to cell membrane receptors.

4.2 Materials

The RAD16 peptide scaffold solution (1% w/v) was purchased as PuraMatrix from BD Bioscience (Bedford, Massachusetts). The designer peptides with active motifs were custom-synthesized (CPC Scientific, San Jose, California). Alternatively, the functionalized designer peptides can also be in-house synthesized with a CEM Liberty Microwave Peptide Synthesizer (Matthews, NC). The peptides were dissolved in water at a final concentration of 1% (w/v) and sonicated for 20 minutes (Aquasonic, model 50T, VWR, New Jersey). Peptides can be easily produced via solid phase F-moc synthesis and purified via standard HPLC techniques.

4.3 Reagents

Standard reagents are commercially available. To maintain the tissue cell lines, penicillin/ streptomycin, the minimal essential medium, and FBS are available from Invitrogen Corp. (Carlsbad, California). Ascorbic acid and β-glycerophosphate, and the Alkaline Phosphatase Fluorescence Assay Kit 85L-2 histological assay is available from Sigma Chemical Co. (St. Louis, Missouri). The PicoGreen dsDNA Quantification Kit (P-7589) and Live/Dead Viability Kit (L-3224) are from Invitrogen (Eugene, Oregon). The Mouse Osteocalcin EIA Kit for Osteocalcin and Calcein-AM Staining is from Biomedical Technologies, Inc. (Massachusetts). Matrigel GF reduced from EHS sarcoma is available from BD Biosciences.

4.4 Methods

4.4.1 Peptide solution preparation

Double lyophilized designer peptides are custom-synthesized by CPC Scientific (San Jose, California).

1. These peptides are dissolved in MilliQ water at a final concentration of 1% w/v (10 mg/ml).
2. They are then sonicated for 30 minutes (Aquasonic, model 50T, VWR, New Jersey).
3. After sonication, they are filter-sterilized (Acrodisc Syringe Filter, 0.22-μm HT Tuffrun Membrane, Pall Corp., Ann Arbor, Michigan) for future use.
4. The designer functionalized peptide solutions (PFS and/or SKP) are mixed in a volume ratio of 1:1, 1:2, 1:4, 1:100 with 1% pure RADA16-I solution to obtain 1% functionalized peptide mixtures.

4.4.2 Designer peptide synthesis and scaffold preparation

Cell viability and differentiation assay tests are carried out.

1. Add 30 μl per well of a 96-well plate of a 1% (w/v) peptide in sterile water solution aqueous solution of either generic or functionalized peptide hydrogel so as to evenly cover the bottom surface of each well, resulting in ~30-μm gel layer thickness (BD Biosciences, Bedford, Massachusetts).
2. Very slowly add 200 μl per each well of basal medium along the side of well.
3. The mix ratio between RADA16 and PRG varied from 100:0 (PRG 0%), 99:1 (1% PRG), 90:10 (10% PRG), 60:40 (40% PRG), 30:70 (70% PRG), up to 0:100 (100% PRG).
4. Allow the peptides to self-assemble at 37°C for 30 minutes and rinse once with medium to wash away any residual acid remaining from peptide synthesis and purification.
5. In the case of SEM imaging both for Matrigel and the peptide hydrogels, the total amount of hydrogel scaffold is reduced to 10 μl, and higher concentrations of peptides (2% w/v or 3% w/v) are preferred to guarantee the necessary scaffold stiffness.

4.4.3 Culture cells in plate inserts

Each of the peptide solutions is directly loaded in the tissue culture plate inserts (10-mm diameter, Millicell-CM, Millipore, Massachusetts). The culture medium is added to induce hydrogel formation.

1. Cells are suspended in 10% sucrose just before seeding. Quickly mix 20 μl of cell suspension with 100 μl of peptide solution and then add the mixture into the insert. Very carefully layer the 400-μl medium onto the gel for gelation. Incubate 10 minutes at 37°C and then change medium for another 30 minutes of incubation. Change two more times to equilibrate the gel to physiological pH for 3D cell culture.
2. When culture cells are on the inserts, the peptide scaffolds in the inserts are washed twice using PBS to remove any residual acid remaining from peptide synthesis and purification and rise to pH 7.4.
3. For cell staining and visualization, a 4-μM calcein AM solution is added to the insert and incubated for 1 hour in the incubator at 37°C.
4. The inserts are rinsed well by PBS twice and the cells are examined via a fluorescence-inverted microscope.

4.4.4 Cell culture system

1. The scaffolds 1% (w/v) are prepared as pure RADA16 or mixed with others at a ratio of 1:1 (v/v) (RADA16: ALK, DGR, or PRG).
2. Each solution is sonicated for 30 minutes, loaded (100 μl) on top of a cell culture insert (10-mm diameter, Millicell-CM, Millipore, Massachusetts), and allowed to form a layer ~3 mm thick.
3. The maintenance medium described later is gently added on the top of the scaffold to induce gelation.
4. The system is incubated at 37°C for an hour.
5. Then the medium inside the insert is exchanged by the maintenance medium and the outside of the insert is filled with the maintenance medium and incubated for half a day within a cell culture incubator at 37°C.
6. Cells are plated at 2×10^4 cells on the hydrogels in the inserts. The cells are cultured in the maintenance medium day 0 through day 2.
7. Then the cells are transferred into the differentiation media supplemented with L-ascorbic acid 50 μg/ml and β-glycerophosphate 10 mM.
8. The media is changed every three days.
9. The gel, cell lysis, and culture medium can be harvested after culturing 14 days for analysis.

4.4.5 Neural cell culture and seeding

1. In the case of adhesion and differentiation tests, cell seeding (at a concentration of 2–8×10^4 cells/cm^2) is performed 2 days after the last mechanical dissociation in order to seed the maximum percentage of stem cells. Cells are seeded on the top surface of each assembled scaffold, where they are able to settle into the nanofiber matrices. Over time, cells migrate into the scaffold.

2. In the case of SEM imaging, cells are thoroughly mixed with 8 μl of aqueous peptide scaffold solution at a final concentration of 5–8 × 10^3 cells/μl in a total final volume of 10 μl per each sample. Self-assembling is then initiated by adding basal medium slowly and placing seeded scaffolds on copper grids (Ted Pella, Inc.) at 37°C for 30 minutes. Cells are thus embedded in the scaffold.
3. For both adhesion and differentiation tests, as well as SEM imaging, cells are cultured with a medium supplemented with βFGF (10 ng/ml), added to enhance neuronal progeny differentiation. After 3 days, the medium is shifted to a medium containing a leukemia inhibitory factor (LIF, Chemicon) (20 ng/ml) and a brain-derived neurotrophic factor (BDNF, Peprotech) (20 ng/ml) to pursue the neuronal and glial population maturation in progeny. Cells are fed every three days with fresh culture medium.
4. Neural precursors isolated from the subventricular zone (SVZ) of 8-week-old CD-1 albino mice striata, at passage 10, are used. Cell proliferation is in Neurocult basal medium (mouse) (Stemcell Technologies, Vancouver), in the presence of basic fibroblast growth factor (βFGF from PeproTech, Rocky Hill, New Jersey) and epidermal growth factor (EGF from PeproTech) at final concentrations of 10 ng/ml and 20 ng/ml, respectively.
5. The medium without growth factors is used as a basal medium. Bulk cultures are generated by mechanically dissociating neurospheres and plating cells in untreated flasks at the appropriate density (1 × 10^4 cells/cm^2) every 4–5 days in the same growth medium.
6. Cell counting and viability examination is required at every passage, using Trypan-Blue exclusion method.

4.4.6 Preparation of MC3T3-E1 cells

Mouse preosteoblast cell line MC3T3-E1 (subclone 4) (ATCC, Virginia) can be purchased.

1. Cells are in modified medium with 10% FBS and 1.5% penicillin/streptomycin.
2. The medium is changed every 3 days.
3. When the cells become subconfluent, they are detached from the flask by treatment with aqueous solution of 0.25% trypsin for 5 minutes at 37°C.
4. The cells are subcultured at a density of 5 × 10^3 cells/cm^2.

4.4.7 Cell culture of human umbilical vein endothelial cells (HUVECs)

Primary isolated HUVECs are commercially available from Lonza Inc. (Walkersville, Maryland) and can be routinely grown in endothelial growth media EGM-2 (Lonza Inc.) on regular tissue culture plates. Subconfluent (~6 × 10^4 cells/insert) of HUVECs is seeded on the top of the scaffolds for 2D cell culture. Approximately 1 × 10^5 of HUVECs is suspended in 100 μl of peptide solution for 3D cell culture.

4.4.8 Cell proliferation assay

To assess the viability of cells seeded on scaffolds made of various peptides, a quantitative method, MTT assay (Sigma), was used. Four independent experiments comprising three replicates each are required. For this viability test, the direct proportional linearity between the optical density and the viability/metabolic activity of the cell populations is assessed by verifying the linearity of 5 different standard curves at 6 increasing cell concentrations, ranging from 5×10^3 to 5×10^5 cells/well. Results are expressed as percent increase in cell population from the population seeded on day one.

Cell proliferation is determined following the manufacturer's protocols:

1. MTT (3-(4,5-dimethylthiazol-2yl)-2,5 diphenyl tetrazolium bromide) is prepared in a 5mg/ml stock solution in PBS and added to the culture medium in a ratio of 1:100.
2. Incubate at 37°C for ~60 minutes.
3. The MTT solution is removed.
4. The insoluble formazans crystals are dissolved by soaking scaffolds and cells for 15 minutes in 250 μl of dimethylsulfoxide (DMSO).
5. The absorbance at A_{550nm} is measured using a Vmax microplate reader (Molecular Devices, Sunnyvale California).

4.4.9 DNA content measurement

The number of cells on the scaffold is determined by the fluorometric quantification of the amount of cellular DNA.

1. The cell-seeded scaffold is rinsed with PBS and recovered by Na citrate buffer solution containing 50 mM Na citrate and 100 mM NaCl and stored at –80°C until assay.
2. After thawing, the cells are lysed in the Na citrate solution with occasional mixing.
3. The 10 μl of cell lysate (400 μl/insert) is mixed with Na Citrate buffer (100 μl) and DNA binding fluorescent dye solution (0.5-μl Picogreen reagent in 100-μl TE buffer).
4. The scaffolds with cells are collected for DNA purification (QIAamp DNA Mini Kit, QIAGEN). 100 μl of purified DNA sample was mixed with 100-μl DNA binding fluorescent dye solution (0.5-μl Picogreen reagent in 100-μl TE buffer, Quant-iT PicoGreen dsDNA Reagent and kits, Invitrogen).
5. The fluorescent intensity of the mixed solution is measured on a fluorescence spectrometer (Wallace Victor2, 1420 Multi-label counter, Perkin-Elmer, Massachusetts, Ex 485 nm/Em 510 nm).
6. The calibration curve between the DNA and cell number is prepared by use of cell suspensions with different cell densities.

4.4.10 Boundary-sandwiched cell migration assay

Peptide scaffolds were prepared as described earlier. Approximately 8×10^4 cells were seeded on the top of peptide scaffold A and then incubated 6 hours at 37°C with 5% CO_2 for cell attachment. The trimmed quadrate peptide scaffold A with attached cells was inversely placed on the surface of peptide scaffold B with cells between two types of scaffolds. The scaffolds with cells were cultured at 37°C for 2 days and then examined with fluorescence microscopy after nuclei staining.

4.4.11 Fluorescence microscopy

Following the experiments, cells on the hydrogels were fixed with 4% paraformaldehyde for 15 minutes and permeabilized with 0.1% Triton X-100 for 5 minutes at room temperature. Fluorescent Rhodamin phalloidin and SYTOX Green (Molecular Probes, Eugene, Oregon) were used for labeling F-actin and nuclei, respectively. Images were taken using a fluorescence microscope (Axiovert 25, ZEISS) or Laser Confocal Scanning Microscope (Olympus FV300).

4.4.12 Immunocytochemistry

Cell differentiation of neural lineage is assessed by double and single immunostaining with lineage-specific antibodies: nestin (1:150, Chemicon) for progenitor cells, rabbit anti-β-Tubulin (1:500, Covance) for neurons, mouse anti-Glial Fibrillary Acidic Protein (1:200, Chemicon) for astrocytes. Primary antibodies were then stained with secondary ALEXA 488 goat antimouse (1:1,000 Molecular Probes) and CY3 AffiniPure $F_{ab'}2$ antirabbit IgG antibodies (1:100 Jackson Immuno Research). Cell nuclei were counterstained with DAPI (Molecular Probes). The samples are then examined by inverted fluorescence microscope. Quantitative analyses are carried out by counting 100–300 cells for each of 10 nonoverlapping (and randomly chosen) fields. Four independent experiments comprising of five or more replicates each are analyzed.

4.4.13 SEM sample preparation

After seeding cells within the self-assembled scaffolds, cells are usually cultured between 1–14 days. Samples are prepared as follows:

1. The scaffold is soaked in 5% glutaraldehyde at 4°C for 2 hours.
2. It is then washed in MilliQ water.
3. It is then subjected to sequential dehydration steps in 10%, 20%, 30%, 40%, 50%, 60%, 70%, 80%, 90%, and 100% of ethanol for 5 minutes each.
4. Samples are then placed in pressurized liquid CO_2/siphon for 1 hour using a CO_2 critical point dryer (Tousims).
5. Scaffold samples with and/or without cells are sputter-coated with gold-palladium particles (~10-nm gold coating thickness).
6. When examination the scaffold containing cells, the 3D culture systems are placed on an EM copper grid at the beginning of the experiments. The sample are prepared as steps 1–5 and examined using a JOEL JSM 6060 SEM at 2,000–100,000× magnification, 6-KV acceleration voltage, 29–32 spot size, and 12-mm electronic working distance.

4.4.14 Circular dichroism (CD)

Far-UV CD spectra are recorded between 190–260 nm at room temperature on an Aviv 62DS spectrometer.

1. All measurements were carried out in 1-mm quartz cuvette in PBS, pH 7.4. Spectra are from the accumulation of four scans. Blank spectra of the buffer without the sample are subtracted.
2. CD spectra of peptide samples at concentrations 5 μM or 10 μM in PBS are collected and compared.
3. Spectra are recorded in 1-nm steps and averaged over 2 seconds.

4.4.15 Structural study using atomic force microscopy (AFM)

1. Peptide from stock solutions (0.5%) was diluted to a working concentration of 0.01% (w/v), after a 30-minute sonication and a 2-hour stationary incubation at room temperature.
2. Atomic force microscopy (AFM) images were collected with a silicon scanning probe (FESP, Vecco Probe Inc., California) with a resonance frequency of 75 kHz, spring constant 2.8 N/m, tip curvature radius 10 nm, and 225-μm length.
3. Images are obtained with a multimode AFM microscope (Nanoscope IIIa, Vecco, Santa Barbara, California) operating in tapping mode. Typical scanning parameters were as follows: RMS amplitude before engage 1–1.2V, set point 0.7–0.9V, integral and proportional gains of 0.2–0.6 and 0.4–1.0, respectively, and scan rate 1.51 Hz.

4.4.16 Biomechanical study using rheology

The mechanical properties of the assembled hydrogels were studied with a TA Instruments AR2000 rheometer. Storage moduli were measured at frequencies from 1 to 10 rad/sec using a 20 mm, 0.5° stainless steel cone with a truncation gap of 9 μm while the strain was held constant at 1%. Each measurement was performed with 35 μl of gel assembled with 70 μl of PBS solution after allowing 1 hour for assembly.

4.4.17 Alkaline phosphatase (ALP) staining for MC3T3-E1 cells

ALP staining is conducted using an Alkaline Phosphatase Staining Kit (85L-2, Sigma, Missouri) according to the manufacturer's protocol.

1. Cells on the scaffold in the inserts are washed twice in saline, fixed for 6 minutes at room temperature in citrate fixative solution contained in the kit.
2. Wash using Mill-Q water. AS-MX solution in the kit is added to the insert and incubated at room temp for 30 minutes.
3. The scaffold in insert is rinsed well using Mill-Q water three to four times and the cells are observed under a light microscope.

4.4.18 Biochemical assays for alkaline phosphatase (ALP) activity for MC3T3-E1 cells

ALP activity in the cells on hydrogel is determined by fluorometric quantification.

1. The cell-seeded hydrogel scaffold is rinsed with saline and recovered by ALP lysis buffer containing 2 mM $MgCl_2$ and 0.05% Triton X-100 and then stored with at –80°C until assay.

2. After thawing, the cells are lysed in the ALP lysis solution with occasional mixing. The 20 μl of cell lysate (300 μl/insert) is mixed with 20-μl $MgCl_2$ solution and 150-μl fluorescent assay buffer, both provided in the Alkaline Phosphatase Fluorescence Assay Kit (Sigma, Missouri).
3. Then 1 μl of suspended substrate (4-methylumbelliferyl phosphate, 10 mM) is added and incubation occurred at room temperature for 1 hour.
4. The fluorescent intensity of the mixed solution is measured on a fluorescence spectrometer (Wallace Victor-2, 1420 Multi-label counter, Perkin-Elmer, Massachusetts, Excitation 355 nm-Emission 460 nm).
5. The calibration curve between the ALP activity and fluorescent is prepared by use of alkaline phosphatase (control enzyme) with different concentration.

4.4.19 Low protein release from the peptide scaffold

In order to combine protein in the scaffold that stimulate cell proliferation, differentiation and migration, we develop method for slow release the proteins.

Peptide hydrogel scaffold is formed using well-established protocols (see Sections 4.1 and 4.2).

1. The Ac-$(RADA)_4$-$CONH_2$ peptide solution or other functionalized sapeptides is mixed with phosphate-buffered saline (PBS, pH7.4) containing protein at a final concentration of 5 nM and 5 μM, respectively.
2. An aliquot 40 μl of the solution is transferred into the wells of a 384-well plate and gelation occurred within 15 minutes.
3. Subsequently, 70 μl of PBS was slowly added to the 40 μl of the hydrogel, so as to satisfy the perfect-sink conditions and allow for the determination of the protein release profile.
4. Another aliquot 40 μl of the supernatant is replaced with the same volume of fresh PBS at frequent time points. The hydrogel volume does not change and, therefore, protein release is not attributed to hydrogel degradation or swelling.

4.5 Data Acquisition, Results, and Interpretation

4.5.1 Designer self-assembling peptide nanofiber hydrogel scaffold

We have shown that this matrix encapsulates several cell types in a manner similar to the extracellular matrix, the peptide hydrogel scaffold system can be used for 3D cell culture, slow protein release, tissue engineering, and tissue regeneration applications.

A single molecule of the ionic self-complementary peptide RADA16-I is shown in Figure 4.5. Millions of peptide molecules self-assembled into individual nanofibers that further form the nanofiber scaffold (Figure 4.5). The nanopores range from a few nanometers to a few hundred nanometers; the scales are similar in size to most biomolecules. The scaffold hydrogel is completely transparent, which is a very important requirement for accurate image collections for uses in 3D tissue cell cultures.

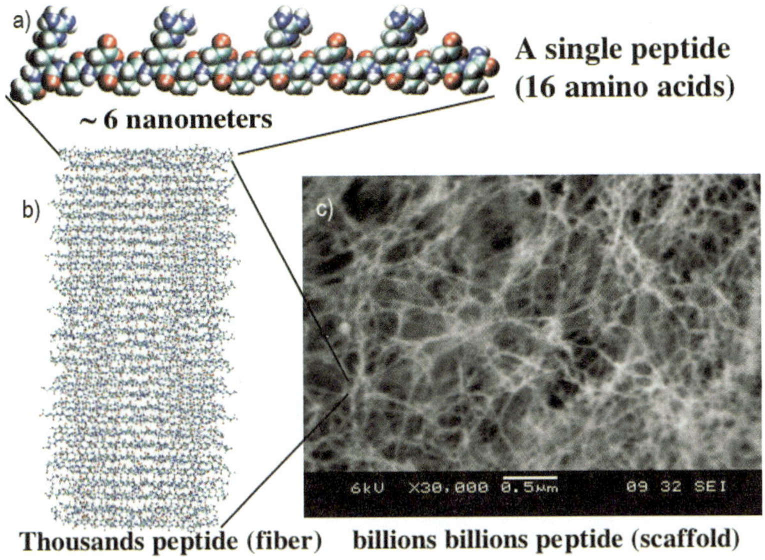

Figure 4.5 Self-assembling peptide RADA16-I nanofiber scaffold hydrogel. (a) Amino acid sequence of RADA16-I, molecular model of a single RADA16-I nanofiber—the dimensions are ~6 nm long, 1.3 nm wide, and 0.8 nm thick; (b) hundreds of thousands of individual peptides self-assemble into a nanofiber; and (c) SEM images of RADA16-I nanofiber scaffold. Note the scale bar, 0.5 μm or 500 nm.

4.5.2 3D cell cultures

The designer self-assembling peptide nanofiber scaffolds have been shown to be an excellent biological material for 3D cell cultures (Figure 4.6), not only capable of stimulating stem cell differentiation [5] and cell migration into the scaffold [6, 7] but also for repairing tissue defects in animals (results not shown).

We developed several peptide nanofiber scaffolds designed specifically for osteoblasts [6]. We designed one of the pure self-assembling peptide scaffolds RADA16-I through direct coupling to short biologically active motifs. The motifs included osteogenic growth peptide ALK (ALKRQGRTLYGF) bone-cell secreted-signal peptide, osteopontin cell adhesion motif DGR (DGRGDSVAYG), and 2-unit RGD binding sequence PGR (PRGDSGYRGDS).

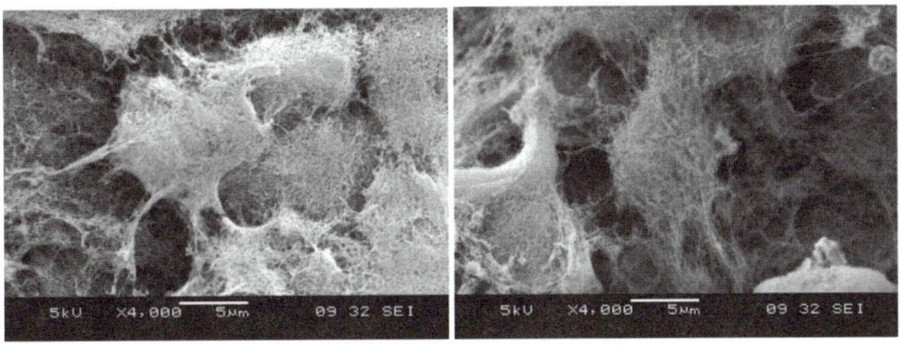

Figure 4.6 Mouse adult neural stem cells are embedded in designer self-assembling peptide scaffold. Note the cells are totally surrounded by the scaffolds and interact directly with both the peptide nanofibers and extracellular matrix that share similar scales, which are indistinguishable based on their sizes. This microenvironment is closer to the reality in the body.

The bioactive peptide scaffolds is made by mixing the pure RADA16-I and designer peptide solutions together. The molecular integration of the mixed nanofiber scaffolds is examined using AFM. Compared to pure RADA16-I scaffold, these designer peptide scaffolds significantly promote mouse preosteoblast MC3T3-E1 cell proliferation. Moreover, alkaline phosphatase (ALP) activity and osteocalcin secretion, which are early and late markers for osteoblastic differentiation, were also significantly increased, thus demonstrating that the designer, self-assembling peptide scaffolds promoted the proliferation and osteogenic differentiation of MC3T3-E1. Under the identical culture medium condition, confocal images showed that the designer PRG peptide scaffold stimulated cell migration into the 3D scaffold (Figure 4.7) [6]. Without the modified motif, cells did not migrate in 3D.

4.5.3 Cell migration in peptide scaffolds

In order to study the preferences of endothelial cells' migration in response to the components of surrounded scaffolds and the importance of functional peptide motif for guiding cells migration, we designed the clear-boundary sandwich assays to assess endothelial cell migration between two types of peptide scaffolds. As shown in Figure 4.8(b), endothelial cells plated on the scaffolds RAD/PRG [Figure 4.8(b), parts a and e] and the RAD/KLT [Figure 4.8(b), parts b and f] settled in these scaffolds and no visible migration towards the RADA16-I scaffold was observed. In contrast, cells seeded on RADA16-I scaffold directionally migrated towards functionalized peptide scaffolds [Figure 4.8(b), parts c, d, g, and h]. These experiments unambiguously show the biological importance of the designer functionalized peptide scaffolds that induce cell directional migrations. This is a very important observation since there are no additional soluble growth factors in these scaffolds. These observations suggest the adhesion peptide motif alone can induce cell migrations without extract-soluble factors.

Many factors are involved in cell unidirectional migration, such as soluble chemoattractants and attachments on the surrounding matrix. In literature reports, endothelial cell migration is mostly stimulated by growth factors such as VEGF and bFGF, and also is activated in response to integrins binding to the ECM component. Our results demonstrated unequivocally that the adhesive interactions governed mainly by the functional motif of PRG alone promote cell attachment and migration from

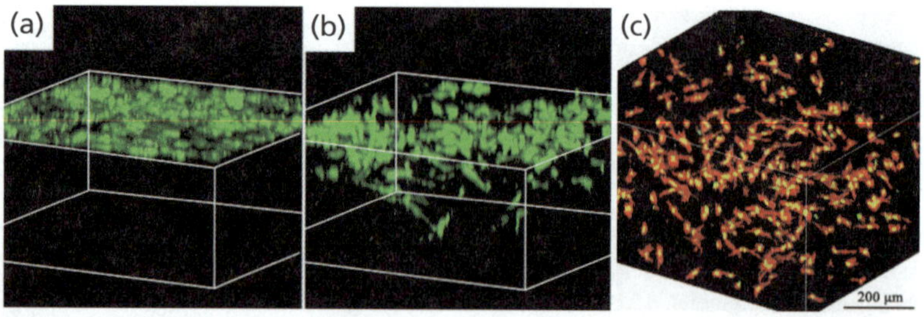

Figure 4.7 Reconstructed image of 3D confocal microscopic image of cells culturing on the different scaffolds consisting of different mix ratio of RADA16 1% (w/v) and PRG 1% (w/v) using calcein-AM staining. (a) 1-part PRG: 9-parts RADA16. (b) 7-part PRG: 3-part RADA16. In the case of 1-part PRG scaffold, the cells attach on the surface of the scaffold, whereas in the case of 7-part PRG scaffold, the cells migrate ~300–400 μm into the scaffold. There is a drastic cell migration into the scaffold with a higher concentration of PRG motif. (c) Endothelial cell morphologies in 3D peptide RADA16/PRG scaffolds. It is evident that cells migrate ~400–500 μm into the scaffold.

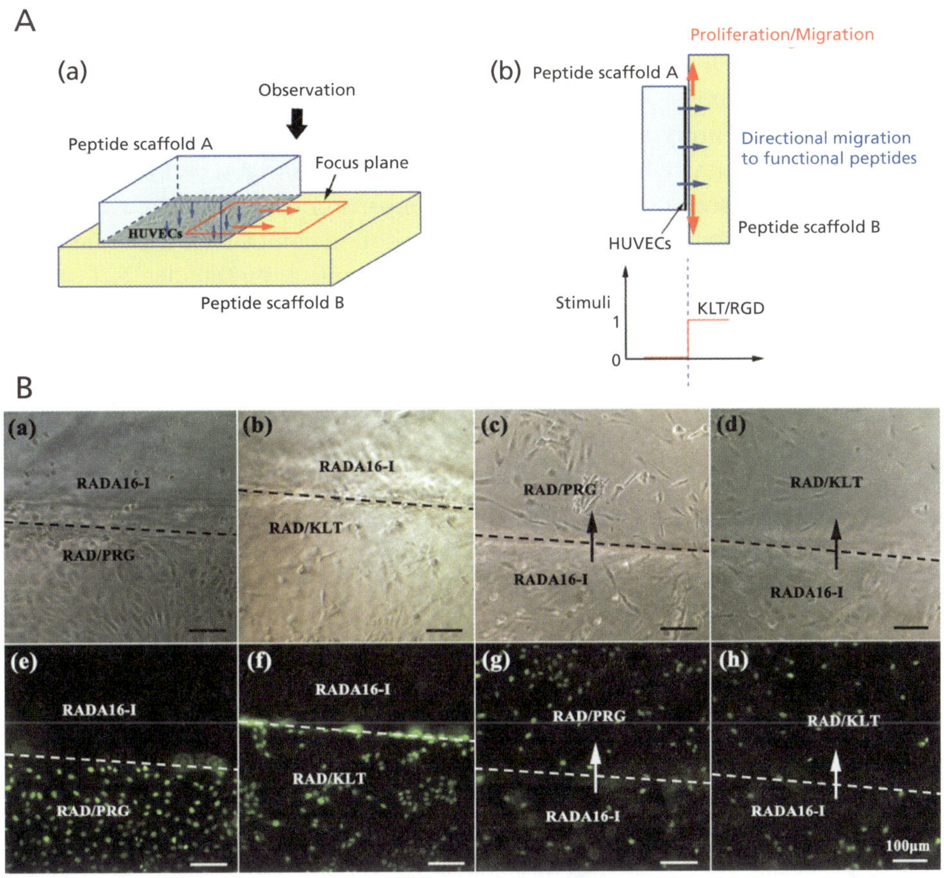

Figure 4.8 Endothelial cell unidirectional migration in response to functional peptide scaffolds. (a) Schematic illustrations of cell directional migration. a. Clear-boundary-sandwich cell migration assay. b. Directional migration induced by functional motifs. (b) Phase contrast microscopy images of HUVECs seeded on peptide scaffolds: a. RAD/PRG; b. RAD/KLT; c. and d. RADA16-I, and fluorescent SYTOX Green nuclear staining for e. RAD/PRG; f. RAD/KLT; g. and h. RADA16-I. Cells directionally migrated from RADA16-I to RAD/PRG (c and g) and RAD/KLT (d and h). The scale bar is 100 μm for all panels.

RADA16-I to RAD/PRG scaffold, whereas the VEGF mimicking sequence of KLT may mainly serve the similar function of VEGF to regulate endothelial cell migration. Cells seeded on RADA16-I were probably induced by the functional motifs of PRG and KLT and migrated to/on these functionalized peptide mixtures scaffolds [Figure 4.8(a), part b)]. More systematic experiments will be carried out to further address these questions.

4.5.4 Rheology of peptide hydrogel scaffold

Rheology was used as a method for comparison of the relative mechanical stiffness of the assembled peptides. The storage moduli (G′) were measured at low frequencies where the loss moduli (G″) were too low to be of consequence. Therefore, the average G′ over the frequency range of 1 to 10 radians/sec is used to compare the relative stiffness of the scaffolds. This information is useful in describing the type of mechanical environment that seeded cells are presented with and can serve as a macroscopic measure of the extent of interactions formed between assembled peptides. The functionalized peptides were generally found to exhibit reduced storage moduli when compared to RADA16-I (G′ = 1,630 Pa), however, peptide RADA16-GGFLGFPT (G′ = 2,320 Pa) showed an increase in stiffness. This is perhaps due to the relatively high degree of hydrophobicity of the added motif (illustrated in Figure 4.3). Peptides of greatest interest for neural stem cell cultures, RADA16-GGSKPPGTSS (G′ = 762 Pa) and RADA16-GGPFSSTKT (G′ = 53.5 Pa), show reduced storage moduli in comparison with RADA16. All of the assembled peptides exhibit relatively low storage moduli in comparison with Matrigel (G′= 5,408 Pa), which was used as a positive control in the cell culture studies. The time required for the self-assembly process to occur was also examined through rheological analysis. Peptide RADA16-GGPFSSTKT was found to have a fairly linear increase in storage modulus with time for approximately one hour, at which point the G′ values stabilized at 762 Pa.

4.5.5 Tissue regeneration and tissue engineering

The importance of nanoscale becomes obvious in 3D cell culture. It is clearly visible in the images that the cells are embedded in the self-assembling peptide nanofiber biological scaffolds in the truly 3D culture (Figure 4.9). Here, the cells and cell clusters intimately interact with the extracellular matrix cells that they produce. Since the scaffolds are made mostly of water, ~99% water at 1% peptide solid, cells can migrate freely without hindrance, similar to fish swimming freely in a seaweed forest in the sea.

These self-assembling peptide nanofiber biological scaffolds have become increasingly important not only in studying the spatial behaviors of cells, but also in developing approaches for a wide range of innovative medical technologies including regenerative medicine (Figure 4.9). Some examples include: neurite growth and differentiation, neural stem cell differentiation, cardiac myocytes, bones, cartilage cells, human umbilical vein endothelial cells, and keratinocytes cultures. The peptide scaffolds from RADA16-I and RADA16-II forms a nanofiber scaffold in physiological solutions, which stimulated extensive rat neurite outgrowth and successfully achieved active synapse formation on the peptide scaffold [3].

4.5.6 Protein releases from the peptide nanofiber hydrogel scaffold

In order to effectively improve long-term cell cultures, we also developed a method to embed a wide spectrum of proteins within the peptide scaffolds, allowing them to release slowly. This method is not only useful for 3D cell culture, but also for delivering a wide range of therapeutic protein medicine including enzymes, growth factors, and monoclonal antibodies.

We have demonstrate that the Ac-$(RADA)_4$-$CONH_2$ peptide hydrogel is an efficient slow delivery carrier not only for small molecules, but also for a variety of proteins including lysozyme, trypsin inhibitor, BSA, and IgG with differing physicochemical properties (pI4.6 – pI8.5, MW 14.3 kDa – 146 kDa) and morphologies, which are encapsulated within the Ac-$(RADA)_4$-$CONH_2$ peptide hydrogel (Figure 4.10).

It is crucial to determine if the processes involved in incorporating and releasing proteins from the peptide hydrogel adversely affect their conformation and function. To this end, the released protein structure was analyzed using circular dichroism (CD) and fluorescent spectroscopy and bioassays were conducted to verify protein functionality. The presentation of functional proteins and the elucidation of crucial protein-hydrogel

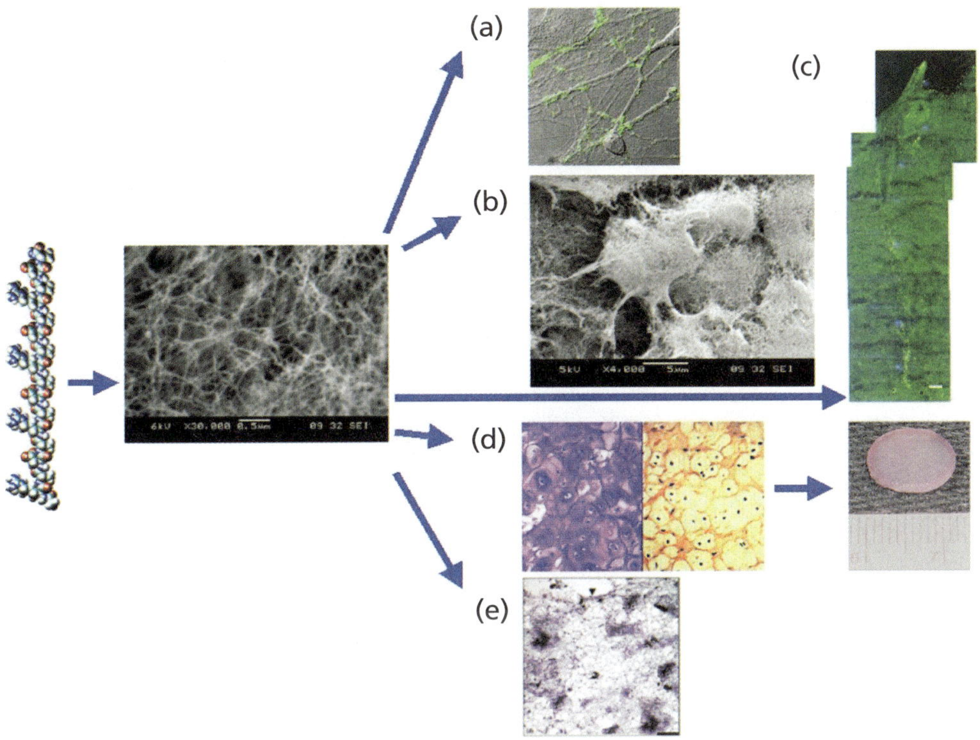

Figure 4.9 From designer peptides to scaffolds to tissues. (a) Active synapses on the peptide surface. Primary rat hippocampal neurons form active synapses on peptide scaffolds. The confocal images show bright discrete green dot labeling indicative of synaptically active membranes after incubation of neurons with the fluorescent lipophilic probe FM-143. FM-143 can selectively trace synaptic vesicle turnover during the process of synaptic transmission. The active synapses on the peptide scaffold are fully functional, indicating that the peptide scaffold is a permissible material for neurite outgrowth and active synapse formation. (b) Adult mouse neural stem cells embedded in 3D scaffold. (c) Brain damage repair in a hamster. The peptide scaffold is injected into the optical nerve area of brain that is first severed with a knife. The injury site is sealed by the migrating neural cells after two days. A great number of neurons form synapses (image courtesy of Rutledge Ellis-Behnke). (d) Peptide KLD12 (KLDLKLDLKLDL), chondrocytes in the peptide scaffold, and cartilage. The chondrocytes stained with TB show abundant GAG production (left panel) and the antibody to type II collagen demonstrates abundant type II collagen production (right panel). A piece of premolded cartilage with encapsulated chondrocytes in the peptide nanofiber scaffold. The cartilage formed over a 3–4-week period after the initial seeding of the chondrocytes (image courtesy of John Kisiday). (e) Von Kossa staining showing transverse sections of primary osteoblast cells on the HA-PHP-RADA16-I self-assembling peptide nanofiber scaffold. Scale bar = 0.1 mm. The intensely stained black areas represent bone nodules forming. (Image courtesy of Maria Bokhari.)

events are considered as significant advances that are required for furthering designer peptide nanofiber hydrogel scaffold for various nanomedicine applications.

An efficient controlled release system should yield biologically active proteins. We tested the released proteins and found that encapsulation and release do not affect the secondary or tertiary structure of the proteins studied, nor is their functionality diminished. These results lay the foundation for creating new tailor-made peptide hydrogels for controlled release of proteins.

Peptide hydrogel scaffolds can be easily designed and synthesized to control the release of proteins and other therapeutic compounds by varying the density of the

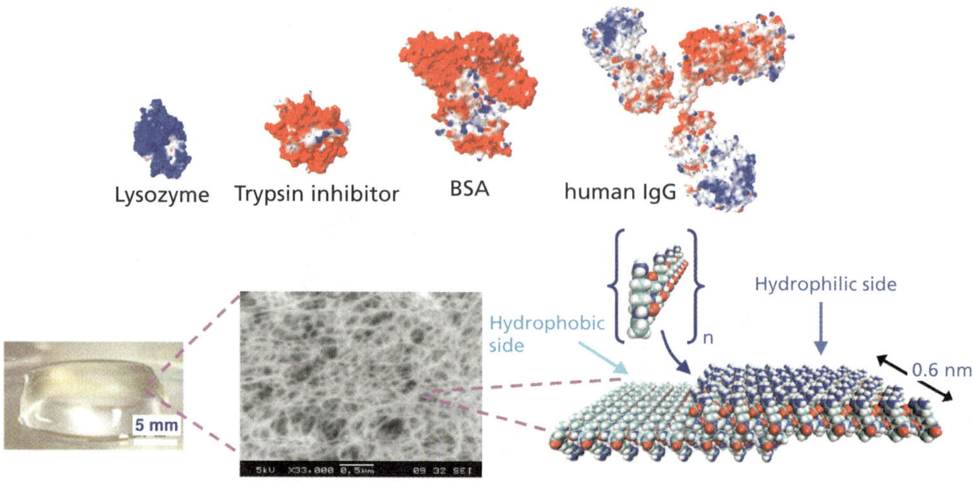

Figure 4.10 Molecular size models of lysozyme, trypsin inhibitor, BSA, and IgG as well as of the Ac-$(RADA)_4$-$CONH_2$ peptide monomer and of the peptide nanofiber. Color scheme for proteins and peptides: positively charged (blue), negatively charged (red), hydrophobic (light blue). Protein models were based on known crystal structures.

nanofibers of the hydrogel or by changing the charge of the nanofibers simply by adding amino acids with positively or negatively charged side groups. Overall, this system would allow the release of diffusing molecules in a sustainable and highly efficient way. We anticipate that further fine-tuned systems will have a wide range of applications in biomedical technology and clinical medicine.

It is possible to combine the 3D culture system with the slow releases of both small molecules and proteins to forge a powerful technology not only for effective 3D cell culture but also for accelerating tissue regeneration.

4.6 Discussions and Commentary

Flat glass and plastic surfaces are not representative of the real cellular environment of living organisms. Tissue-specific architectures, mechanical forces, and cell-cell interactions are usually not represented in 2D inert surfaces. Monolayer cell cultures often modify the cellular intrinsic signal pathways, thus 2D studies are not realistic and result in flawed models, which deviate from the conditions found in tissues where cells interact through chemical and mechanical stimuli with adjacent cells and with extracellular matrix.

Biologically derived biomaterials such as Matrigel from the mouse sarcoma and different types of collagen have been used as a template for 3D cell studies. However, their biological source not only prevents them from any applications in humans but also results in studies, which are not reproducible because their composition may vary from lot to lot. Furthermore, the fact that they contain residual growth factors and other nonquantified impurities results in ambiguous conclusions.

The biologically inspired nanoscale designer self-assembling peptide scaffolds mimic the in vivo environment and serves as permissive substrates for cell growth, differentiation, and biological function. Self assembling peptide nanofiber scaffolds are useful not only for furthering our understanding of cell biology in 3D environment, but also for advancing medical technology, tissue engineering, regenerative biology, and medicine. The self-assembling peptide scaffolds are inert, nonimmunogenic, and nontoxic, consisting of natural amino acids. Peptide hydrogel scaffolds are increasingly important not only in studying the cell behavior in a realistic 3D environment, but also in developing innovative technologies in biomedicine.

Troubleshooting Table

Problem	Explanation	Potential Solutions
Self-assembling peptide solution is viscous.	Limited peptide association is possible during storage.	Ultrasonication facilitates peptide nanofiber dissociation and enables easy pipetting.
Hydrogel is very soft.	The peptide nanofiber density is probably too low; more nanofibers are required to reinforce the hydrogel structure.	Increase the concentration of self assembling peptides; increase the salt concentration of the medium to at least 100 mM.
	The electrolyte concentration may be low resulting in incomplete assembly.	
Cells do not migrate.	The peptide nanofiber density is too high preventing cell migration.	Use lower density peptide hydrogel scaffolds.
Cell do not proliferate.	The peptide nanofiber density is too high and the encapsulated cells cannot grow and proliferate.	Lower density gel is required.
Hydrogel appears fragmented.	The self assembly process which leads to sol-gel transition is not complete.	Allow at least 15 minutes to complete the sol-gel transformation.
	The peptide hydrogel is a soft biomaterial with elastic properties; however, excessive force will cause macroscopic ruptures.	Avoid contact of the gel surface with the pipette tips; change medium gently.
Poor quality microscope images.	Tissue cell cultures in the peptide hydrogel scaffold result in 3D morphologies where focusing may be difficult.	3D tissue culture imaging is facilitated by using confocal microscope techniques.
Poor cell immunostaining.	Staining of the cells requires sufficient time for the antibodies and other fluorescent probes to diffuse through the peptide hydrogel and interact with the cells.	Longer incubation times are necessary to allow for the PFA and antibodies to penetrate the gel and interact with cells.

4.7 Application Notes

The sol-gel transformation of the self-peptides occurs in response to external stimuli when the individual peptide monomers are brought in contact with an electrolyte solution having a composition similar to that of most biological fluids. This harmless triggered self-assembling and the fact that sapeptide hydrogel scaffolds are biocompatible, nontoxic, and nonimmunogenic are the major advantages of this nanotechnology inspired system and allow for numerous applications in bioengineering via a number of different methods.

4.7.1 In vivo injectable self-assembling peptides

It has been shown that injection of the peptide solution in the damaged tissue may be used for regeneration of the heart muscle and of the optical tract in mice as well as for wound healing and hemostasis. In these cases, the self-assembling peptide solution alone or mixed with progenitor cells and growth factors was delivered through a small diameter needle in the injured spot. This methodology may be applied in many in vivo tissue regeneration applications of internal organs where the site of injury is focalized and where a minimally invasive treatment is required.

The RADA16-I self-assembling peptide has been used for neural regeneration in optic nerve lesions. Hamster pups with an injured optical tract are treated by injecting RADA16-I self-assembling peptides into the wound. Control animals with the same brain lesion were treated with an injection of isotonic saline solution in the injured tissue. Animals were sacrificed at various time frames for brain examinations where it was shown that animals treated with self-assembling peptide scaffold the brain tissue was healed and new axons connecting to the retina were grown beyond the tissue lesion. In all animals treated with the peptide scaffold, a significant functional improvement in their sight capabilities was observed using specifically developed behavioral tests.

4.7.2 In vitro multicell system for tissue engineering

Although significant advances have been made in the field, the final goal to engineer and form a tissue in vitro has not been reached yet. Many studies using the self-assembling peptide nanofiber hydrogel scaffold can support the proliferation of numerous mammalian cells including endothelial cells for angiogenesis applications and tissue vascularization, neural stem cells for neural tissue regeneration, mesenchymal stem cells for bone regeneration, chondrocytes for cartilage regeneration, fibroblasts for wound healing and skin graft therapies, and cardiac myocytes for heart muscle regeneration. Hydrogel scaffolds porosity ranges from 100 nm to 500 nm, and the scaffold mechanical properties matches with biomechanical requirements necessary for cells to branch, differentiate, migrate, and establish new functional cytoarchitectures inside the scaffold matrix. This may allow for in vitro formation of a functional, fully vascularized tissue, which may then be transplanted into the host.

4.7.3 Mixed peptide hydrogel with polymer composites

Self-assembling peptides may be used alone or mixed with known compatible biopolymers to generate novel materials where the biocompatibility of the peptide hydrogel is combined with the mechanical properties of polymers. This may be achieved simply by mixing the two components so as to integrate the peptide hydrogel within the volume of the stiff polymer, or by developing advanced hybrid peptide-polymer materials as in the case of the peptide-polymer conjugates. Both of these approaches result in the formation of peptide-based materials with increased mechanical properties that can be used for implantation in the reconstruction of hard tissues such as bone and cartilage.

The possibilities are limitless, thus offering numerous alternative strategies for generating tailor-made biomaterials for biomedical applications with desired properties and characteristics.

4.8 Summary Points

1. The 3D cell culture studies are advantageous over the traditional less reliable 2D studies where cells are cultured on the flat surface of a plastic or glass material.

2. Designer self-assembling peptides are nontoxic, nonimmunogenic, and biocompatible, while the degradation products are natural amino acids.
3. The peptide assembly process into nanofibers occurs in the presence of an electrolyte solution or biological fluids.
4. Designer self-assembling peptide hydrogel scaffolds support cell growth, proliferation, migration, and differentiation of a number of cell types and can be used for tissue engineering and tissue regeneration applications.
5. The new generation of designer self-assembling peptides consists of active peptide motifs that carry cell adhesion and cell differentiation activities; thus, they can be fairly considered as more efficient scaffolds for both in vitro cell culture and in vivo tissue regeneration.

Acknowledgments

We would like to thank the members of our laboratories, past and present, for making discoveries and developing 3D culture research. We gratefully acknowledge the supports of grants from the Whitaker Foundation; Olympus Corp., Japan; CARIPLO Foundation; and NIH BRP Grant EB003805. Sostirios Koutsopoulos is a HighQ Foundation fellow. Shuguang Zhang gratefully acknowledges the John Simon Guggenheim Foundation for providing a Guggenheim fellowship for the pursuit of freedom of research.

References

[1] Zhang, S., et al., "Zuotin, a Putative Z-DNA Binding Protein in Saccharomyces Cerevisiae," *EMBO J.*, Vol. 11, 1992, pp. 3787–3796.

[2] Zhang, S., et al., "Self-Complementary Oligopeptide Matrices Support Mammalian Cell Attachment," *Biomaterials*, Vol. 16, 1995, pp. 1385–1393.

[3] Holmes, T., et al., "Extensive Neurite Outgrowth and Active Neuronal Synapses on Peptide Scaffolds," *Proc. Natl. Acad. Sci. USA*, Vol. 97, 2000, pp. 6728–6733.

[4] Kisiday, J., et al., "Self-Assembling Peptide Hydrogel Fosters Chondrocyte Extracellular Matrix Production and Cell Division: Implications for Cartilage Tissue Repair," *Proc. Natl. Acad. Sci. USA*, Vol. 99, 2002, pp. 9996–10001.

[5] Gelain, F., et al., "Designer Self-Assembling Peptide Nanofiber Scaffolds for Adult Mouse Neural Stem Cell 3-Dimensional Cultures," *PLoS ONE*, Vol. 1, e119, 2006.

[6] Horii, A., et al., "Biological Designer Self-Assembling Peptide Scaffolds Significantly Enhance Osteoblast Proliferation, Differentiation, and 3D Migration," *PLoS ONE*, Vol. 2, e190, 2007.

[7] Wang, X., A. Horii, and S. Zhang, "Designer Functionalized Self-Assembling Peptide Nanofiber Scaffolds for Growth, Migration, and Tubulogenesis of Human Umbilical Vein Endothelial Cell," *Soft Matter*, Vol. 4, 2008, pp. 2388–2395.

CHAPTER

5

Chip-Based Tissue Engineering in Microbioreactors

Brigitte Altmann,[1] Stefan Giselbrecht,[1] Matthias Rieke,[2] Alexander Welle,[1] Tim Scharnweber,[1] Karl-Friedrich Weibezahn,[1] and Eric Gottwald[1]

[1]Institute for Biological Interfaces, Karlsruhe Institute of Technology (North Campus), Germany
[2]Institute of Zoology, Technische Universität Darmstadt, Darmstadt, Germany, Corresponding author: Eric Gottwald, address: Institute for Biological Interfaces-1, Karlsruhe Institute of Technology (North Campus), Hermann-von-Helmholtz-Platz 1, 76344 Eggenstein-Leopoldshafen, Germany, Phone: +49-7247-82-2504, Fax: +49-7247-82-5546, e-mail: eric.gottwald@kit.edu

Abstract

We present a method to generate three-dimensional tissues with defined geometries by means of a micromachined chip capable of housing up to $1*10^7$ cells in 1,156 microcontainers on an area of 2 cm^2. The so-called KITChip with its design variants is intended to serve as a platform technique to either generate organotypical tissue constructs from differentiated cells for basic science applications as well as a tool to develop artificial niches for all kinds of stem cell applications. The polymer membrane of the KITChip can be chemically micropatterned to guide cell adhesion. The patterning technique is also useful for conventional 2D cell culture substrates. For an optimal nutrient and gas supply the KITChip is inserted into a microbioreactor housing that can be perfused, superfused, or even both. The bioreactor can be equipped with all kinds of sensors, like fiber-optic oxygen sensors, that monitor the oxygen consumption of the cells during the culture period, which typically ranges from a few days to several weeks.

Key terms chip-based tissue engineering, hot embossing, microbioreactor, microinjection molding microthermoforming, perfusion culture, surface modification, 3D culture

5.1 Introduction

Probably the Petri dish will be one of the most frequent answers when you ask biologists what will be the most important item in a cell culture laboratory. This is for good reason: there is no comparable culture technique that is as simple and convenient in daily cell culture routine. This is why for more than 120 years after Julius Richard Petri published his methodology of growing bacteria in flat glass dishes in 1887 [1], indefinite numbers of scientists have used this culture format for growing not only prokaryotes but also all kinds of eukaryotic cells and tissues.

With the introduction of three-dimensional culture techniques as early as 1912 [2], the most simple one being the aggregate culture, scientists have noticed that cells behave more organotypic when cultured in higher density. One of the most successful developments, introduced by Knazek and colleagues [3], was the hollow fiber system termed artificial capillaries. The system allowed nourishment of the cells that were cultivated three-dimensionally on the porous outside of the capillaries by using the inside of hollow fibers for the supply of medium and oxygen. However, because of the chosen configuration in the areas most distant from the capillaries necrosis occurred. In addition to the radial gradients that may cause problems in hollow fibers, also longitudinal gradients in the medium may occur in cases where fibers are too long and/or the cell numbers on the fibers are too high, which eventually may lead to necrosis towards the outflow tract.

Common to all of the 3D culture techniques, although to a different extent, is the gain of function to the expense of ease of use and costs. In this unequal struggle between the famous and the inconvenient we introduced the KITChip system [4]. Although the system is equally as inconvenient as other 3D systems, an environment can be realized that for many cells resembles very closely the organ of origin [5]. This is achieved by using polymeric scaffolds with microcontainers (usually $300 \times 300 \times 300\ \mu m\ w \times l \times h$). Routinely, polycarbonate (PC), polystyrene (PS), and polymethylmethacrylate (PMMA) are used as nonbiodegradable polymers, whereas polylactic acid (PLA) is used as a biodegradable polymer for chip production. The manufacturing process is realized either by microinjection molding, hot embossing, or microthermoforming. Depending on the chip design, the bottom of the KITChip features a pyramid-like structure (p-KITChip), a flat surface (f-KITChip), or consists of a thermoformed membrane with round cavities (r-KITChip) (Figure 5.1) [6, 7]. In the p- and f-KITChip only the bottom of the chip contains pores whereas the r-KITChip is porous throughout the whole chip area. Depending on the pore-forming process, which can be a laser-based process or ion track technology, a pore density of 45×10^3 to 2×10^6 pores per cm^2 is achieved. The polymer membrane of the KITChip can be chemically micropatterned to guide cell adhesion and/or differentiation. The patterning technique is also useful for conventional 2D cell culture substrates.

Although many kinds of cells show tendencies to adhere to unmodified PC, PS, or PMMA, it is desirable to guide not only cellular adhesion but also cellular behavior in general. For hepatocytes this can be greatly enhanced if the substrate is conditioned with collagen as described.

Several surface modification techniques are compatible with the used materials and technologies. If structures for spatially defined cell adhesion are desired, a resist-free deep-UV lithography can be used, which renders the irradiated surfaces of otherwise cell-repellent polystyrene more attractive for cells [8]. The irradiation of polystyrene

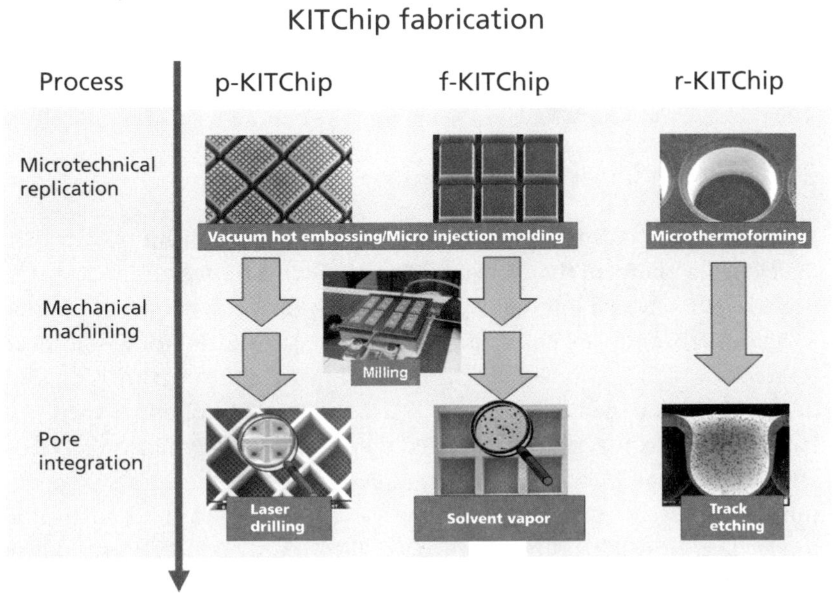

Figure 5.1 Process scheme for the fabrication of the 3 KITChip variants: p-, f-, and r-chip. The p- and f-chip are replicated by vacuum hot embossing. Before pore integration, both variants have to be mechanically machined by a milling process. Pores are generated by a laser drilling process (p-chips) or by a solvent vapor welding process (f-design). r-chips are produced by microtechnical thermoforming of thin polymer films, and pores are generated according to the SMART technology by combining microthermoforming with ion track technology [process sequence: irradiation with accelerated heavy ions (not shown), microthermoforming, and track etching].

with UV at $\lambda = 185$ nm (emitted by a low pressure mercury lamp with quartz windows) yields peroxides, which decompose upon storage; stable carboxylic groups for irradiation doses around 1 J/cm^2; and finally, at high doses, slow surface ablation due to full photo-oxidation. Since the obtained hydrophilic surfaces exhibit a higher affinity towards the adsorption of cell adhesion stimulating proteins from serum containing media, cell patterns readily develop on the patterned surfaces. It should be noted here that the carboxylates tolerate the microthermoforming process, and therefore a pattern created on a flat membrane by usual quartz/chromium masks in direct contact can be converted into a patterned 3D structure (r-KITChip). If more sophisticated cellular reactions are required, the photopatterned polymer surface can be further modified by controlled adsorption of laminin or by coupling growth factors to it [9, 10]. For optimal nutrient and gas supply the KITChip is inserted into a bioreactor housing that is actively perfused or superfused and thus avoids unintended gradient formation. Depending on the experimental purpose, a multitude of bioreactors is available. For basic science applications, single- or double-unit bioreactors are used that can house one and two chips, respectively [5, 6]. Especially for microscopic applications, a bioreactor in microscopic slide format has been developed whose superior optical quality allows for time lapse laser scanning microscopy. When higher cell numbers are available, or when scarce populations are to be expanded, a 32 KITChip-containing bioreactor can be used [6]. Its eight compartments can be independently connected to pumps and medium reservoirs so that it is possible to adjust the cell to a medium volume ratio according to the culture's needs. The bioreactor system can be equipped with all kinds of sensors, like for oxygen, temperature, and/or pH; thus, online monitoring of the culture is possible.

5.2 Experimental Design

Since 3D tissue culture is often more organotypic than monolayer cultures, we have developed a platform that consists of a chip with a bioreactor and periphery that can be used to cultivate cell lines as well as primary cells, be it stem cells or differentiated cells, in an actively perfused chip-based bioreactor. The bioreactor is connected to a medium reservoir, which is connected to a gas mixing station to ensure proper oxygen and CO_2 delivery into the medium. The sterile, closed circulation loop is then placed in an incubator where it is run for the intended duration, which typically lasts from 7 to 42 days. During the experiment, medium samples can be drawn in a sterile way to determine metabolites secreted into the medium. Every 2 to 3 days a half medium exchange is made. The bioreactor run is compared with monolayer cultures that were inoculated with the same cell count in 6-cm Petri dishes at the beginning of the experiment and serve as controls. A further control includes a chip culture that is not inserted into a bioreactor housing but instead is placed in a Petri dish. This control represents the 3D culture without active perfusion and is called the stationary chip culture (Figure 5.2).

5.3 Materials and Equipment

5.3.1 Fabrication of p- and f-chips

- Semifinished product: PMMA film, a bit thicker than the final chip (thickness: approximately 1.2 mm)
- Porous membranes: for example, track etch polycarbonate membranes, at least 2×2 cm^2
- Mold with inverse geometry: for example, brass mold micromachined with diamond tools
- Counter plate with increased surface roughness (e.g., produced by sandblasting)
- Conventional vacuum hot embossing machine (WUM02, Jenoptik Mikrotechnik, Jena, Germany)
- Diamond mill
- UV excimer laser (248 nm, 15 Hz)
- Freeze clamping device for molded chips
- Cooling device
- Custom-made solvent vapor welding apparatus: heatable vacuum chamber with pressing unit consisting of an elastomeric stamp and a porous steel frit

5.3.2 Fabrication of the r-chip

- Thin polymer films with thicknesses of 20–100 μm; wherever applicable, use films that are already irradiated with accelerated heavy ions. Tool consisting of two brass plates (diameter 116 mm) mounted into a conventional hot embossing

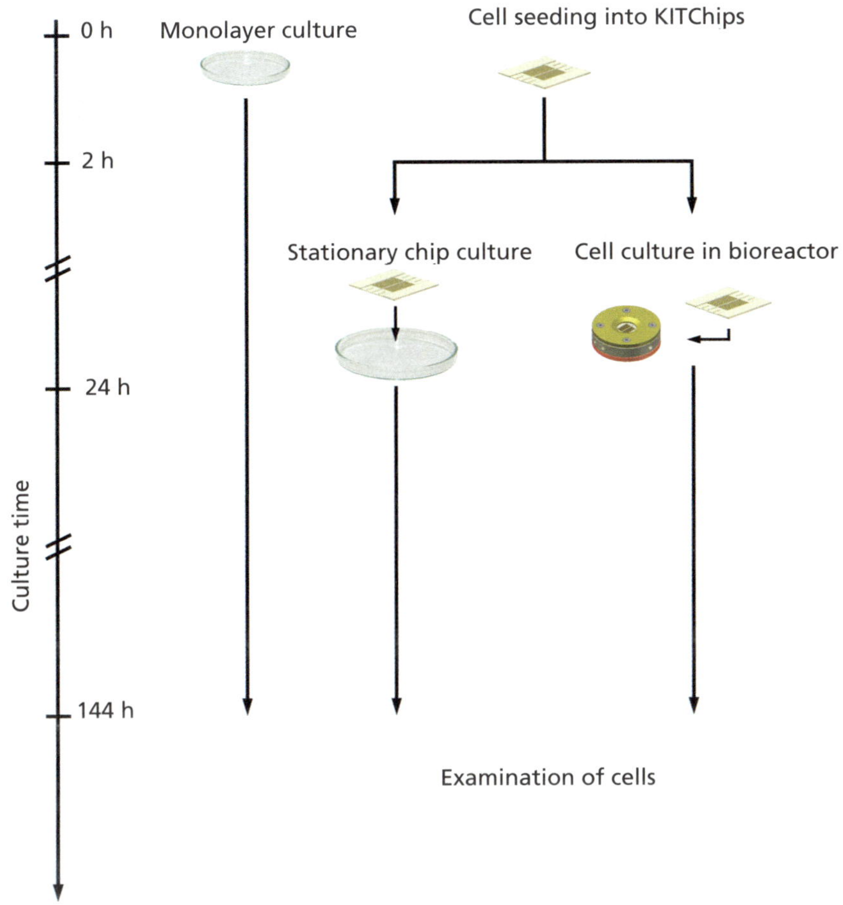

Figure 5.2 Illustration of an experimental setup for the 3D cultivation of cells in KITChips with active medium supply in a bioreactor and the corresponding controls in the stationary chip culture as well as monolayer culture.

machine—one plate is provided with an array of micromolds (for the chip 25 × 25 cavities with 300 μm in depth and 350 μm in diameter) micromachined with diamond end mills; the other plate is equipped with a sealing and connectors for the application of gas pressure and for evacuation of the tool

- Conventional vacuum hot embossing machine (WUM02, Jenoptik Mikrotechnik, Germany) without vacuum chamber or a simple heatable press adapted for the microtechnical thermoforming process
- Sodium hydroxide + methanol
- Hot plate/magnetic stirrer
- Glass beaker
- Support for the polymer films (e.g., Teflon or Teflon-coated forceps)

5.3.3 Bioreactor assembly

- Bioreactor tubing: Tygon ST R3607 and R3603 (Ismatec Laboratoriumstechnik GmbH, Wertheim-Mondfeld, Germany).

- Custom-made bioreactor [Figure 5.3(a)].
- MILLEX HV Filter Unit 0.45 μm (Millipore GmbH, Schwalbach, Germany).
- Luer-lock adapter (neoLab Migge Laborbedarf-Vertriebs GmbH, Heidelberg, Germany).
- Collagen type I from rat tail (Roche Diagnostics GmbH, Mannheim, Germany).
- Phosphate-buffered saline (PBS, PAA Laboratories GmbH, Cölbe, Germany).

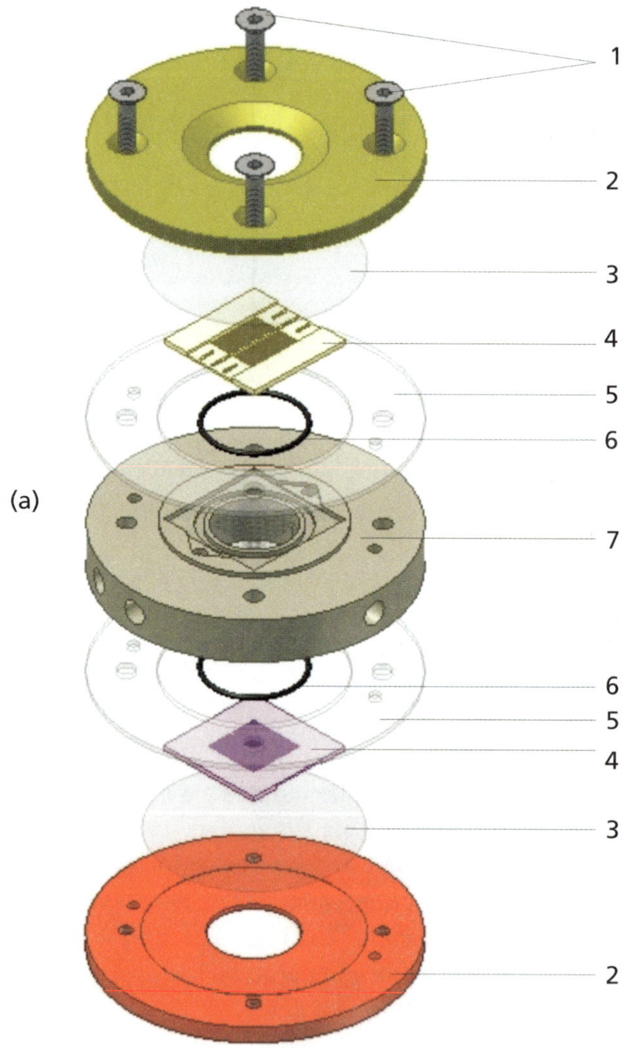

Figure 5.3 Description of the bioreactor assembly, the circulation, and fluid flow of the medium in a KITChip-equipped bioreactor setup. (a) Exploded view of the bioreactor assembly. 1 = screws, 2 = lids, 3 = microscope cover slip, 4 = chip, 5 = outer gasket, 6 = inner gasket, 7 = bioreactor body. (b) Setup of the closed circulation system comprising a bioreactor, a tubing pump, and a medium reservoir with gas supply with the two typical operation modes perfusion (red) and superfusion (green). Numbers indicate the port numbers for the connection of the tubings. The gas supply is realized via sterile filters connected to the bottle top so that the space in the bottle above the medium serves as a gas reservoir. (c) Cross section of a bioreactor housing operated in perfusion mode (fluid flow shown through the bottom of the chip in red). (d) Cross section of a bioreactor housing operated in superfusion mode (fluid flow above the chip in green). (e) Inoculation of an f-KITChip with a 150-μl cell suspension. (f) Schematic illustration of an f-KITChip with a magnification of the microstructured area showing the superfusion and perfusion setup.

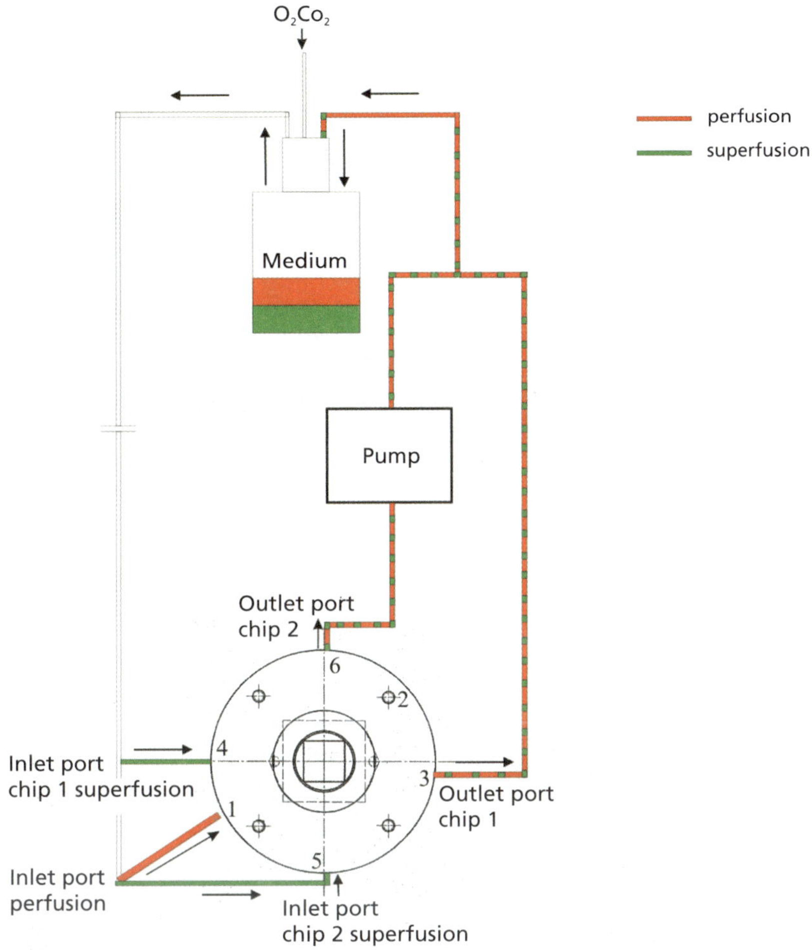

(b)

Perfusion

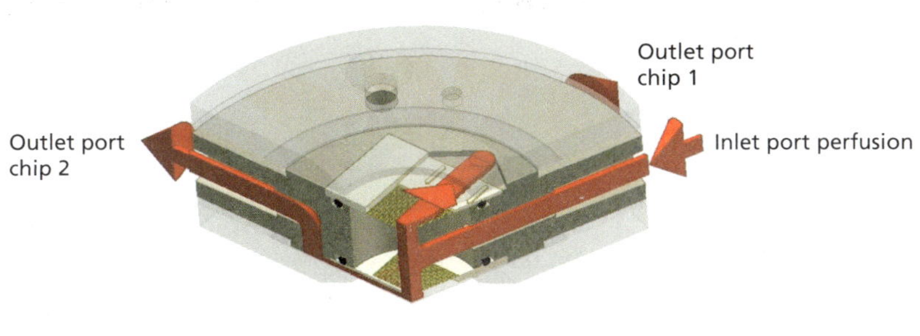

(c)

Figure 5.3 continued

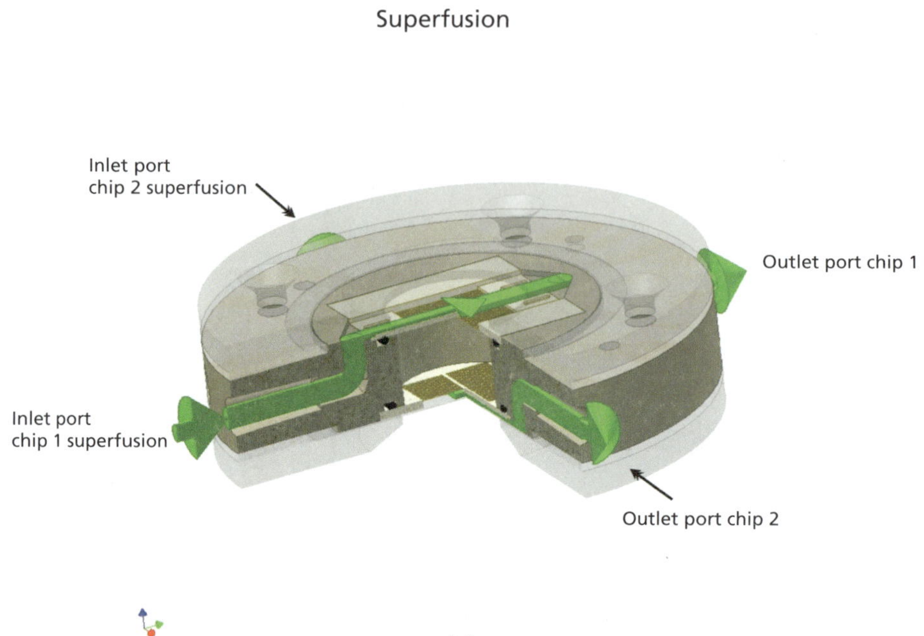

(d)

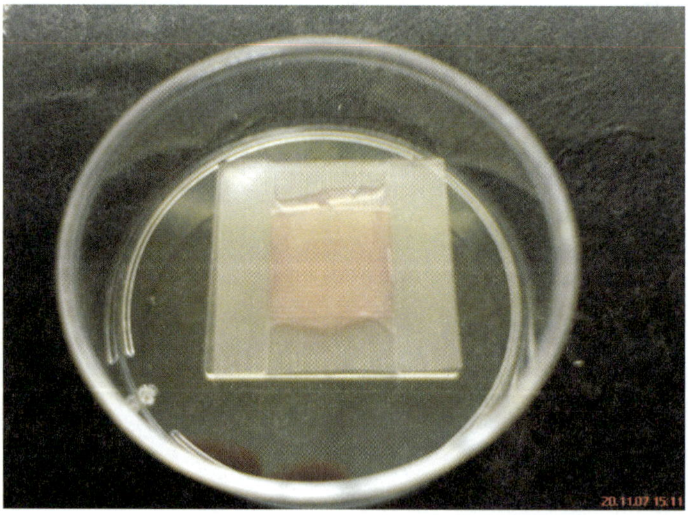

(e)

Figure 5.3 continued

- Medium reservoir (glass flask) that should be connectable under sterile conditions with the tubing of the bioreactor to allow continuous medium flow through the closed circuit system. Furthermore, it should provide two additional connections for the gas inlet and outlet, respectively. In our laboratory we usually interconnect sterile filter units between the gas mixer and medium reservoir, as well as at the gas outlet.

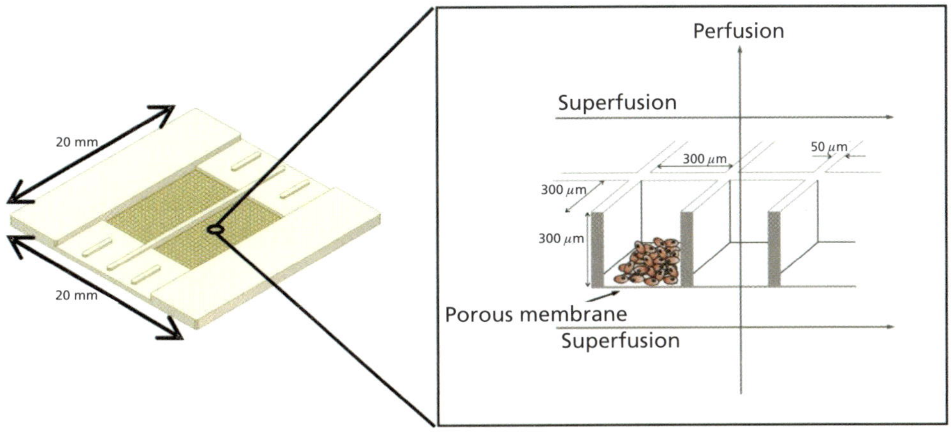

(f)

Figure 5.3 continued

- Peristaltic pump (Ismatec Laboratoriumstechnik GmbH, Wertheim-Mondfeld, Germany) for continuous medium flow through the bioreactor, which is compatible with the used tubing and features flow rates ranging from 60 to 500 μl/min for a hepatocyte cell culture. However, flow rates must be optimized for each individual cell type.
- Gas mixing station or premixed gas for the supply with oxygen (21%), CO_2 (5%), and nitrogen (74%).
- Adaptor for sterile sampling and medium exchange (Ultrasite valve, B. Braun Melsungen AG, Melsungen, Germany).
- Optional: fiber-optic oxygen sensors (Oxy10, PreSens, Regensburg, Germany) for monitoring oxygen concentrations in the system.

5.4 Methods

5.4.1 KITChip fabrication (p- and f-chip)

For both p- and f-chip (microcontainer array with pyramidal and flat porous bottom), vacuum hot embossing is used to produce piece numbers in a small batch, whereas microinjection molding (not described) can be applied to manufacture larger quantities of the chip.

5.4.1.1 Microtechnical polymer replication (vacuum hot embossing)

1. Load the tool with semifinished product (Plexiglas 8N, Evonik Industries, Essen, Germany).
2. Close vacuum chamber and evacuate tool.
3. Heat to forming temperature (approximately 140°C).
4. Replicate the mold geometry by applying force of up to 70,000N.

5. After a dwell time of a few seconds start with cooling down to the demolding temperature of approximately 100°C.
6. Demold.

5.4.1.2 Mechanical machining

1. Cut the overlapping lateral parts of the residual layer.
2. Freeze clamp the chips upside down with deionized water at approximately −10°C.
3. Mill the back of the molded chips (diamond tools are preferred).
4. p-chip: thin the bottom layer to a final thickness of less than 80 μm.
5. f-chip: mill until the residual layer is completely removed and the containers are opened at the back.
6. Separate, deburr, and clean (sonicate with deionized water added with some 2-propanol).

5.4.1.3 Pore integration

p-chip

1. Clamp chip upside down and adjust laser focus and mask.
2. Pores smaller than 3 μm in diameter are drilled by a mask-based excimer laser process through the remaining thin back of the chip (248 nm, 150 pulses per hole, 4 J/cm^2, 15 Hz, projection 1:10, laser machined steel mask with pore sizes of 20–30 μm).
3. By 9 × 9 positioning steps of the mask, up to 45,000 pores per chip are generated.

f-chip

1. Cut a porous membrane (e.g., commercially available track etch membrane, polycarbonate, appropriate pore diameter) to an appropriate size (for embossed KITChip 20 × 20 mm).
2. Bond the porous membrane to the back of the molded chip by solvent vapor welding [11, 12].
3. Load the vacuum chamber with the molded chip and porous membrane.
4. Close and evacuate chamber.
5. Inject acetone vapor and expose to chip and porous membrane until a saturated acetone vapor (duration and temperature controlled: 10 seconds at 30°C) has developed.
6. Press chip and membrane with their softened surface layers together by an elastomeric stamp.
7. Evacuate and eliminate the solvent vapor to create irreversible and permanent heterogeneous bonds.

5.4.2 r-chip (SMART technology)

Substrate modification and replication by thermoforming (SMART) is a recently developed technology to produce functionalized microstructures from thin polymer films. In principle, the technology consists of three major steps: preprocess, microtechnical thermoforming or microthermoforming, and postprocess. Due to a permanent material coherence of the polymer film during the thermoforming process, the polymer film can be locally modified by various means in the preprocess, for example by lithographic methods with high resolution, and the (patterned) modifications are preserved. In the postprocess, the membrane-like microstructures can be further treated with isotropic methods such as wet chemical treatments [13, 14].

This technology is applied to produce porous r-chips by a combination of ion track technology and microthermoforming.

5.4.2.1 Microthermoforming of preprocessed films

1. Load tool with preprocessed polymer film (e.g., irradiated with accelerated heavy ions—see Section 5.3.
2. Close tool without pressing the film between the plates and evacuate the micromold.
3. Press plates together (at least 50 kN) and thus clamp the film.
4. Heat the tool to softening temperature of used polymer by contact heating. (Caution: Irradiation can cause a decrease of softening temperature and an increase in mold sticking.)
5. Stretch softened polymer film into evacuated microcavities by applying gas pressure (e.g., nitrogen with up to 5 MPa).
6. Cool down the tool to demolding temperature (at least 10–20°C below the forming temperature).
7. Relieve gas pressure and subsequently open the tool.
8. Finally, demold the thermoformed part.

5.4.2.2 Pore integration

1. Immerse film samples in agitated etchant with chemically inert forceps. Porous polycarbonate microstructures are produced by etching latent tracks with sodium hydroxide solution. Pores in the range of approximately 1–3 μm are produced in polycarbonate with an etching time of approximately 2–4 hours in 5N NaOH with 10 v/v% MeOH at 40°C.
2. Stop etching process by rinsing the sample thoroughly with deionized water.
3. Dry samples with compressed air or nitrogen.

5.4.3 Preparation of KITChips and bioreactors for cell culture

5.4.3.1 Sterilization of the KITChips and bioreactors

1. Place one or more chips into a Petri dish and seal the Petri dish with Parafilm.
2. Assemble the bioreactor and connect tubes for medium and gas supply via luer-lock adapter with the bioreactor housing depending on experimental setup and flow conditions [Figure 5.3(a–d)].
3. Pack the bioreactor with the corresponding tubings and connectors as well as the chips placed in a Petri dish into a heat sealable film, and close the package with a bag sealer.

4. The chips and bioreactors are sterilized by γ-irradiation (the minimum dose for medical devices is 25 kGray) or ethylene oxide. After applying the latter, degas appropriately.

5.4.3.2 Deaeration and hydrophilization of the chips

Before using the KITChip it is necessary to remove the air from the cavities of the chip to achieve a complete wetting of the microstructured area with fluid [15]. Perform all steps under sterile conditions.

1. Prepare the following dilutions of 2-propanol with sterile deionized water in 50-ml beakers: 100%, 70%, 50%, and 30% solution.
2. Dip the chip into the serial dilution for up to 30 seconds for each dilution starting with the 100% solution.
3. Wash the chip three times with sterile deionized water and place the chip into a sterile Petri dish for further handling. In order to avoid the formation of air bubbles inside the cavities of the chip, for all downstream process steps it is important to keep the microstructured area wet.

5.4.3.3 Coating the chips with collagen type I

After hydrophilization by an alcohol series, the chip can be coated with extracellular matrix proteins depending on the cell type used. We use collagen type I from a rat tail for the hepatocyte culture.

1. Dilute a stock solution of collagen type I (2 mg/ml in 0.2% acetic acid) in sterile deionized water to the required collagen concentration in a final volume of 150 μl per chip. We usually coat the chip surface with 10 μg collagen/cm^2. The surface area depends on the type of the KITChip used. For the f-KITChip with 506 micro-containers the surface area averages 2.85 cm^2. Hence, the collagen solution should contain 28.5 μg of collagen in a final volume of 150 μl.
2. Pipette 150 μl of the appropriately diluted collagen solution on the top of the microstructured area of the chip and incubate for 2 hours at room temperature or alternatively at 4°C overnight. Afterwards, the KITChip is ready to use for cell culture.

5.4.4 Cell culture

1. After coating the chip with collagen type I or other extracellular matrix proteins, aspirate the collagen solution, wash the chip once with PBS, and put the chip back into the Petri dish. It is important to dry the frame of the microstructured area as good as possible, as in the next step the drop with the cell suspension should spatially be restricted to the microstructured area of the chip during the cell seeding process [Figure 5.3(e)] [15].
2. Cell seeding is performed by pipetting 150-μl cell suspension onto the micro-structured area of the chip following 2–4 hours incubation at 37°C. Cell density and adhesion time should be optimized for each individual cell type. We recommend starting with a cell density typical for standard cell culture conditions of the

respective cell type. In our laboratory we cultivate 6×10^6 HepG2 cells in one f-KITChip.

3. After completion of the adhesion phase the chip is placed in a sterile Petri dish and submerged with culture medium for nonperfused cell culture or can be integrated into a bioreactor for active medium supply of the cells.
4. For three-dimensional cell culture with active medium supply all presented bioreactor types are suitable for superfusion or perfusion conditions. Figure 5.3(b–f) shows the difference between superfusion and perfusion of a KITChip. As already mentioned, the choice of the bioreactor type depends on the experimental purpose. Furthermore, the optimal culture configuration (superfusion or perfusion) depends on the chosen cells and should be optimized for each cell type.

5.4.5 Data analysis

The chip culture can be characterized by a variety of methods during the run and thereafter. Analytical methods during the bioreactor run include sampling of probes via the sterile ports to detect all those components that are secreted into the medium as well as online detection of the parameters of interest via the sensors connected to the circulation. Furthermore, microscopical analysis via the built-in microscopic slides for the observation of the living culture is possible. After the run, the bioreactor is disassembled and the chip is amenable to all kinds of analysis. For the isolation of intracellular components, like DNA, RNA, and protein, the cells can be lysed either on-chip or after trypsination. The advantage by using the latter technique is that the cells can be subjected to, for example, conventional FACS analysis. If microscopical techniques shall be applied, the chip is removed from the bioreactor and can be subjected to standard immunostaining protocols and can be evaluated via laser scanning microscopy.

5.5 Anticipated Results

By means of the KITChip and the corresponding periphery, of which for a minimum setup a medium reservoir, a bioreactor and a pump is required [Figure 5.3(b)], tissue like organoid structures shall be constructed. The geometry of the chip and the easy to realize culture configurations, like perfusion or superfusion, lead to a defined microenvironment for the cells. Different kinds of surface modification techniques can be used to guide cellular behavior and development, which will be especially useful for the guidance of stem cells, either with the aim of differentiation or most importantly, stem cell expansion. Due to the incorporation of microscopic cover slips into the bioreactor the chip is amenable to microscopic observation, be it bright field or laser scanning microscopy. The KITChip is also well suited for the isolation of principle cellular components after the experiment has been terminated, either by on chip-lysis or after removal of the cells from the chip. By this it is possible to make use of standard analytical techniques, like gene expression profiling via microarrays and real-time PCR, on lysates that are equally easily produced like those derived from monolayer cultures.

5.6 Discussion and Commentary

The KITChip-based culture system for three-dimensional cell culture applications represents a platform for a variety of applications in tissue engineering and stem cell research, as has already been shown for hepatic tissue engineering [5–7, 16] and photoreceptor differentiation from retina stem cells [17]. The culture system is suitable for all types of cells that require high-density 3D culture conditions to obtain and/or retain their tissue-specific function in vitro. Furthermore, the culture system allows the development of chemically defined niches for all kinds of stem cell applications such as identification, isolation, expansion, proliferation, and subsequent differentiation.

In contrast to other 3D culture substrates like sponge-like structures or hollow fibers, the KITChip allows a uniform cell distribution with a defined surface area. Thus, the system allows coating of the chip with a defined amount of extracellular matrix proteins per unit surface area and the cultivation of cells with a defined cell density in the chip, thereby making the experiments reproducible and comparable. In addition, a variety of analytical methods, for instance determination of total protein content or mRNA isolation for gene expression analysis, can be performed to characterize the cells in chip culture. Beyond that, the KITChip allows the performance of fluorescence staining and immunfluorescence labeling of the adherent cells inside the chip and the subsequent high-resolution optical analysis using laser scanning microscopy. The use of reporter gene transfected cells to determine effects resulting from altered 3D culture conditions might easily be judged.

With respect to organotypic culture of hepatocytes, we could show that not only primary hepatocytes, but also the hepatic cell line Hep G2 expresses a more differentiated phenotype in 3D chip culture compared to conventional monolayer culture [6]. Another investigation performed by Rieke et al. [17] showed that the KITChip system is suitable for the reaggregation and tissue formation of dissociated retinal progenitor cells from neonatal gerbils. Immunohistochemical analysis of the retinal aggregates in the chip revealed Müller glia cells, ganglions, amacrine and bipolar cells, as well as photoreceptors. The differentiation of photoreceptors was slightly further developed on the motionless KITChip [Figure 5.4(a)], compared to their counterparts in rotation cul-

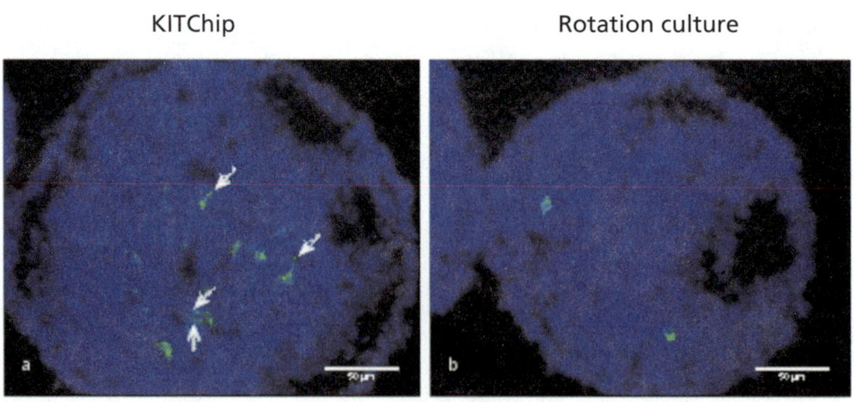

Figure 5.4 Differentiation of (a) photoreceptors (PR, green) in retinal reaggregates derived on the KITChip is further advanced, compared to (b) their counterparts cultured in classical rotation culture. Increased numbers of PR have been found in the KITChip reaggregates; note their histotypic morphology showing features like prolonged rhodopsin⁺ processes (arrows) corresponding to developing outer segments.

tures [Figure 5.4(b)], discernible by their well developed morphology with rhodopsin$^+$ processes [Figure 5.4(a), arrows].

Although spheroid size and proliferation rates of the cells were almost identical in the chip culture and the reference culture, a classical rotation culture system, apoptosis became insignificant in the KITChip culture after 5 days in vitro, while apoptosis increased in the conventional rotation culture.

Troubleshooting Table

Problem	Explanation	Potential Solutions
Empty microcontainers on the chip.	Entrapped air bubbles.	De-aerate properly by increasing the duration of the alcohol series steps.
Cells float off the chip.	Inappropriate cell counts due to initially too high cell numbers or too long cultivation periods with proliferating cells. Inappropriate surface modification or ECM deposition.	Predetermine optimal cell numbers for each cell type separately prior to the experiment. For UV-based surface modifications, determine the optimal irradiation dose.
Entrapped air bubbles in the bioreactor circulation.	After transferring the bioreactor system to the 37°C chamber, dissolved gases in the medium outgas.	Switch the three-way connectors of the bioreactor circulation to superfusion. This leads to the export of the air bubbles.
During long term experiments the medium in the reservoir will decrease.	The use of dry gas mixtures will lead to an evaporation of medium through the sterile filters.	Incorporate a wash flask into the gas inlet tract containing sterile water.
Generation of small bubbles on top of the chip.	Accumulation of cellular respiration products.	Switch the three-way connectors of the bioreactor circulation to superfusion. This leads to the export of the air bubbles.

5.7 Application Notes

The chip-based platform for 3D cell culture has a multitude of possible applications. Besides the ones that we have already introduced with our own investigations, we also have used the system to build more sophisticated culture models to mimic, for example, the first pass effect for drugs and drug candidates. For this, the hepatocyte cell line Hep G2 was cultivated inside the microcontainers of the chip whereas the human adenocarcinoma cell line CaCo-2 was cultivated on the backside of an f-KITChip. The chip was mounted in a bioreactor and perfused as described. The system may also be parallelizable in a way that a 96-well plate incorporates all necessary features to carry out 96 bioreactor experiments with an independent medium supply. This platform could be used for high-throughput 3D cell culture experiments. The chip with its up to 1,156 microcontainers can also be used as a microtiter plate itself because with pipetting robots each microcontainer can be addressed separately. Due to the fact that one microcontainer can house up to 10,000 cells this micro 3D cell culture would nevertheless generate meaningful results due to the 3D culture with active perfusion, which is much more organotypic than monolayers.

By the inside-outside coculture configuration, where two or more different cells are separated by the bottom membrane of the chip, it is possible to create highly relevant tissue models where the effects on the cells inside the microcontainers of either metabolites or secreted factors in general can be evaluated. This configuration can also be very useful for tissue models where the tissue of origin is comprised of at least two different populations of cells that face two different fluidic compartments. This situation occurs for example in blood vessels with endothelial cells facing the blood and the smooth muscle cells facing interstitious fluids. By cultivating endothelial cells in a monolayer on the bottom membrane and smooth muscle cells in the microcontainers, mass transport through the blood vessel wall can be mimicked.

This setup is also important in the generation of structured tissues for transplantation. The KITChip in cross section resembles the cross section of the skin with its layered structure of epidermis, dermis, and subcutis with respect to the saw tooth-like connection between epidermis and dermis. Most likely the microcavities of the chip can be used to generate epidermal structures that upon removal from the chip can be transplanted by retaining the morphological structure of the chip and thereby being perfectly shaped for an optimal skin integration. Moreover, when biodegradable materials for the chip manufacturing processes are used this configuration is useful with regard to transplantation. By seeding different cells on the two sides of an r-KITChip membrane a structured tissue can be grown in vitro. During the differentiation process the scaffold is degraded and replaced by extracellular matrix components synthesized by the cells. Eventually, the in vitro grown tissue can be transplanted. Because the manufacturing process is highly variable regarding the overall size of the microstructured area as well as to the size of the microcontainers, the system is ideally suited to adapt the chip structure to the shape and size of tissue defects. This will lead to in vitro grown tissues that perfectly matches the recipient's site of injury.

5.8 Summary Points

1. We have developed a microstructured chip that is intended to serve as a 3D cell culture platform. For an active nutrients and gas supply the chip can be inserted in a variety of bioreactor housings. Most of the bioreactors can be perfused or superfused or even both, depending on the cell type and/or experimental design.
2. Depending on the design variant, the chip is manufactured by injection molding, hot embossing, or microthermoforming. The latter process can be combined with surface modification techniques that result in the substrate modification and replication by thermoforming (SMART) process.
3. The KITChip is amenable to all kinds of current standard analytical techniques of which laser scanning microscopy is especially valuable because the cells in the microcontainers can be characterized in all spatial directions thereby making it possible to detect changes in protein expression in a 3D environment.
4. Besides the applications already described by us there is a plenty of possible future applications, like stem cell identification, isolation, expansion, differentiation, and transplantation.

Acknowledgments

We would like to thank Anke Dech, David Thiele, Anja Becker, Alex Gerwald, Siegfried Horn, Hartmut Gutzeit, Jörg Bohn, and Christina Trautmann for their excellent technical assistance.

References

[1] Petri, R. J., "Eine kleine Modification des Koch'schen Plattenverfahrens," *Centralblatt für Bacteriologie und Parasitenkunde*, Vol. 1, 1887, pp. 279–280.

[2] Carrel, A., "On the Permanent Life of Tissue Outside of the Organism," *J. Exp. Med.*, Vol. 15, No. 3, 1912, pp. 516–528.

[3] Knazek, R. A., et al., "Cell Culture on Artificial Capillaries: An Approach to Tissue Growth In Vitro," *Science*, Vol. 178, 1972, pp. 65–67.

[4] Weibezahn, K. F., et al., *Cell Culture Substrate,* Germany: International patent, WO 93/07258, 1993.

[5] Eschbach, E., et al., "Microstructured Scaffolds for Liver Tissue Culture of High Cell Density: Morphological and Biochemical Characterization of Tissue Aggregates," *J. Cell Biochem.*, Vol. 95, 2005, pp. 243–255.

[6] Altmann, B., et al., "The Three-Dimensional Cultivation of the Carcinoma Cell Line HepG2 in a Perfused Chip System Leads to a More Differentiated Phenotype of the Cells Compared to Monolayer Culture," *Biomed. Mater.*, Vol. 3, No. 3, 2008, p. 034120.

[7] Gottwald, E., et al., "A Chip-Based Platform for the In Vitro Generation of Tissues in Three-Dimensional Organization," *Lab Chip*, Vol. 7, No. 6, 2007, pp. 777–785.

[8] Welle, A., and E. Gottwald, "UV-Based Patterning of Polymeric Substrates for Cell Culture Applications," *Biomedical Microdevices*, Vol. 4, No. 1, 2002, pp. 33–41.

[9] Welle, A., et al., "Photo-Chemically Patterned Polymer Surfaces for Controlled PC-12 Adhesion and Outgrowth," *J. Neurosci. Meth.*, Vol. 142, 2005, pp. 243–250.

[10] Welle, A., A. Chiumiento, and R. Barbucci, "Competitive Protein Adsorption on Micro Patterned Polymeric Biomaterials, and Viscoelastic Properties of Tailor Made Extracellular Matrices," *Biomolec. Eng.*, Vol. 24, 2007, pp. 87–91.

[11] Giselbrecht, S., et al., "Microthermoforming as a Novel Technique for Manufacturing Scaffolds in Tissue Engineering," *IEE Proc. Nanobiotechnol.*, Vol. 151, No. 4, 2004, pp. 151–157.

[12] Giselbrecht, S., et al., "Microfabrication of Chip-Sized Scaffolds for Three-Dimensional Cell Cultivation," *Journal of Visualized Experiments JoVE*, Vol. 15, 2008, http://www.jove.com/index/Details.stp?ID=699.

[13] Giselbrecht, S., et al., "3D Tissue Culture Substrates Produced by Microthermoforming of Pre-Processed Polymer Films," *Biomed. Microdev.*, Vol. 8, 2006, pp. 191–199.

[14] Truckenmüller, R., et al., "Flexible Fluidic Microchips Based on Thermoformed and Locally Modified Thin Polymer Films," *Lab Chip*, Vol. 8, No. 9, 2008, pp. 1570–1579.

[15] Gottwald, E., et al., "Chip-Based Three-Dimensional Cell Culture in Perfused Micro-Reactors," *JoVE*, Vol. 15, 2008, p. 15.

[16] Knedlitschek, G., et al., "A Tissue-Like Culture System Using Microstructures: Influence of Extracellular Matrix Material on Cell Adhesion and Aggregation," *J. Biomech. Eng.*, Vol. 121, 1999, pp. 35–39.

[17] Rieke, M., et al., "Tissue Reconstruction in 3D-Spheroids from Rodent Retina in a Motion-Free, Bioreactor-Based Microstructure," *Lab Chip*, Vol. 8, 2008, pp. 1570–1579.

CHAPTER

6

Affinity-Binding Alginate Scaffolds for the Controlled Delivery of Multiple Heparin-Binding Proteins

Sigalit Amitay-Shaprut, Inbar Freeman, and Smadar Cohen

Department of Biotechnology Engineering, Ben-Gurion University of the Negev, Beer Sheva, Israel, Corresponding author: Smadar Cohen, address: Department of Biotechnology Engineering, Marcus Campus, Building 39, Room 222, Ben-Gurion University of the Negev, 84105 Beer Sheva, Israel, phone: +972 8 6461798, fax: +972 8 6472915, e-mail: scohen@bgu.ac.il

Abstract

We present here procedures for the fabrication of macroporous alginate scaffold, suitable for stem cell culture and for tissue engineering applications and with a capability of precisely controlling the delivery of multiple heparin-binding proteins. Examples of such biosignals include angiogenic-related factors for inducing and enhancing scaffold vascularization, and signal molecules controlling stem cell maintenance, differentiation, and recruitment. Specifically, we describe the detailed preparation of alginate-sulfate/alginate scaffold, wherein vascular endothelial growth factor (VEGF), platelet-derived growth factor-BB (PDGF-BB), and transforming growth factor-β1 (TGF-β1) are bound to alginate-sulfate with binding affinities similar to that realized upon their binding to heparin. The release rate from such scaffolds was correlated with the equilibrium binding constants of the factors to matrix, resulting in the sequential delivery of VEGF, PDGF-BB, and TGF-β1 and elicitation of mature, dense blood vessel network in implanted scaffolds. We expect that the platform developed herein will be applied for the presentation and delivery of combinations of growth factors active in different tissue regeneration processes.

Key terms
affinity binding scaffold
alginate
alginate-sulfate
controlled delivery
stem cells
tissue engineering

6.1 Introduction

Tissue engineering has emerged as a promising strategy to develop functional tissues for the purpose of replacing or regenerating tissues damaged by injury or disease. Ideally, the engineered tissue should recapitulate the normal structure and function of the tissue to be replaced, and remodel in response to environmental factors, growth, and aging. Engineering of a functional tissue usually involves seeding of polymeric scaffolds with donor primary or stem cells and growth factors, then culturing and implanting the cell constructs to induce and direct the growth of new, healthy tissue [1]. The role of the polymeric scaffold in tissue engineering is critical. It provides the seeded cells with a biomechanical support until they produce their own extracellular matrix (ECM) and it can guide cell differentiation and organization into a functional tissue. Additionally, the scaffold can incorporate and release, in a controlled manner, a variety of angiogenic and antiapoptotic factors, cytokines, and signals that are important for maintenance of cell and tissue viability, for directing stem cell differentiation and maturation, and for inducing scaffold vascularization.

Our group has developed a macroporous alginate scaffold and explored it for versatile tissue engineering applications due to its cell compatibility, nonimmunogenicity, and its hydrogel nature [2, 3]. We showed that the macroporous structure ($> 90\%$ porosity, controllable pore size in the range of 30–200 μm) and the biomechanical properties of the alginate scaffold provide excellent matrix for cultivating hepatocytes [4–10], cardiomyocytes [11–14], and human embryonic stem cells [15] while inducing their organization into functional organoids. Further, the macroporous structure was beneficial following implantation, allowing vascularization of the scaffold without obstruction [16–18]. While the alginate scaffold is a promising cell matrix, the release profiles of biosignal molecules, such as the heparin-binding proteins, from such a scaffold has been frequently unpredictable, being mediated by dissolution of the nonspecific ionic binding between the positively charged growth factors and the polyanionic alginate and their subsequent diffusion.

To enable a precise control over factor release and to allow the release of combinations of growth factors, we recently developed alginate scaffolds with affinity binding sites for heparin-binding proteins by sulfation of the uronic acid monomers in alginate [19, 20] (Figure 6.1). Taking an example from nature, many growth factors, chemokines, and cell adhesion molecules, collectively known as heparin-binding proteins, bind the proteoglycans heparin and heparan sulfate [21], via high affinity, specific electrostatic interactions with low- and high-sulfated sequences in these glycosaminoglycans (GAG) [22]. We showed by surface plasmon resonance (SPR) analysis that of the 14 examined proteins, only the 11 heparin-binding proteins revealed strong binding to alginate-sulfate (Table 6.1) [19]. Examples for bound proteins to the alginate-sulfate/alginate matrix are the angiogenic factors basic fibroblast growth factors (bFGF), vascular endothelial growth factor (VEGF), platelet-derived growth factor BB (PDGF-BB) and transforming growth factor β1 (TGF-β1), as well as others listed in Table 6.1 [19]. We then showed that the affinity-binding alginate scaffold is capable of sequentially delivering multiple heparin-binding proteins, at a rate reflected by their equilibrium binding constants to the matrix [20].

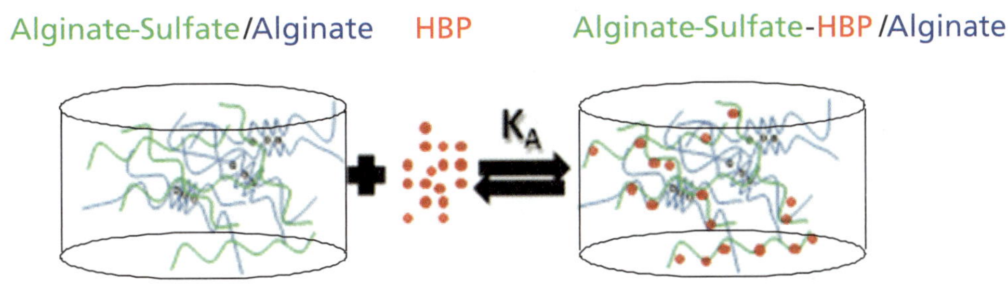

Figure 6.1 The concept of affinity-binding alginate scaffolds for controlled delivery of heparin-binding proteins. The scaffold fabricated from alginate-sulfate/alginate can bind multiple heparin-binding proteins (HBP) via specific affinity sites on alginate-sulfate. The release rate from such scaffolds is correlated with the equilibrium binding constants (K_A) of the factors (Table 6.1).

Table 6.1 Equilibrium Binding Constants (K_A) Calculated from the Interactions of Alginate-Sulfate with Proteins (SPR Analysis) [19, 20]

K_A (M^{-1})	Protein (Abbreviated)	Protein	#
6.98×10^6	VEGF	Vascular endothelial growth factor	1
3.53×10^7	PDGF-BB	Platelet-derived growth factor-BB	2
6.63×10^7	TGF-β1	Transforming growth factor-β1	3
2.57×10^6	b-FGF	Basic fibroblast growth factor	4
2.8×10^7	a-FGF	Acidic fibroblast growth factor	5
1.38×10^7	IL-6	Interleukin 6	6
1.81×10^6	TPO	Thrombopoietin	7
2.06×10^8	SDF-1	Stromal cell derived factor-1	8
5.36×10^7	HGF	Hepatocyte growth factor	9
9.93×10^6	EGF	Epidermal growth factor	10
1.01×10^8	IGF	Insulin growth factor	11
Not bound	FLT-3	FLT (not HBP)	12
Not bound	SCF	Stem cell factor (not HBP)	13
Not bound	OCM	Oncostatin (not HBP)	14

Here, we describe in detail the fabrication of an affinity-binding alginate scaffold, suitable for stem cell culture and for tissue engineering applications and with a capability of precisely controlling the release of multiple heparin-binding proteins. As an example, we focus on fabrication of a scaffold capable of a sequential delivery of three common angiogenic factors, namely VEGF, PDGF-BB, and TGF-β1. In vasculogenesis and angiogenesis, these factors serve as key biosignaling molecules for inducing stable and functional networks of blood vessels [23–26]. The factors are attached to the extracellular matrix via specific interactions with heparan sulfate and act in spatiotemporal gradients to regulate vessel density, size, and distribution [27]. We found that the sequential delivery of VEGF, PDGF-BB, and TGF-β1 from the scaffold mimics the signal cascade acting in angiogenesis, namely the initiation of the process by VEGF, followed by vessel stabilization by PDGF-BB-mediated SMC and pericyte recruitment, and finally, vessel remodeling with ECM induced by TGF-β1 [20].

The affinity-binding scaffold described herein may serve as a platform for the controlled delivery of a combination of different heparin-binding proteins, which are active in versatile biological processes, from cell proliferation, to differentiation, to maturation. Once the alginate-sulfate/alginate scaffold is ready to use, the process of protein loading onto the scaffold is rather simple—incubating an aqueous solution of the protein with the dry scaffold—until the equilibrium binding is reached (usually 30 minutes, at 37°C). Researchers working in stem cells and tissue engineering fields would be able to adopt and optimize this platform according to their needs.

6.2 Experimental Design

The fabrication of an affinity-binding alginate scaffold was motivated by the concept that "nature does it best." Thus, to gain a precise control over factor release from the macroporous alginate scaffold, we aimed to mimic the specific interactions between heparin-binding proteins and heparin/heparan sulfate, by the sulfation of alginate and incorporation of the sulfated product into the scaffold.

The key experimental steps in fabrication and in vitro characterization of the affinity-binding alginate scaffolds [19] are:

1. Perform *O*-sulfation of the uronic acid on an alginate chain by the carbodiimide chemistry.
2. Characterize the product in terms of percentage sulfation and location on uronic acid by spectroscopic, chromatographic, and biochemical assays.
3. Fabricate the alginate-sulfate/alginate scaffolds by a freeze-dry technique [2] and characterize matrix porosity and stability as a function of the percentage of incorporated alginate-sulfate into the scaffold.
4. Load heparin-binding proteins into the affinity-binding scaffold by incubating aqueous solutions of a single or multiple factors with the dry scaffold, until equilibrium binding is reached (30 minutes at 37°C).
5. Conduct a release study in a physiological solution (pH 7.2–7.4, 37°C) and analyze the quantity and biological activity of the released factor or factors by their specific enzyme-linked immunosorbet assays (ELISA) and in cell cultures.
6. Correlate the actual in vitro release patterns with patterns calculated from the equilibrium binding constants of the factor/s to alginate-sulfate as determined by SPR analysis (Table 6.1).

In vivo, the implications of having a tissue engineering scaffold capable of a sequential delivery of three angiogenic factors (VEGF, PDGF-BB, TGF-β1) on its vascularization after implantation were investigated. Vascularization was evaluated by two quantitative parameters as a function of time: the density of the newly formed vessels and the extent of vessel coverage by pericytes/smooth muscle cells as indication of vessel maturation. The experimental design of the in vivo study included implantation in 3 groups of 10 rats each; group 1 was implanted with the triple angiogenic factors as affinity-bound to alginate-sulfate/alginate scaffolds, group 2 was implanted with the triple factors as adsorbed to alginate scaffolds (shown to release the 3 factors mostly at burst), and group 3—the negative control—was implanted with an alginate-sulfate/alginate scaffold without factor supplementation. The inclusion of group 2 in the study intended to reveal the effect of the sequential factor delivery (VEGF followed by PDGF-BB and finally TGF-β1) as compared to the burst release of all 3 factors at the same time. Vascularization of the scaffold was examined at 1 and 3 months after implantation. The explanted scaffolds were paraffin embedded and cross-sectioned from different thickness of the scaffold. The sections were evaluated to follow the extent of vessel ingrowth. The sections were immuno-stained by antilectin for endothelial cell-containing vessels and by smooth muscle actin to detect vessel coverage by pericytes and smooth muscle cells. The key steps for evaluating vascularization are presented in detail in Section 6.4.

6.3 Materials

6.3.1 Materials for alginate sulfation

- Alginate-sodium salt, LVG, > 65% guluronic acid content (NovaMatrix, FMC Biopolymers, Drammen, Norway)
- Cold double-distilled water (DDW, 2–8°C)
- Dowex 50W-X8 ion exchange resin (20–50 mesh, H+ polycation, Bio-Rad)
- Tributylamine—purum grade, = 98% GC (TBA, Fluka)
- Sulfuric acid (Sigma)
- Dimethylformamide (DMF, Sigma)
- N, N′ -Dicyclohexylcarbodiimide (DCC, Sigma)
- Sodium hydroxide (Sigma)
- Dichloromethane (Sigma)
- Filter paper—Grade 1, 70 mm qualitative (Fisher Scientific)
- Dialysis bag—3,500 MWCO (Spectra/Por Biotech)
- Liquid nitrogen

All Sigma reagents and salts are analytical grade.

6.3.2 Materials for scaffold fabrication and factor loading

- Alginate-sodium salt, LVG, > 65% guluronic acid content, MW ~100 kDa (NovaMatrix, FMC Biopolymers, Drammen, Norway)
- Alginate-sulfate manufactured as described in Section 6.4.1
- D-gluconic acid-hemi calcium salt (Sigma)
- Recombinant VEGF, PDGF-BB, and TGF-β1 (Cytolab, Rehovot, Israel)
- Filter polyvinylidene fluoride (PVDF, 0.22 μm, Millipore Millex-GY, United States)

6.3.3 Materials for immunohistochemistry

- Ethanol (analytical grade)
- Xylene (analytical grade)
- Formalin (Sigma)
- Paraffin wax (Paraplast Plus, Thermo Scientific)
- Microscope slides—Superfrost Plus (Menzel-Glazer, Thermo Scientific)

- Tissue processing embedding cassettes
- Stainless steel base molds—size 24 × 24 × 5 mm (Leica)

6.4 Methods

6.4.1 General procedure

Approximate time (~8 days).

6.4.1.1 Sulfation of alginate

1. TBA-alginate formation, 40 minutes
2. Lyophilization* of TBA-alginate, 2 days
3. *O*-sulfation by carbodiimide chemistry, 4 hours
4. Dialysis to remove nonreacted reagents, 3 days
5. Lyophilization* of alginate-sulfate, 2 days

6.4.1.2 Scaffold fabrication

1. Preparation of alginate/alginate-sulfate solution, 1 hour
2. Calcium cross-linking of alginate, 1 hour
3. Freezing of cross-linked alginate, 12 hours
4. Lyophilization to get scaffold, 2 days (lyophilization time can be shortened by accelerating the sublimation rate and also depends on the equipment)
5. Factor loading, 1 hour

6.4.2 Preparation of alginate-sulfate and characterization of product

Alginate sulfation consists of two major steps:

1. Conversion of the sodium alginate salt to a tertiary amine salt;
2. *O*-sulfation of the uronic acid monomer with carbodiimide (DCC) and sulfuric acid.

A probable mechanism for the reaction involves the formation of a solvolyzed, protonated DCC–H_2SO_4 intermediate, followed by a hydroxyl nucleophilic attack to produce monosulfated alginate and dicyclohexylurea (Figure 6.2).

The reaction scheme of the sulfation of uronic acids in alginate involves the formation of protonated DCC–H_2SO_4 intermediate, followed by a hydroxyl nucleophilic attack to produce sulfated alginate and dicyclohexylurea. The latter is removed by extensive dialysis [19].

6.4.2.1 Step 1: conversion to TBA-alginate salt

1. Prepare 0.2 (%, w/v) alginate solution by dissolving 0.3g sodium alginate salt in 150-mL cold DDW.
2. Add 20g ion exchange resin [(13.3%, w/v), Dowex 50W-X8] into the alginate solution and stir for 5 minutes [room temperature (RT)].

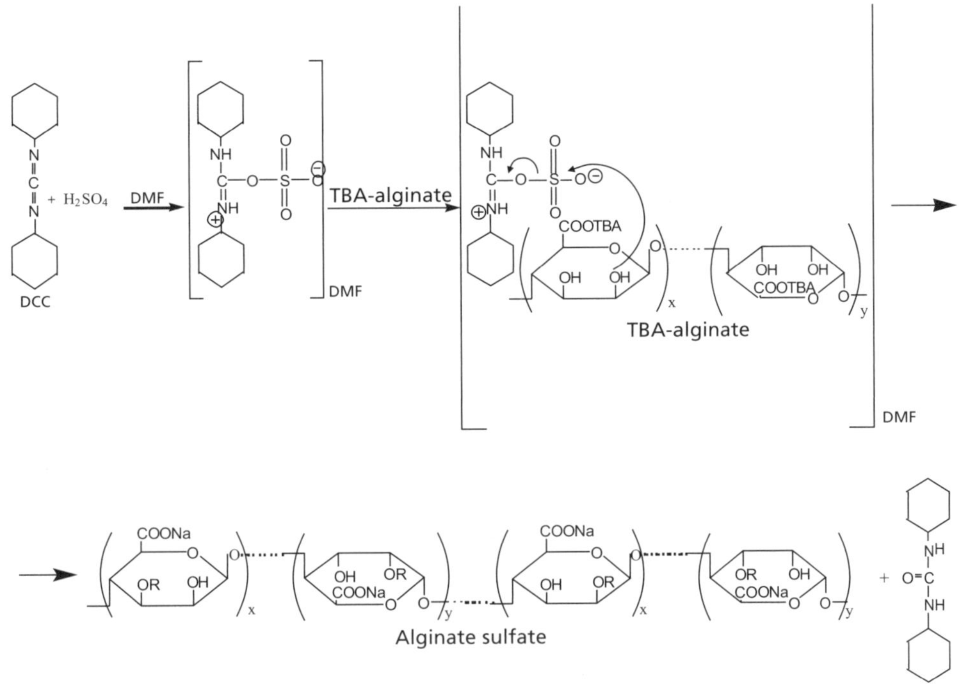

R= SO_3Na or H

Figure 6.2 *O*-sulfation of the uronic acid on alginate. The reaction scheme of the sulfation of uronic acids in alginate involves the formation of protonated DCC–H_2SO_4 intermediate, followed by a hydroxyl nucleophilic attack to produce sulfated alginate and dicyclohexylurea. The latter is removed by extensive dialysis [19].

3. Remove the ion exchange resin by centrifugation (2,500g, 5 minutes, room temperature) and collect the supernatant. (In this stage the resin seems like a gel and the suspension is very viscous.)
4. Wash the resin with DDW a few times, until the resin retains its initial texture—clean and granular. After each washing, centrifuge and collect the supernatant.
5. Filter the resin using filter paper under vacuum and merge the filtrates collected. (The resin can be recycled by washing the resin with DDW and then with 0.5N HCl and dry by filtration under vacuum.)
6. Titer the filtrate until the pH reaches to 6.0–6.5 using tributylamine (diluted: 1:10 in DDW)
7. Freeze the solution in boiling flask (250 mL) using liquid N_2.
8. Lyophilize till dryness. It takes about 2 days to dry.

6.4.2.2 Step 2: O-sulfation via carbodiimide chemistry

1. Cool 100-mL DMF on ice within closed boiling flask (250 mL). The flask should be completely dry and closed with open glass tube with spherical head containing $CaCl_2$ salt for humidity absorption (Figure 6.3).
2. Dissolve 3g of sulfuric acid in 100-mL DMF. Be careful of an exothermic reaction. Therefore, the DMF should be cooled and kept chilled on ice. White fumes are expected.
3. Add 0.3g TBA-alginate and stir until the solution is clear.

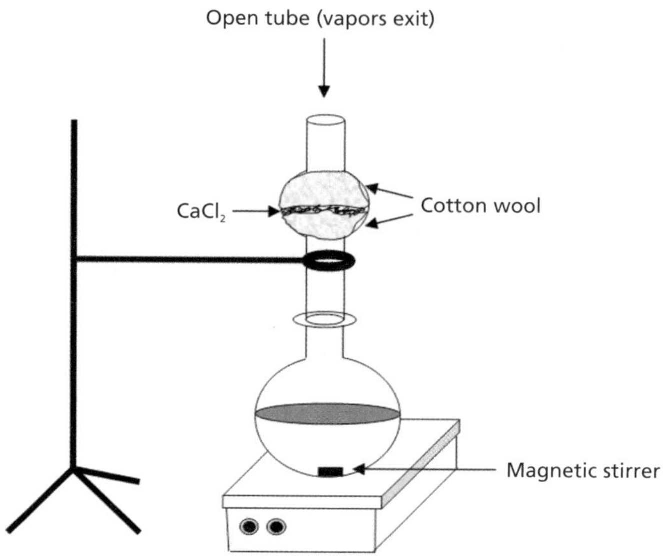

Figure 6.3 The glassware used for *O*-sulfation of alginate. A closed and dry boiling flask (250 mL) with an open glass tube and spherical head and containing $CaCl_2$ salt for minimizing the humidity. The $CaCl_2$ is held between two pieces of cotton wool to avoid its contact with reaction materials.

4. Add and dissolve 6g of DCC. Stir for 2 hours (room temperature).
5. Filter the solution under vacuum and keep the precipitate.
6. Add to the filtrate (~100 mL) three equal volumes of dichloromethane (~300 mL) and wait for 30 minutes. During this time a precipitant is formed.
7. Filter the solution under a vacuum and keep the precipitate.
8. Immerse the precipitants from steps 5–7 in 100 mL of 0.5N NaOH and mix for 30 minutes, until the precipitant is dissolved.
9. Filter the solution under the vacuum to remove the precipitate (DCC-Urea) by vacuum filtration.
10. Insert the filtrate (yellow transparent liquid) into the dialysis bag against 2L DDW. Replace (× 5) with fresh water during 3 days.
11. Split the solution into four polypropylene tubes and freeze with liquid N_2, then lyophilize till dryness (~2 days). (The dry alginate-sulfate has a fluffy fibrous texture.)

6.4.2.3 Step 3: characterization of the product

Characterization of the product in terms of molecular weight (MW), percentage of sulfation, and its location on the uronic acid included [19]:

1. Gel permeation chromatography—multiangle light scattering (GPC-MALLS)
2. Fourier-transformed infrared spectroscopy (FTIR)
3. Solution ^{1}H and ^{13}C nuclear magnetic resonance (NMR)
4. Elemental analysis by scanning electron microscope (SEM) in low-vacuum (20 kV) mode and the analysis carried out by energy dispersive X-ray spectrometry (EDX system by EDAX)
5. Sheniger biochemical assay for sulfur [28]

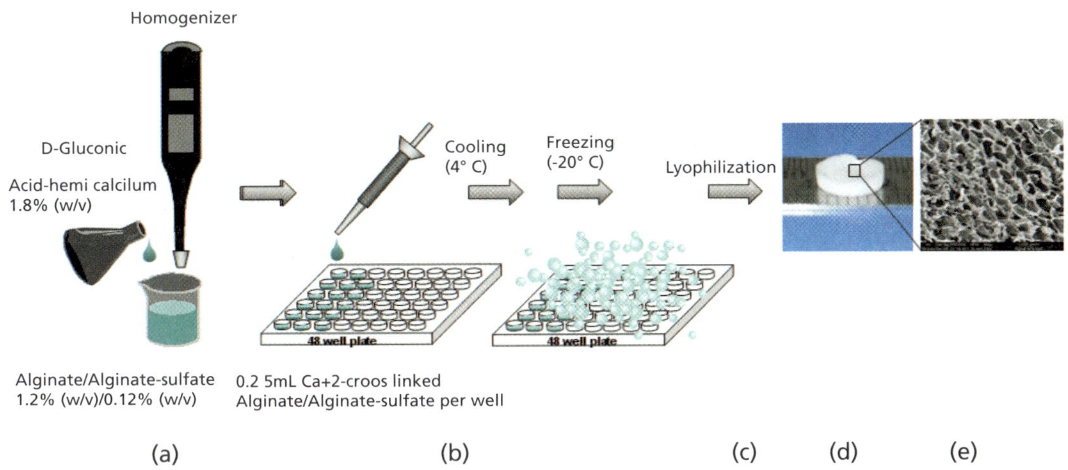

Figure 6.4 Scheme for scaffold fabrication. (a) Cross-linking of a mixture of alginate-sulfate/alginate solution by D-gluconic acid-hemi calcium solution followed by homogenization to spread the dissolved calcium ions and obtain a homogenous cross-linked alginate solution. (b) Pour the cross-linked solution into 48-well plate and chill overnight, at 4°C, the follow by freezing (−20°C). (c) Lyophilization of the frozen plates at < 10 mbar until dry (~2 days). (d) Picture of alginate-sulfate/alginate dry scaffold (11 × 3 mm, $d \times h$). (e) SEM picture of cross-section of the scaffold (pore diameter 120 ± 30 μm).

6.4.3 Scaffold fabrication

The different steps for scaffold fabrication are schematically presented in Figure 6.4. An aqueous solution of alginate (final concentration 1%, w/v) alone or mixed with alginate-sulfate (final concentration 0.1%, w/v) is cross-linked by adding an aqueous solution of D-gluconic acid-hemi calcium salt followed by a homogenization to spread the dissolved calcium ions and obtain a homogenous cross-linked alginate solution. The solution is frozen and lyophilized to obtain macroporous scaffolds. Specifically, the steps are:

1. Prepare aqueous solutions of alginate/alginate-sulfate and cross-linker: A mixture of alginate 1.2 (% w/v) and alginate-sulfate 0.12 (%w/v) solution dissolved in DDW by stirring at room temperature.
2. A cross-linker solution of D-gluconic acid-hemi calcium salt, 1.8 (%w/v) dissolved in DDW and filtered (0.22 μm). The final concentrations of those components after mixing and cross-linking should be: alginate 1 (% w/v), alginate-sulfate 0.1 (%w/v), and D-gluconic acid-hemi calcium salt 0.3 (% w/v). Therefore, the volumetric mixing ratio of the alginate/alginate-sulfate solution with the cross-linker is 5:1, accordingly. The total volume of cross-linked solution depends on the number of prepared scaffolds.
2. Calcium cross-linking is performed while the alginate mixture solution is homogenized, at 26,000 rpm, for 5 minutes for obtaining a uniform cross-linking of alginate.
3. Pour 0.25 mL/well of the cross-linked solution within 48-well plate and chill overnight at 4°C. Then freeze at −20°C overnight.

4. Transfer the frozen plates to vacuum vessel and lyophilize at < 10 mbar until dry. (The scaffold should be kept in a clean and dry place until use.)
5. Sterilize the scaffolds within the plate before use by exposure to UV light in a laminar flow hood for 1 hour.
6. Characterize the porosity and stability of the scaffolds using SEM as described in [2]. Under these conditions, the scaffold size is 11 × 3 mm ($d \times h$) with an average pore size of 120 ± 30 μm. Scaffolds with different overall size and shape can be easily achieved by using different molds and volumes of the cross-linked alginate solution. In addition, by controlling the freezing regime, scaffolds with different porosity and mechanical properties can be achieved [2, 3].

6.4.4 Triple factor loading into scaffolds and release studies

1. Dissolve VEGF, PDGF-BB, and TGF-β1 at a molar ratio 0.6:1:1, in medium.
2. Pour the factor mixture solution onto the dry sterile scaffold then incubate for 30 minutes, at 37°C. The total protein loaded is 100 ng per scaffold in an 80-μL serum-free medium. Loading to the ready-to-use alginate-sulfate/alginate scaffold is simple and takes 1 hour for completion.
3. In vitro release studies: the factor-loaded scaffolds, placed in 24-well plate (one scaffold per well) are suspended in a 1-mL culture medium (DMEM, 1% Pen/Strep) and incubated on a rotating incubator at 37°C. The medium is semireplaced daily (0.5 mL) and the amounts of released growth factors are determined by the appropriate ELISA, preformed according to the manufacturer's instructions. The experiments are performed under sterile conditions.

6.4.5 In vivo studies: immunostaining, imaging, and data acquisition

The scaffolds (two scaffolds per rat) are implanted subcutaneously in the dorsal area of anesthetized rats following removal of the dorsal hair. Each experimental group should include at least three animals per group. After specified time intervals, the implanted scaffolds are explanted and processed for immunohistochemistry.

6.4.5.1 Histology and immunostaining

1. Explant the implanted scaffold with its surrounding tissue and transfer to fixation in 4 (%, v/v) formalin solution in Dulbecco's Modified Eagle's Medium (DMEM, containing Ca^{2+} and Mg^{2+}) overnight at RT.
2. Process the scaffold by transferring it in the order of solutions in Table 6.2.

Table 6.2 Fixation of Explanted Implant: Order of Solutions

Step	Solution	Time	Temperature	Repetition
1	70% Ethanol	30 minutes	RT	—
2	95% Ethanol	60 minutes	RT	×5
3	Absolute ethanol	60 minutes	RT	×3
4	Xylene	30 minutes	RT	—
5	Xylene	60 minutes	RT	—
6	Paraffin wax	90 minutes	60°C	×2

3. Embed the specimen by dipping it into warm paraffin (60°C) within stainless steel base molds and then put the mold on an ice block to allow the wax to harden.
4. Cross-section (5 μm thick) the paraffin blocks and place them onto precoated slides.
5. The samples are deparaffinized and rehydrated gradually prior to immunostaining by immersing the slides in the solutions detailed in Table 6.3.
6. Immunostaining the cross-sections according to the manufacturer's instructions with antibodies against: α-lectin as endothelial marker and α-smooth muscle actin (α-SMA) present in high amounts in vascular SMC used for identification of mature blood vessels.

6.4.5.2 Imaging and quantification of vascularization

1. Microscope images are acquired, at 200× magnification, from 10 different fields in each slide, randomly selected from the slides of α-lectin and α-SMA (n = 6) immunostained cross-sections, using an Olympus light microscope (BX61, motorized system microscope) connected to an Olympus (DD71) digital capture system.
2. Picture analysis is preformed using cell imaging software (Olympus Soft Imaging Solutions GmbH; Munster, Germany).
3. Quantitation of scaffold vascularization should include the following data: vessel density (number of capillaries/mm^2), percentage area occupied by blood vessels, and percentage of mature blood vessels.
4. Statistical significance is determined by two-way analysis of variance (ANOVA) using Tukey' s multiple comparison test or a one-way ANOVA (t-test) utilizing GraphPad Prism software (version 5.0, San Diego, California).

The following example demonstrates our approach for evaluating scaffold vascularization (vessel density and the percentage of vessel maturation). Table 6.4 details the vessel density counts on slides immunostained for α-lectin and SMA (n = 60; 2 scaffolds per animal × 3 animals per group and counting 10 fields per slide). Only mature vessels are stained positive for SMA. Alg-S/Alg indicates a group implanted with alginate-sulfate/alginate scaffold with no factor supplementation; Alg/triple indicates group implanted with triple angiogenic factors (VEGF, PDGF-BB and TGF-β1) adsorbed to alginate scaffold; Alg-S/Alg-triple indicates a group implanted with triple angiogenic factors (VEGF, PDGF-BB and TGF-β1) bound to an alginate-sulfate/alginate scaffold.

The percentage of matured vessels is calculated according to the equation:

$$\%\ \text{Mature vessels} = 100 \times (\text{SMA-positive vessel density})/(\text{lectin-positive vessel density})$$

Table 6.3 Deparaffinzation and Rehydration of the Cross-Section Samples

Step	Solution	Time	Temperature	Repetition
1	Xylene	5 minutes	RT	× 3
2	Absolute ethanol	6 dipping	RT	× 4
3	70% Ethanol	6 dipping	RT	
04	DDW	1 minute	RT	× 2

Table 6.4 Vessel Density Counts on Slides Immunostained for α-Lectin and SMA

		Vessel Density, Number of Vessels/mm^2 Area		
		Alg-S/Alg-triple	Alg/triple	Alg-S/Alg
Lectin	1 month	268.05 ± 119.21	171.94 ± 67.75	69.47 ± 27.78
	3 month	200.60 ± 80.28	98.03 ± 35.15	43.07 ± 27.36
SMA	1 month	120.88 ± 28.90	113.94 ± 22.83	51.41 ± 9.32
	3 month	186.19 ± 47.48	91.70 ± 11.42	36.13 ± 19.89

Figures 6.5 and 6.6 present the results obtained for scaffold vascularization after implantation for 1 and 3 months. Representative immunostained pictures are also presented.

6.5 Anticipated Results

The procedures described herein should lead to the fabrication of an affinity-binding alginate scaffold that can specifically bind multiple heparin-binding proteins and release them at a rate determined by their equilibrium binding constants to the matrix. It is anticipated that researchers working with stem cells and on tissue engineering of biological substitutes would greatly benefit from having such a system with a precise control over the presentation and release of heparin-binding proteins. This family of proteins represents a large number of growth factors, cytokines, and chemokines, which participate in many biological processes, such as cell proliferation, differentiation, and migration. Their controlled presentation at the right time and location should contribute to the normal execution of the biological process in study. For example, we found that bolus delivery of bFGF resulted in the formation of thicker than usual layer of smooth muscle cells around the newly formed blood vessels, while the sequential delivery of VEGF, PDGF-BB, and TGF-β1 induced the formation of what appears to be a normal morphology of mature blood vessels (Figure 6.7).

6.6 Discussion and Commentary

The affinity-binding alginate scaffold represents a controllable delivery system for multiple heparin-binding proteins as well as a supporting matrix for stem cell culture and tissue engineering applications. By virtue of these properties, it can be a valuable platform mimicking the "right" cell microenvironment.

The matrix affinity to heparin-binding proteins was achieved by alginate sulfation using the common carbodiimide chemistry [19]. The reaction comprised of converting sodium alginate into tertiary amine salt to enable its dissolution in the aprotic solvent, dimethylformamide (DMF), and then *O*-sulfation of the uronic acid with carbodiimide and sulfuric acid. The product was characterized by spectroscopic, chromatographic, and biochemical assays. According to ^{13}C NMR spectra, sulfation was mainly confined to the alcoholic hydroxyl groups (C-2 and C-3) of the uronic acids. FTIR spectra revealed a new major peak at ~1,250 cm^{-1}, assigned to S=O symmetric stretching, and a minor peak at 800 cm^{-1}, assigned to S-O-C stretching, indicating sulfation of the uronic acids in

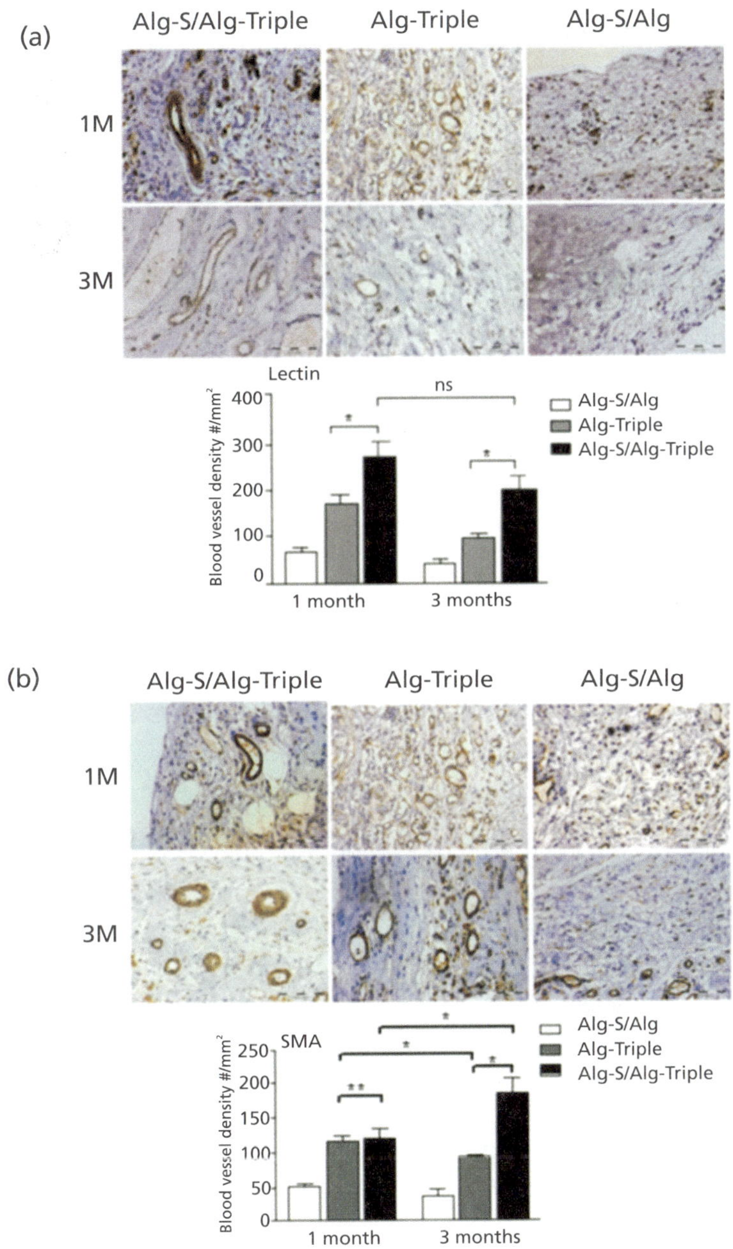

Figure 6.5 Quantification of blood vessel densities by counting (a) lectin-positive vessels or (b) SMC-positive vessels in sections from implanted scaffolds retrieved after 1 and 3 months. Alg-S/Alg-Triple and Alg-Triple are alginate-sulfate/alginate and alginate scaffolds, respectively, loaded with triple factors (VEGF, PDGF-BB, and TGF-β1). Alg-S/Alg is alginate-sulfate/alginate scaffold with no supplemental factors: (*) $p < 0.05$, (**) $p < 0.01$. Values represent the mean and standard deviation. Scale bar 100 μm [20].

alginate (Figure 6.8). SEM-EDX analysis revealed the presence of 11.5 ± 4.0% sulfur in alginate-sulfate (wt. sulfur/wt. alginate), while Sheniger analysis yielded 7.9 ± 0.3% (wt. sulfur/wt. alginate).

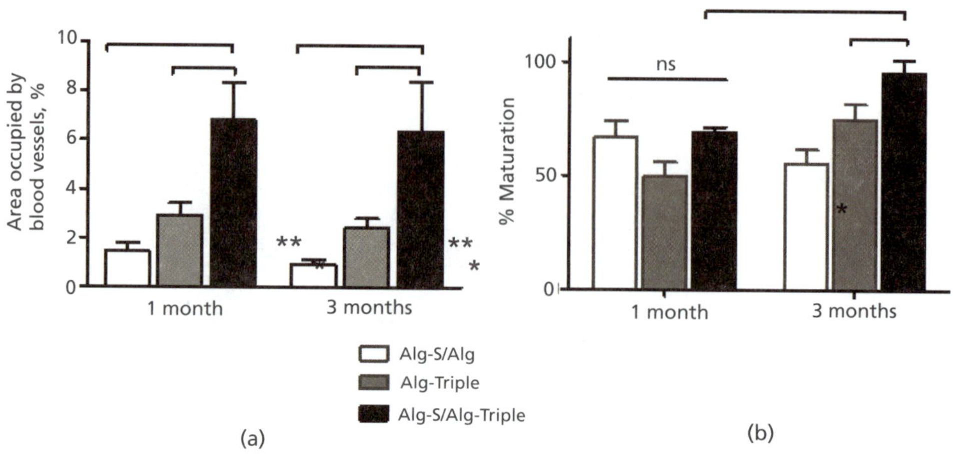

Figure 6.6 Blood vessel size and maturation in the implanted scaffolds as judged by (a) percentage of area occupied by blood vessels determined on lectin-stained sections, and (b) percentage of matured vessels (i.e., the ratio of SMA-positive vessel density to lectin-positive vessel density × 100). Alg-S/Alg-Triple and Alg-Triple are alginate-sulfate/alginate and alginate scaffolds, respectively, loaded with triple factors (VEGF, PDGF-BB, and TGF-β1). Alg-S/Alg is alginate-sulfate/alginate scaffold with no supplemental factors. (*) $p < 0.05$, (**) $p < 0.01$. Values represent the mean and standard deviation [20].

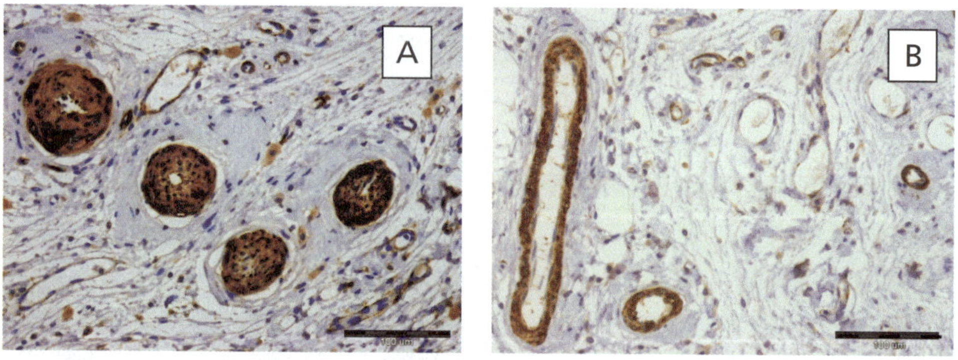

Figure 6.7 Visualization of mature blood vessels by SMA-positive immunostaining on cross-sections from subcutaneously implanted scaffolds—retrieved after 3 months. (a) Abnormal vessels, having a very thick smooth muscle cell layer are presented in alginate scaffold delivering bFGF in burst. (b) Mature vessels with a normal smooth muscle cell layer, after a sequential delivery of VEGF, PDGF-BB, and TGF-β1 from alginate-sulfate/alginate scaffold. Scale bar 100 μm.

Notably, we found that alginate-sulfate does not undergo phase transition from sol-to-gel in the presence of calcium ions. We performed several studies to elucidate the causes for this behavior. By NMR spectroscopy, we found that alginate-sulfate maintained its initial ratio of guluronic acid/mannuronic acid (G/M). However, alginate sulfation caused a 30% decrease in the apparent viscosity of its aqueous solution. Attempts to measure the molecular weight (MW) of alginate-sulfate by GPC-MALLS were inconclusive, revealing greater MW values than expected. Interestingly, according to rheol-

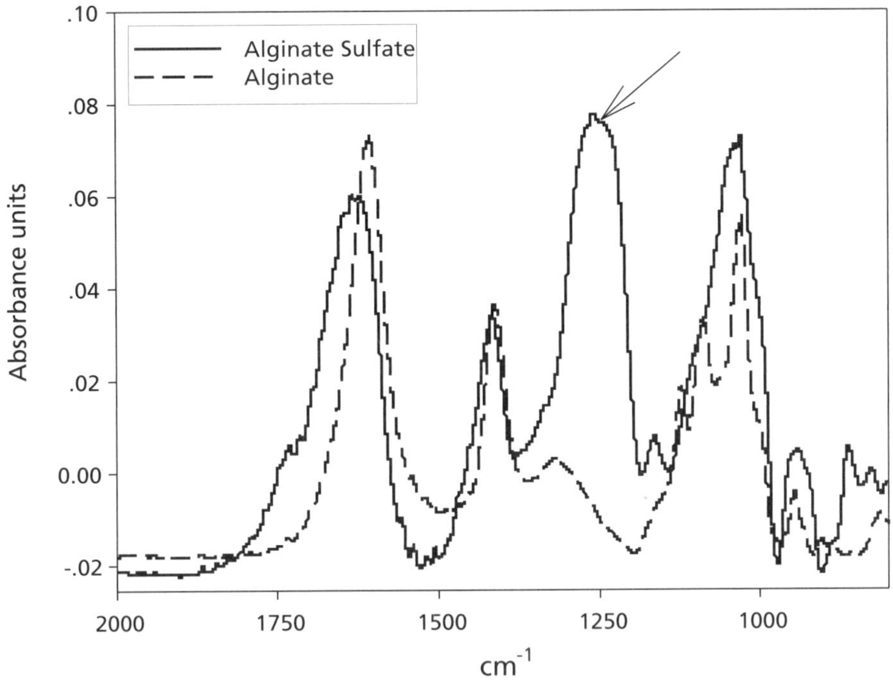

Figure 6.8 FTIR spectra of alginate-sulfate and raw sodium alginate. The arrow points towards the new peak at ~1,250 cm^{-1} assigned to S=O symmetric stretching formed as a result from alginate sulfation [19].

ogy, G′—the elastic modulus—increased after alginate sulfation, suggesting processes such as cross-linking. At present, we are still exploring this issue. Nevertheless, since alginate-sulfate constitutes only up to 10% wt of the alginate scaffold, its presence does not affect the stability or internal structure/porosity of the scaffold, as we have previously shown [20].

Another issue worth noting is our limited ability to precisely control the degree of alginate sulfation using the carbodiimide chemistry. Of the 10 batches produced under the same conditions, the degree of alginate sulfation ranged between 7–20%, according to FTIR analysis. In this analysis, we used the unchanged peak (COC) at ~1,030 cm^{-1} as a reference peak and determined the ratio between the areas under the peaks of S=O and COC in the FTIR spectrum, after reducing the ratio of the unmodified alginate (Figure 6.8). Nevertheless, since the range of sulfation degree is still reproducible, we do not see this issue as critical. In the future, we plan to examine an enzymatic method to achieve sulfation.

Perhaps the most important feature of the affinity-binding scaffold composed of alginate-sulfate/alginate is its capability to specifically bind multiple heparin-binding proteins (Table 6.1) and then to release them, at a rate reflected by their equilibrium binding constants to alginate-sulfate. Thus, combinations of heparin-binding proteins, selected according to their binding constants, may be released at different rates from one device, such as exemplified by the sequential delivery of the triple angiogenic factors, VEGF, PDGF-BB, and TGF-β1 from the scaffold [20].

As a proof-of-concept of our system utility to enhance angiogenesis and scaffold vascularization, three common angiogenic factors, VEGF, PDGF-BB, and TGF-β1, were affinity-bound to the scaffold. In vitro release studies revealed the sequential delivery of first VEGF, then PDGF-BB, and finally TGF-β1. In contrast, in alginate scaffolds lacking alginate-sulfate, release of the adsorbed proteins was instantaneous. The sequential delivery of the angiogenic factors resulted in the elicitation of a mature and dense network of blood vessels in the implanted scaffold and its surroundings (after subcutaneous implantation in rats for 1 and 3 months) (Figure 6.5). Vessel formation and extent of maturation was followed by immunostaining of cross-sections for α-lectin (endothelial cells) and α-smooth muscle actin (smooth muscle cells and pericytes). To ensure the extent of ingrowth, the cross-sections were dissected from different locations in the implanted scaffold and the vessel count was performed on both lectin- and SMA-stained slides to quantify the extent of vessel maturation.

The results of implantation studies in terms of scaffold vascularization were conclusive, revealing that the sequential delivery of the three angiogenic factors is optimal for inducing mature blood vessels. The vascularization pattern and the vessel shape and structure were normal compared to when the factor was delivered at burst. For example, when bFGF was delivered at burst, the blood vessels appeared to be abnormal, showing extensive coverage by SMC after 3 months (Figure 6.7).

The tool described herein for attaining a sequential delivery of three angiogenic factors, presents a significant advancement over the systems described so far, wherein different release patterns were achieved by combining different types of devices [29], for example, by combining microencapsulation of the different factors in polyester microspheres and hydrogels. Our method is simpler, relying on the different affinities of factor binding to alginate-sulfate. The affinity-binding scaffolds can be loaded with more than two factors and the loading process is simple while maintaining maximal activity of the factors.

As already indicated in this chapter, the affinity-binding scaffold may exhibit a platform mimicking the "right" cell microenvironment and may be used as a testbed tool for investigating the growth and differentiation of stem cells. Different stem-cell–related factors, such as those promoting proliferation/self-renewal or differentiation to specific lineages, can be delivered from the scaffold and locally presented to the seeded stem cells.

Troubleshooting Table

Problem	Explanation	Potential Solutions
Alginate scaffold dissolves after wetting.	1. Low MW and G-content alginate is used for scaffold preparation.	1. Use sodium alginate with > 65% G-content and MW of 100–150 kDa.
	2. The cross-linker solution is not properly dispersed.	2. Use homogenization for distributing the cross-linking calcium ions.
	3. Solution contains chelators for calcium ions (e.g., citrate or phosphate ions).	3. Avoid using solutions with chelators of calcium ions.
During O-sulfation, the alginate-TBA solution in DMF turns black after addition of sulfuric acid.	The order of reactant addition is important.	Sulforic acid should be added to a cooled DMF prior to alginate-TBA.
Low yield of alginate-sulfate.	Anhydrous conditions are not maintained.	Use oven to dry dishes and solution prior to their use.
	Dialysis bag is not properly sealed.	Ensure sealing of dialysis bags.

6.7 Application Notes

The affinity-binding scaffold should be a useful tool in tissue engineering applications, enhancing the vascularization and integration of thick tissue-engineered cell constructs after their implantation. Promoting rapid vascularization in implanted cardiac patches for treating myocardial infarction (MI) or heart defects, for example, is one of the most challenging tasks for a tissue engineer. We recently used the affinity-binding alginate scaffolds for the controlled presentation of a mixture of prosurvival and proangiogenic factors (stromal-cell derived factor-1 (SDF-1); insulin-like growth factor-1 (IGF-1); and VEGF [30]. Cardiac cells, seeded in the affinity-binding scaffold and supplemented with the factor mixture, developed ex vivo into cardiac muscle tissues. To induce prevascularization in the cardiac patches prior to their implantation on the a-vascular scar tissue, they were first implanted on the omentum for 7 days and then were explanted and reimplanted on the scar tissue, 6 days after inducing MI in rats. The successful prevascularization of the cardiac patch on the omentum and the formation of mature vessel network enabled its structural and electrical integration into infracted myocardium. By echocardiography performed 28 days after implantation into the scar, the vascularized patch induced thicker scars, and prevented further dilatation of the chamber and ventricular dysfunction. Interestingly, similar beneficial results were obtained when the omentum-generated patch was constructed from an affinity-binding scaffold that was supplemented with only the mixture of prosurvival and angiogenic factors and without seeded cardiac cells. These results indicate that prevascularization of the cardiac patch on the omentum contributes to enhanced angiogenesis and to the preservation of remaining resident cardiac tissue at the infarct zone after MI. This has been attributed to the fact that the patches are affinity-bound and deliver angiogenic and cardioprotective factors at a controlled manner and for the time period needed to induce angiogenesis in the scar tissue [30].

6.8 Summary Points

1. We developed a macroporous alginate scaffold for stem cell culture and tissue engineering applications, capable of precisely controlling the delivery of multiple heparin-binding proteins.
2. The heparin-binding proteins are affinity-bound to the scaffold via specific interactions with alginate-sulfate, mimicking their interactions with heparin/heparan sulfate.
3. Scaffolds composed of alginate-sulfate/alginate (i.e., the affinity-binding scaffolds) release their bound proteins at a rate determined by their equilibrium-binding constants.
4. The sequential delivery of VEGF, PDGF-BB, and TGF-β1 from alginate-sulfate/alginate scaffolds induces the formation of a mature, dense blood vessel network in implanted scaffolds.
5. The simplicity of macromolecules loading into a preformed alginate-sulfate/alginate scaffold while maintaining their biological activities makes this system attractive for protein delivery.

Acknowledgments

The research was supported by grants from the Israel Science Foundation (793/04 & 1368/08). Dr. Smadar Cohen holds the Claire & Harold Oshry professor chair in biotechnology.

References

[1] Langer, R., and J. P. Vacanti, "Tissue Engineering," *Science,* Vol. 260, No. 5110, 1993, pp. 920–926.

[2] Shapiro, L., and S. Cohen, "Novel Alginate Sponges for Cell Culture and Transplantation," *Biomaterials,* Vol. 18, No. 8, 1997, pp. 583–590.

[3] Zmora, S., et al., "Tailoring the Pore Architecture in 3-D Alginate Scaffolds by Controlling the Freezing Regime During Fabrication," *Biomaterials,* Vol. 23, 2002, pp. 4087–4094.

[4] Glicklis, R., et al., "Hepatocyte Behavior Within Three-Dimensional Porous Alginate Scaffolds," *Biotechnol. Bioeng.,* Vol. 67, No. 3, 2000, pp. 344–353.

[5] Dvir-Ginzberg, M., et al., "Liver Tissue Engineering Within Alginate Scaffolds: Effects of Cell-Seeding Density on Hepatocyte Viability, Morphology, and Function," *Tissue Eng.,* Vol. 9, No. 4, 2003, pp. 757–766.

[6] Glicklis, R., et al., "Modeling Mass Transfer in Hepatocyte Spheroids Via Cell Viability, Spheroid Size, and Hepatocellular Functions," *Biotechnol. Bioeng.,* Vol. 86, No. 6, 2004, pp. 672–680.

[7] Dvir-Ginzberg, M., et al., "Ultrastructural and Functional Investigations of Adult Hepatocyte Spheroids During In Vitro Cultivation," *Tissue Eng.,* Vol. 10, No. 11–12, 2004, pp. 1806–1817.

[8] Elkayam, T., et al., "Enhancing the Drug Metabolism Activities of C3A: A Human Hepatocyte Cell Line by Tissue Engineering Within Alginate Scaffolds," *Tissue Eng.,* Vol. 12, No. 5, 2006, pp. 1357–1368.

[9] Dvir-Ginzberg, M., et al., "Induced Differentiation and Maturation of Newborn Liver Cells Into Functional Hepatic Tissue in Macroporous Alginate Scaffolds," *FASEB Journal,* Vol. 22, No. 5, 2008, pp. 1440–1449.

[10] Shvartsman, I., et al., "Perfusion Cell Seeding and Cultivation Induce the Assembly of Thick and Functional Hepatocellular Tissue-Like Construct," *Tissue Eng.,* Vol. 15, No. 4, 2009, pp. 751–760.

[11] Dar, A., et al., "Cardiac Tissue Engineering–Optimization of Cardiac Cell Seeding and Distribution in 3D Porous Alginate Scaffolds," *Biotechnol. Bioeng.,* Vol. 80, No. 3, 2002, pp. 305–312.

[12] Dvir, T., et al., "A Novel Perfusion Bioreactor Providing a Homogenous Milieu for Tissue Regeneration," *Tissue Eng.,* Vol. 12, No. 10, 2006, pp. 2843–2852.

[13] Schwarzkopf, R., et al., "Autospecies and Post-Myocardial Infarction Sera Enhance the Viability, Proliferation, and Maturation of 3D Cardiac Cell Culture," *Tissue Eng.,* Vol. 12, No. 12, 2006, pp. 3467–3475.

[14] Dvir, T., et al., "Activation of the ERK1/2 Cascade Via Pulsatile Interstitial Fluid Flow Promotes Cardiac Tissue Assembly," *Tissue Eng.,* Vol. 13, No. 9, 2007, pp. 2185–2193.

[15] Gerecht-Nir, S., et al., "Three-Dimensional Porous Alginate Scaffolds Provide a Conducive Environment for Generation of Well-Vascularized Embryoid Bodies from Human Embryonic Stem Cells," *Biotechnol Bioeng.,* Vol. 88, No. 3, 2004, pp. 313–320.

[16] Leor, J., et al., "Bioengineered Cardiac Grafts: A New Approach to Repair the Infarcted Myocardium?" *Circulation,* Vol. 102, No. 3, 2000, pp. III56–III61.

[17] Perets, A., et al., "Enhancing the Vascularization of Three-Dimensional Porous Alginate Scaffolds by Incorporating Controlled Release Basic Fibroblast Growth Factor Microspheres," *J. Biomed. Mat. Res.,* Vol. 65A, No. 4, 2003, pp. 489–497.

[18] Kedem, A., et al., "Vascular Endothelial Growth Factor-Releasing Scaffolds Enhance Vascularization and Engraftment of Hepatocytes Transplanted on Liver Lobes," *Tissue Eng.,* Vol. 11, No. 5–6, 2005, pp. 715–722.

[19] Freeman, I., et al., "The Effect of Sulfation of Alginate Hydrogels on the Specific Binding and Controlled Release of Heparin-Binding Proteins," *Biomaterials,* Vol. 29, No. 22, 2008, pp. 3260–3268.

[20] Freeman, I., and S. Cohen, "The Influence of the Sequential Delivery of Angiogenic Factors from Affinity-Binding Alginate Scaffolds on Vascularization," *Biomaterials,* Vol. 30, No. 11, 2009, pp. 2122–2131.

[21] Chen, B. L., et al., "Strategies to Suppress Aggregation of Recombinant Keratinocyte Growth Factor During Liquid Formulation Development." *J. Pharm. Sci.,* Vol. 19, No. 11, 2001, pp. 1029–1034.

[22] Casu, B., and U. Lindahl, "Structure and Biological Interactions of Heparin and Heparan Sulfate," *Adv. Carbohydr. Chem. Bioch.,* Vol. 57, 2001, pp. 159–206.

[23] Carmeliet, P., "Mechanisms of Angiogenesis and Arteriogenesis," *Nat. Med.,* Vol. 6, No. 4, 2000, pp. 389–395.

[24] Conway, E. M., et al., "Molecular Mechanisms of Blood Vessel Growth," *Cardio. Res.,* Vol. 49, No. 3, 2001, pp. 507–521.

[25] Darland, D. C., and P. A. D'Amore, "Blood Vessel Maturation: Vascular Development Comes of Age," *J. Clin. Invest.,* Vol. 103, No. 2, 1999, pp. 157–158.

[26] Yancopoulos, G. D., et al., "Vascular-Specific Growth Factors and Blood Vessel Formation," *Nature,* Vol. 407, No. 6801, 2000, pp. 242–248.

[27] Dor, Y., et al., "Making Vascular Networks in the Adult: Branching Morphogenesis Without a Roadmap," *Trends Cell. Biol.,* Vol. 13, No. 3, 2003, pp. 131–136.

[28] Bock, R., *A Handbook of Decomposition Methods in Analytical Chemistry*, Glasgow, Scotland: International Textbook Co., 1979.

[29] Chen, R.R., et al., "Spatio-Temporal VEGF and PDGF Delivery Patterns Blood Vessel Formation and Maturation," *Pharm. Res.,* Vol. 24, No. 2, 2007, pp. 258–264.

[30] Dvir, T., et al., "Pre-Vascularization of Cardiac Patch on the Omentum Improves Its Therapeutic Outcome," *PNAS*, Vol. 106, No. 35, 2009, pp. 14990–14995.

CHAPTER

7

Self-Assembly of Cell-Laden Hydrogels on the Liquid-Air Interface

Behnam Zamanian,[1,2] Nezamoddin N. Kachouie,[1,2] Mahdokht Masaeli,[1,2,3] Jason W. Nichol,[1,2] and Ali Khademhosseini[1,2]

[1]Department of Medicine, Center for Biomedical Engineering, Brigham and Women's Hospital, Harvard Medical School, Cambridge, MA, [2]Harvard–MIT Division of Health Sciences and Technology, Massachusetts Institute of Technology, Cambridge, MA, [3]Department of Electrical and Computer Engineering, Northeastern University, Boston, MA, corresponding author: Ali Khademhosseini, address: Partners Research Building, Room 252, 65 Landsdowne Street, Cambridge, MA 02139, e-mail: alik@mit.edu, Phone: (617) 768-8395, Fax: (617) 768-8477

Abstract

The microarchitecture surrounding cells can have a substantial impact on cell function. Therefore in designing complex engineered tissues, improved control of the cellular microarchitecture can greatly improve the function of engineered tissues. The proposed procedure describes a bottom-up approach for fabrication of three-dimensional (3D) tissue constructs with the capability to better control the cellular microarchitecture. This platform can be used to fabricate 3D tissues through self-assembly of cell-laden hydrogels with tunable microarchitectural features. The fabrication process is controlled by the surface tension forces at the liquid-air interface. As a result, cell-laden hydrogels with a broad range of different sizes, shapes, and cell densities can be used to construct macroscale engineered tissues with specific microarchitectures in a rapid, high-throughput approach.

Key terms
bottom-up approach
controllable microenvironment
hydrogel
self-assembly
tissue engineering

7.1 Introduction

Tissue engineering is a promising way to address the limited supply of donor tissue. Many of the current approaches to engineer tissues are based on seeding cells on 3D scaffolds [1, 2]. However, some of the major disadvantages of this top-down approach are a lack of control of microarchitectural features, poor spatial control over cell seeding, and the inability to direct cell coculture seeding and function [3]. An alternative approach, the bottom-up technique, focuses on designing building blocks with specific microarchitectural features and assembling these blocks into macroscale engineered tissues [3]. While the major advantages of this technique are better control of cell seeding, and microarchitecture than with top-down approaches, one of the major challenges is in creating assembly techniques to make engineered tissues with clinically relevant length scales and mechanical properties.

The cellular microenvironment, such as soluble factors, extracellular matrix (ECM), and cell-cell interactions can control cell behavior in vivo; therefore, improved control over these interactions can better direct the development and function of engineered tissues [4]. Microfabrication technologies have been applied to tissue engineering to mimic the complex in vivo spatiotemporal microenvironment leading to engineered tissues with biomimetic properties and microarchitectures [5]. The bottom-up approach mimics natural tissue structures, such as in the liver, in which repeating functional units arranged in an organized manner [6]. Cell-laden hydrogels are well suited for this process as their biological, physical, and chemical characteristics are similar to many of the tissues of interest [7–11].

For the proposed assembly process, we assemble engineered tissues through control of hydrophilic/hydrophobic interactions of cell-laden hydrogels. First, a biodegradable hydrogel prepolymer is mixed with a photoinitiator. Cell viability of the system can be optimized by the type and the concentration of the photoinitiator [12]. UV light is then passed through a photomask to cross-link the prepolymers and to construct cell-laden building blocks with specific microarchitectures. The UV light passes only through the desired pattern, causing only those regions to polymerize. The building blocks are randomly placed on a hydrophobic surface and are attracted to and move towards each other due to the surface tension on the liquid-air interface [13, 14]. The blocks continue to move towards each other, creating aggregates, the mechanics of which can be directed to some extent by control of external factors, such as the solution and polymer characteristics and agitation [15]. A stir plate or rotary shaker can be used, for example, to improve the movement of the building blocks toward the center of the container directing aggregation. To minimize the surface free energy, the constructed self-assembled cell-laden scaffold remains aggregated on the surface of hydrophobic component [14, 16]. The scaffold is eventually harvested by exposing the system to the UV light for a short time period to polymerize the blocks into one large scale unit.

This method can be used to fabricate cell-laden scaffolds for engineering complex tissues within a range of micro- to mesoscale [13]. Using these techniques it is possible to create engineered tissues on a clinically relevant length scale with precise control over the microarchitecture of the building blocks. In general, it is possible to create centimeter scale tissues with microscale resolution. In addition, this system provides significant chemical (mixing specific growth factors within building blocks) [17, 18], biological (encapsulating specific cell types within the pre-polymer) and geometrical (using photo masks with different patterns) control on the final product.

7.2 Experimental Design

This procedure is proposed for direct fabrication of self-assembled engineered tissue constructs of clinically relevant length scales with control over the microarchitectural features. In this method cells are encapsulated in hydrophilic, biodegradable polyethylene glycol diacrylate (PEG) hydrogels. These hydrophilic PEG building blocks are randomly placed on the surface of a high-density hydrophobic solution (CCl_4) where they will migrate towards each other by surface tension forces to construct an aggregated scaffold. Aggregation of various building blocks leads to the construction of tissue constructs through a secondary UV cross-linking step (Figure 7.1). This method can be performed with minimal necessary expertise or expensive customized equipment. In addition, as the hydrophobic-hydrophilic interface plays a critical role in this process, any material with these characteristics is applicable for this process. For instance, perfluorodecalin could be used in place of CCl_4 or methacrylated hyaluronic acid could replace PEG for cell encapsulation. Preliminary experiments in our lab have shown these to be viable alternatives, and there are likely many other solutions and polymers that would work in this system.

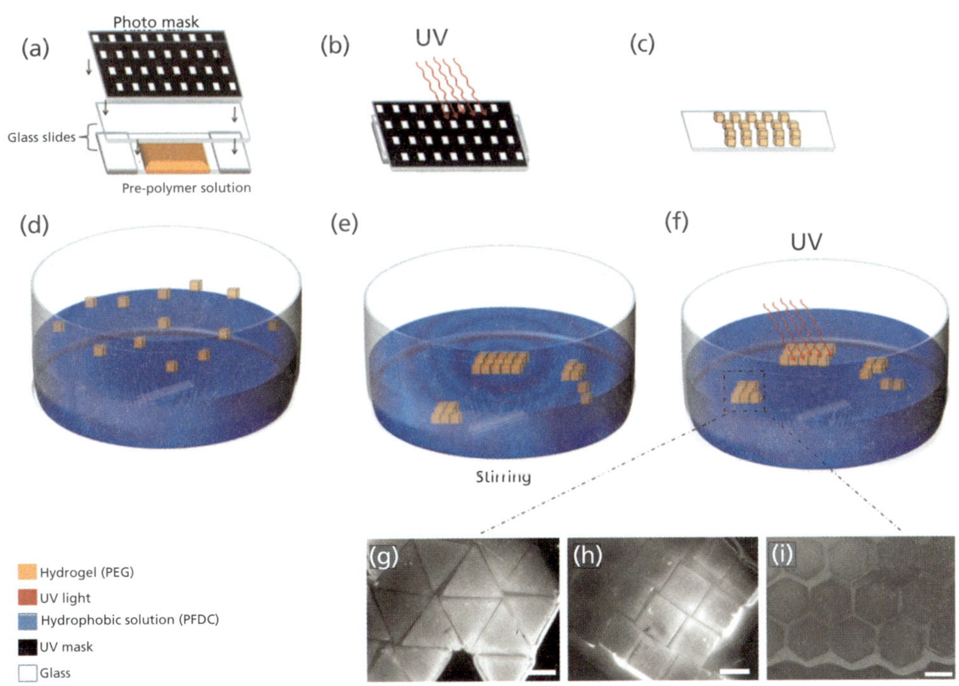

Figure 7.1 Schematic illustration of proposed self-assembly technique. (a) PEG solution containing cells was placed on top of the OTS treated glass slide between the mask and spacers. (b) UV light exposed through the mask, which gel the PEG-cell solution. (c) The PEG-cell mixture is gelled on top of OTS treated glass. (d) The hydrogel units are randomly placed on the surface of carbon tetrachloride (CCl_4). (e) Stirring the solution produced a centripetal force to mimic the scaffold. (f) Aggregates form because of the tendency to reduce the surface free energy of the hydrogel particles. (g–i) Pictures of fabricated hydrogels through the presented methods. Scale bar: 1 mm.

7.3 Materials

- Ethanol (Fisher Scientific)
- Polyethylene glycol diacrylate (PEG), mw = 4,000 (Polyscience)
- Irgacure-2959 (I-2959) photoinitiator (Ciba)
- Dulbecco's phosphate-buffered saline (DPBS, GIBCO)
- Ocadecyltrichlorosilane 90%, OTS (Alrich)
- Hexane 95% (Aldrich)
- Photomask with desired design
- Microscope slide, 25 mm × 75 mm × 1 mm (Fisherbrand)
- Microcover glass, 18 mm × 18 mm (VWR)
- UV light source 365 MM source for polyethylene glycol diacrilate gel polymerization

7.4 Method

7.4.1 Preparation of 1 ml of 20% poly (ethylene glycol) diacrylate prepolymer

PEG (with molecular weights 1,000 or greater) is a hydrophilic, photopolymerizable hydrogel that has been shown to maintain cell viability in many cell encapsulation applications [19–21]. The first step is to make the prepolymer solution; in this instance we use 20% PEG, but lower percentages may be acceptable for different applications, as could other acrylated polyethelene glycol.

1. Mix 0.2g PEG powder with 0.79-ml DPBS.
2. Add 0.01g photoinitiator to the solution.
3. Use vortex to thoroughly mix the solution.
4. Leave the sample in 80°C oven for 10 to 15 minutes.
5. Remove the sample from the oven and allow sample to reach equilibrium with room temperature (25°C).

Note that the sample is UV sensitive; therefore, it is necessary to either keep the sample covered or contained in a dark glass container at all times following addition of the photoinitiator.

7.4.2 Cell preparation (NIH 3T3)

Cell encapsulation in PEG hydrogels can be performed on a wide variety of cells. In this instance we use NIH 3T3 cells; however, any number of cell types could be used. Internal protocols for removing cells from flasks may be used in place of this step.

1. Aspirate the media from cell flask.
2. Based on size of the flask add 10 ml (T-75) or 15 ml (T-175) DPBS to wash reservoir media from cells.
3. Aspirate the PBS from the flask.
4. Add 1× trypsin to the flask, using 5 ml for T-75 or 10 ml for T-175 flasks.
5. Leave the flask in 37°C incubator for 3 to 5 minutes.

6. Rotate the solution a few times in the flask to make sure all the cells are detached.
7. If the majority of cells are detached, add an equal amount of media to the inactive trypsin. Otherwise, repeat steps 5–6 until cells are detached and then proceed with this step.
8. Remove the cell suspension from flask and add to an appropriate sterile centrifuge tube.
9. Centrifuge the solution for 5 minutes to separate the cells; speed = 1,000 rpm.

7.4.3 Storage of PEG

PEG is a photosensitive solution; therefore, it is advisable to keep it in colored containers or cover all exposed surfaces with aluminum foil.

1. The prepared PEG solution should be stored at 4°C.
2. It is better to use PEG after reaching equilibrium with room temperature (25°C).

7.4.4 Mixing PEG solution with cells

The cells must be mixed in the PEG prepolymer solution prior to polymerization, all while maintaining sterility.

Within a laminar flow hood:

1. Remove media from the cell pellet container.
2. Add appropriate amount of PEG solution to the container to obtain desired cell density.
3. Rotate the PEG solution a few times gently to make sure it is well mixed.

7.4.5 Glass OTS treatment

Treating the glass slides with OTS prevents the hydrogels from attaching to the slides upon polymerization with UV, making it easier to harvest the cell-laden gels intact.

1. Wash the glass slide with ethanol two to three times.
2. Mix 0.25-ml OTS in 4.75-ml hexane, to make a 5% OTS solution.
3. Cover the surface of cleaned glass slides with a 5% OTS solution, making sure to mark to which side the treatment was applied.
4. Incubate the glass slides at room temperature for 30 minutes in a chemical hood.
5. Aspirate the 5% OTS solution from the glass slides.
6. Put the slides in an 80°C oven for 2 hours.
7. Remove the sample from the oven.
8. Wash the sample with ethanol.
9. Remove any remaining solution from the surface of the glass slides.

7.4.6 Photolithography

To cross-link the cell-laden PEG in the desired shapes, UV light is passed through a photomask. The photomask should be clear in the desired pattern to pass UV light through, and opaque everywhere else. Features as small as 100 μm can typically be reproduced with good fidelity. The photomask should be printed on a high resolution printer and designed in a CAD program—typical office printers do not often have sufficient resolution to produce these transparencies. Note that to maintain sterility, all components (slides, photomasks, and so forth) must be handled either with sterile gloves, sterilized forceps, or something similar.

Within a laminar flow hood:

1. Sterilize the OTS-treated microscope slides and cover slips by spraying with 70% ethanol and allow to dry.
2. Pipette a 35-μl PEG-cell solution on treated slide surface.
3. Adjust the desired height by stacking glass cover slips on top of the slide glass on each side of the PEG-cell solution. (Each cover slip typically has a thickness of 150 μm, but this can vary. Read manufacturers specifications carefully prior to use.)
4. Place a clean glass slide on top of the cover slips, such that the PEG-cell solution is located between the two slides and on the OTS-treated surface of both.
5. Place the desired photo mask on top of the uppermost treated slide.
6. Place entire assembly into a sterile Petri dish.
7. Sterilize the UV area with ethanol.
8. Shine the UV through the assembly in the Petri dish to polymerize the PEG cell solution.
9. Optimized conditions for UV exposure:
   - Height of 78 mm;
   - UV power of 12.5 ω/cm^2;
   - Time = 27 seconds. It is important to have some prepolymer left on each sample.
10. Return to hood.
11. Remove the Petri dish cover and then the microscope slide glass.
12. Wash away the remaining ungelled PEG-cell solution with DPBS.

7.4.7 Aggregation process

To aggregate the cell-laden particles it is necessary to add them to an appropriate volume of dense, hydrophobic solution in a sterile container in a laminar flow hood or a sealed container.

Within a laminar flow hood:

1. Adjust the height of solution in the sterile container (in this case, 3 cm).
2. The shape of the vertex created due to stirring speed is a direct function of the height of carbon tetrachloride. Therefore the suggested numbers are only applicable for a 3-cm height.
3. Place the cell-laden hydrogel blocks randomly on the surface of the carbon tetrachloride. Cover before using stir plate outside of hood.
4. Adjust the stirring speed to find the optimized speed (in our case 200 rpm). One minute should be enough time for particles to aggregate. Do not keep the particles for more than 10 minutes in the CCl_4 solution to maintain viability.
5. Turn off the stirring motion and allow the construct to become motionless.
6. Place the construct under UV light to initiate secondary cross-linking (to freeze particles in the aggregated form) for 5 seconds.
7. Return to hood.
8. Using a glass slide, remove the particles from carbon tetrachloride solution.

7.4.8 Data analysis

To quantify the particle aggregation, we introduced an *aggregation factor* (AF). The aggregation factor was calculated and normalized based on the surrounding area of the aggregated particles as: $A_f = 1 - a_r/a_s$, where A_f is the aggregation factor, a_r is the resultant surrounding area, and a_s is the surrounding area of all aggregated particles while they are detached.

7.5 Anticipated Results

Following these steps, the final product will be a 3D tissue-like construct composed of individual building blocks. However to optimize the system, it is necessary to characterize the effects of the potential cell toxins such as CCl_4 and UV exposure. To characterize these effects, cell viability was tested in a study designed to simulate each step of the procedure using the live/dead assay (Figure 7.2). Cell viability is roughly 95% in control cells mixed in the PEG prepolymer only, 87% in cells/PEG exposed to UV light for 27 seconds, 80% following a 1-minute agitation in CCl_4, and 52% following secondary UV exposure in CCl_4 for 5 seconds. As the end goal is to create engineered tissues with controlled microarchitectural features, improvement of cell viability is critical to achieving the final goal. Recently published results in our group have demonstrated excellent viability after 7 days of culture by substituting CCl_4 with perfluorodecalin [22]. Investigation into use of other dense, hydrophobic solutions with improved cell compatibility, as well as optimization of the techniques to minimize exposure to potential cell toxins, could potentially further optimize this technique.

Building blocks with any desired geometry can be fabricated in the proposed platform; however, symmetric particles are more favorable than asymmetric ones. Increasing the thickness of the building blocks increases the aggregation factor by increasing of the surface energy, but also would affect the UV exposure time, potentially affecting the viability. Moreover, increasing the number of the particles in each experiment can improve the hydrogel aggregation process. The number of the particles and the thickness of the building blocks are linearly related to the aggregation factor; however, the aggregation factor can also be optimized by the stirring speed. The relation between the speed and the aggregation factor is depicted in Figure 7.3.

7.6 Discussion and Commentary

Current approaches to fabricate 3D tissues are typically based on seeding cells on 3D scaffolds with random pore structures, leaving little control over the cellular microenvironment and structure. Cell-cell and cell-ECM interactions can direct the morphogenesis to control the cell proliferation and construct a functional tissue, making control of the microarchitecture paramount to controlling tissue morphogenesis. To control the complex spatiotemporal microenvironment and mimic the ECM, microfabrication technologies have been applied to in vitro systems to encapsulate cells in specific microarchitectural arrangements. Tissue engineering methods with the capability of controlling the microarchitecture are desired to fabricate tissue structures with controlled cell behavior. This was the main motivation to design the

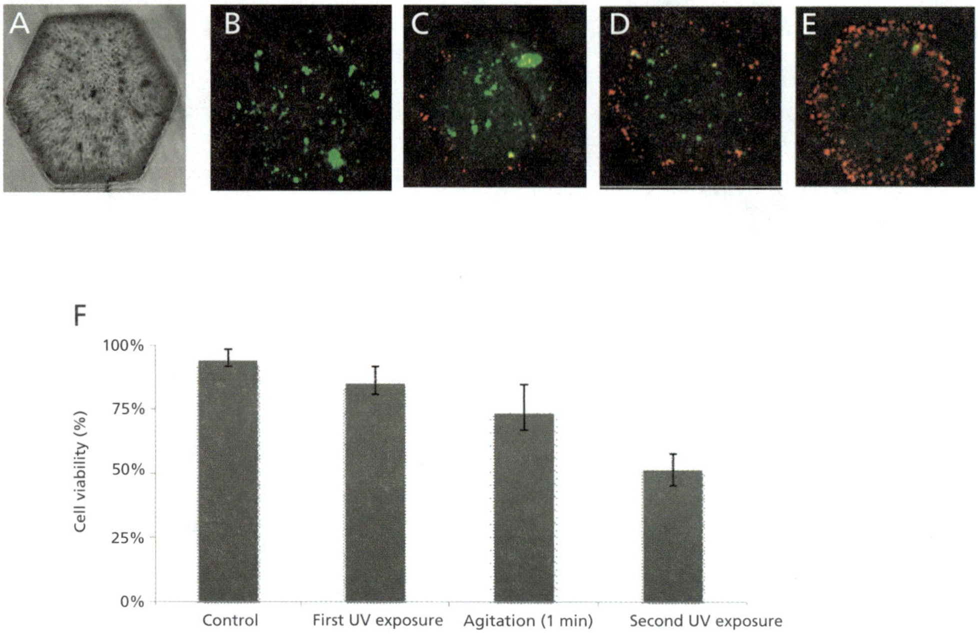

Figure 7.2 Cell viability following UV and CCl_4 exposure. (a) Phase contrast image of individual cell-laden microgel. Live/dead images of cell-laden microgels (b) prior to exposure, (c) following the first UV exposure, (d) after agitation in CCl_4, and (e) following the second UV exposure. (f) Quantification of live/dead imaging demonstrating the percentage of living cells.

proposed technique with the capability of fabrication of cell-laden tissue constructs by applying 2D self-assembly on a surface.

Employing surface tension as a driving force enables application of this method in a broad range from the nano- to the mesoscale [13]. Furthermore, control of external factors to the system, such as the centripetal forces caused by stirring, can better control the macrostructure of the final construct. The final product of this process will be a cell-laden tissue layer, composed of building blocks potentially consisting of multiple cell types and growth factors with specific microarchitectural features specific to the desired tissue type. The final shape of the fabricated layer is not fully predictable; however, in order to increase the control over the final shape of the construct, a series of system characteristics such as thickness of building blocks, PEG molecular weight, initial number of particles, and the stirring speed were optimized.

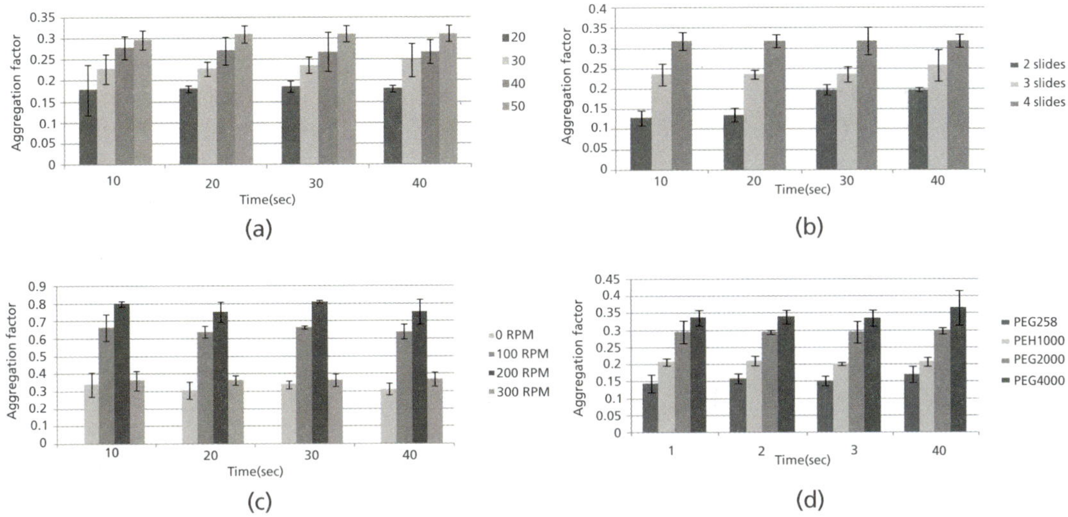

Figure 7.3 Characterization of the aggregation factor. (a) Effect of initial number of particles on aggregation factor. (b) Effect of building block thickness on aggregation factor. (c) Effect of stirring speed on aggregation factor. (d) Effect of PEG molecular weight on aggregation factor.

Troubleshooting Table

Problem	Explanation	Potential Solution
Effect of UV exposure on viability.	Excess UV is lethal for cells.	The overall UV exposure time should not be more than 30 seconds.
Poor aggregation or dissociation of aggregates.	Shape of vortex produced by stirring should be optimized.	Adjust stirring speed and/or height of CCl4.
No aggregation.	Dust may disturb the surface tension.	It is recommended to run the process under the hood.
Poor cell viability, hydrogel drying.	It is possible for the hydrogels to be dehydrate, affecting the cell viability.	It is highly recommended to manage the process such that it will be done within 10 minutes from cell capsulation to second cross-linking.

7.7 Application Notes

This chapter describes the fabrication of 3D tissue-like structures constructed by the self-assembly of cell-laden hydrogels where cell-laden blocks are aggregated by enhancing the hydrophilic-hydrophobic interactions. The proposed technique is an enabling technology to fabricate tissues with repeated building blocks [23] such as the liver, skin, and bladder [24]. This method can potentially be used for in vitro and in vivo research for tissue engineering.

7.8 Summary Points

1. We developed a self-assembly process to fabricate cell-laden tissue-like constructs, which can be applied to fabricate tissues with repeated units.

2. The self-aggregated scaffolds were optimized as a function of PEG molecular weight, thickness of building blocks, number of particles, and stirring speed.
3. The cell viability was quantified and optimized at different stages as a function of different factors, which lead to the cell death.

Acknowledgments

We thank Masoud Khabiri, Dr.Yanan Du, and Dr. Seunghwan Lee who helped us on this work. This work was supported by the National Institutes of Health (EB007249; DE019024; HL092836), the NSF CAREER award, the Institute for Soldier Nanotechnology, and the U.S. Army Corps of Engineers.

References

[1] Koh, H. K., et al., "A Statewide Public Health Approach to Improving Organ Donation: The Massachusetts Organ Donation Initiative," *American Journal of Public Health,* 2007, pp. 30–36.

[2] Langer, R., and J. Vacanti, "Tissue Engineering," *Science*, Vol. 260, No. 5110, 1993, pp. 920–926.

[3] Nichol, J. W., and A. Khademhosseini, "Modular Tissue Engineering: Engineering Biological Tissues from the Bottom Up," *Soft Matter*, Vol. 5, 2009, pp. 1312–1319.

[4] Hamilton, D., K. Wong, and D. Brunette, "Microfabricated Discontinuous-Edge Surface Topographies Influence Osteoblast Adhesion, Migration, Cytoskeletal Organization, and Proliferation and Enhance Matrix and Mineral Deposition In Vitro," *Calcified Tissue International*, Vol. 78, No. 5, 2006, pp. 314–325.

[5] Khademhosseini, A., et al., "Micromolding of Photocrosslinkable Hyaluronic Acid for Cell Encapsulation and Entrapment," *J. Biomed. Mater. Res. A*, Vol. 79, No. 3, 2006, pp. 522–532.

[6] Tsang, V. L., et al., "Fabrication of 3D Hepatic Tissues by Additive Photopatterning of Cellular Hydrogels," *FASEB. J.*, Vol. 21, No. 3, 2007, pp. 790–801.

[7] Ringel, R. L., et al., "The Application of Tissue Engineering Procedures to Repair the Larynx," *Journal of Speech, Language & Hearing Research*, 2006, pp. 194–208.

[8] Allan, S. H., "Hydrogels for Biomedical Applications," *Annals of the New York Academy of Sciences*, Vol. 944, 2001, pp. 62–73.

[9] Dong-An, W., et al., "Multifunctional Chondroitin Sulphate for Cartilage Tissue Biomaterial Integration," *Nature Materials*, 2007, pp. 385–392.

[10] Ifkovits, J. L., and J. A. Burdick, "Review: Photopolymerizable and Degradable Biomaterials for Tissue Engineering Applications," *Tissue Eng.*, Vol. 13, No. 10, 2007, p. 2369.

[11] Lee, K. Y., and D. J. Mooney, "Hydrogels for Tissue Engineering," *Chemical Reviews*, Vol. 101, No. 7, 2001, pp. 1869–1880.

[12] Fisher, J. P., et al., "Photoinitiated Polymerization of Biomaterials," *Annual Review of Materials Research*, Vol. 31, No. 1, 2001, pp. 171–181.

[13] Whitesides, G. M., and B. Grzybowski, "Self-Assembly at All Scales," *Science*, Vol. 295, No. 5564, 2002, pp. 2418–2421.

[14] Kralchevsky, P. A., et al., "Capillary Meniscus Interaction Between Colloidal Particles Attached to a Liquid-Fluid Interface," *Journal of Colloid and Interface Science*, Vol. 151, 1992, pp. 79–93.

[15] Breen, T. L., et al., "Design and Self Assembly of Open, Regular, 3D Mesostructures," *Science*, Vol. 284, 1997, pp. 848–851.

[16] Kralchevsky, P. A., et al., "Energetical and Force Approaches to the Capillary Interactions Between Particles Attached to a Liquid-Fluid Interface," *J. Colloid Interface Sci.*, Vol. 155, 1993, pp. 420–437.

[17] Peppas, N. A., et al., "Hydrogels in Pharmaceutical Formulations," *European Journal of Pharmaceutics and Biopharmaceutics*, Vol. 50, No. 1, 2000, pp. 27–46.

[18] Byrne, M. E., K. Park, and N. A. Peppas, "Molecular Imprinting Within Hydrogels," *Science*, Vol. 54, No. 1, 2002, pp. 149–161.

[19] Revzin, A., et al., "Fabrication of Poly(Ethylene Glycol) Hydrogel Microstructures Using Photolithography," *Langmuir*, Vol. 17, 2001, pp. 5440–5447.

[20] Koh, W. G., A. Revzin, and M. V. Pishko, "Poly(Ethylene Glycol) Hydrogel Microstructures Encapsulating Living Cells," *Langmuir*, Vol. 18, No. 7, 2002, pp. 2459–2462.

[21] Khademhosseini, A., et al., "Molded Polyethylene Glycol Microstructures for Capturing Cells Within Microfluidic Channels," *Lab Chip*, Vol. 4, No. 5, 2004, pp. 425–430.

[22] Zamanian, B., et al., "Interface Directed Self-Assembly of Cell-Laden Microgels into Macroscale Engineered Tissues," *Small*, 2010.

[23] Khademhosseini, A., J. P. Vacanti, and R. Langer, "Progress in Tissue Engineering," *Sci. Am.*, Vol. 300, No. 5, 2009, pp. 64–71.

[24] Costanzo, L., *Physiology,* 3rd ed., Philadelphia, PA: Saunders, 2006.

CHAPTER

8

3D Encapsulation of Cells in Hydrogels Using Radical and Addition Cross-Linking

Sudhir Khetan, Vyas Ramanan, and Jason A. Burdick

Department of Bioengineering, University of Pennsylvania, Philadelphia, PA, Corresponding author: Jason A. Burdick, address: Department of Bioengineering, University of Pennsylvania, 240 Skirkanich Hall, 210 South 33rd Street, Philadelphia, PA 19104, e-mail: burdick2@seas.upenn.edu

Abstract

We present protocols for the encapsulation of cells in hydrogels using addition (through chemical cross-linkers), radical (through photoinitiation), and sequential (incorporating both techniques) cross-linking mechanisms. These techniques are most useful for tissue engineering applications with a wide range of polymers. Depending on the cross-linking mode and polymer chemistry, cell behavior can be controlled, including cellular morphology and interactions with other cells. Here, we outline the protocol for each gelation technique, as well as methods for characterization of acellular gel properties and encapsulated cell behavior. We also describe techniques by which gels can be spatially patterned (properties or chemistry), and methods to assess pattern fidelity.

Key terms biomaterial
encapsulation
hydrogel
tissue engineering

8.1 Introduction

Recent biomaterials research has demonstrated a dynamic interplay of elements of the microenvironment (e.g., substrate mechanics [1, 2] and adhesivity [3]) on cellular outcomes such as differentiation and matrix production. Much of this work has been performed on two dimensional (2D) substrates, which poorly reflects the three-dimensional (3D) tissue environment that is found in vivo. The 3D nature of tissues has motivated the development of biomaterials such as hydrogels (i.e., water swollen, cross-linked polymers) that can form 3D structures in the presence of cells for tissue regeneration applications. A schematic of the design of such networks is shown in Figure 8.1. A polymer functionalized with reactive groups can be cross-linked into a network through either an addition, free radical (as discussed here, by photo-initiation), or as recently demonstrated, a novel sequential cross-linking [4] mechanism. Biodegradable hydrogels are widely used in tissue engineering applications for a range of tissues due to their high water content, tissue-like properties, ability to uniformly encapsulate cells, and versatility in polymer chemistry [5–7].

Although not necessary, addition cross-linking typically imparts some bioactive functionality to the hydrogel; a common example in recent work is covalent tethering of cell-adhesive (pendant) and proteolytically degradable (cross-linking) peptides to functionalized polymers for synthesis of networks that permit encapsulated cell spreading and remodeling [8, 9]. The addition mechanism may be performed as long as

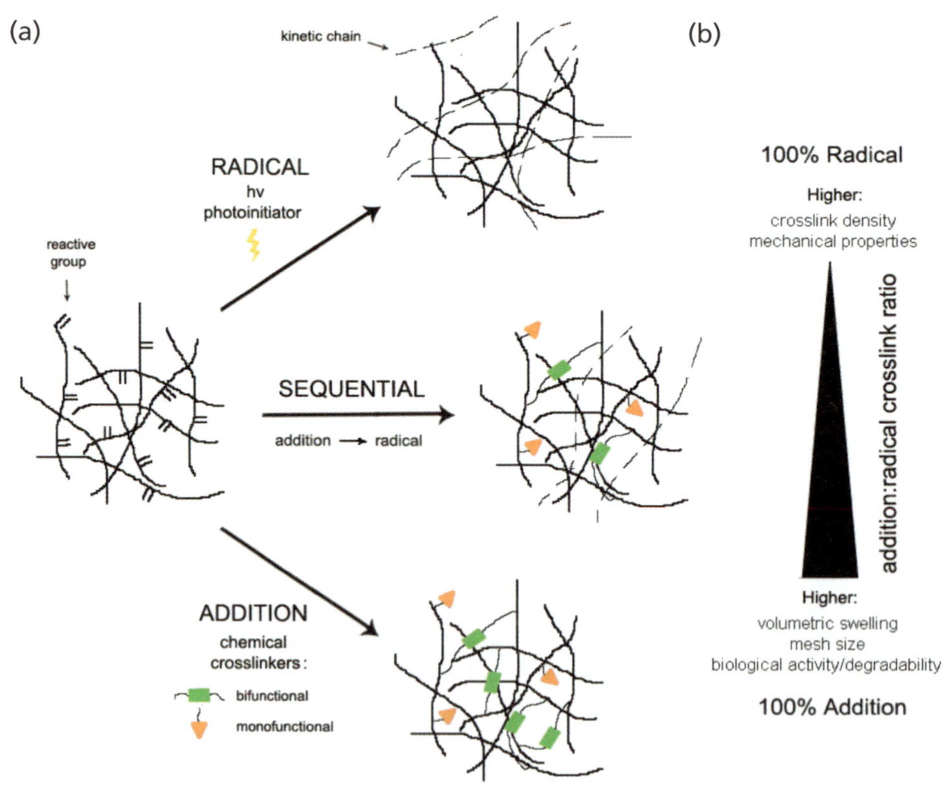

Figure 8.1 (a) Schematic of radical, addition, and sequential cross-linking (addition then radical). (b) Trends in properties of hydrogels versus cross-link type ratio in sequentially cross-linked hydrogels.

gelation occurs in sufficiently short timescales to ensure uniform cell distributions (< 20 minutes). Most commonly, polymers functionalized with reactive groups (e.g., acrylate or vinyl sulfone groups) at high functionality (i.e., at least 2 per macromer unit) are covalently reacted with thiol-containing cross-linkers [8, 10]. Radical cross-linking, which requires relatively short exposure times for network formation (typically < 10 minutes), is a well established paradigm for cell encapsulation toward tissue regeneration [11–15]. As long as parameters (initiator type and concentration, light intensity) are selected appropriately, viable cells are readily encapsulated with this approach.

Cellular encapsulation in radical or addition polymerized hydrogels are now well-established techniques that have been explored for numerous tissue engineering applications. Photopolymerized hydrogels have been synthesized from functionalized derivatives of natural or synthetic polymers including chondroitin sulfate (CS) [15, 16], hyaluronic acid (HA) [12, 17, 18], fibrinogen [19], phosphoesters [20], and poly(ethylene glycol) (PEG) [21, 22]. Addition cross-linked gels, often employing covalent reactivity between vinyl groups and thiols as described earlier, have been formed using polymers including HA [23, 24], PEG [8, 25], and synthetic extracellular matrix (ECM) analogs [26]. In general, cell-encapsulated hydrogels developed for any given regenerative target are designed by parameters including the choice of polymer, cross-linking method, and cell type to give optimal biochemical, mechanical, and degradation properties to induce an encapsulated cellular response to best guide the cells to the desired phenotype. Biodegradation of each type of hydrogel occurs via enzymatic (through enzyme secretion by encapsulated cells or addition of exogenous enzyme in culture) and/or hydrolytic cleavage of covalent bonds located on the polymer backbone or in the cross links. By varying parameters such as those listed above and others including polymer modification, cell density, and macromer concentration, the rate of biodegradation of the network is ideally tuned to match ECM deposition and tissue formation.

Sequential cross-linking incorporating both addition and radical mechanisms can be performed with any functionalized polymer capable of undergoing both mechanisms. In this approach, the fraction of total available reactive groups consumed by the primary addition step can be varied and is followed by secondary free radical cross-linking to consume remaining unreacted groups. The range of cross-linking compositions available, from 100% radical to 100% addition, corresponds to a range of properties and encapsulated cell behavior achievable in single hydrogels [4, 27] [Figure 1(b)]. The differences in the properties shown is due largely to differences in cross-link density between the addition and radical mechanisms, as discussed in further detail in Section 1.5. Additionally, if a photoinitiated system is used for the secondary free radical cross-linking, hydrogels can be spatially patterned via the simple application of a photomask to the gel between the addition and radical cross-linking steps. This technique is motivated by its potential to induce regionally distinct properties or cell behavior in single hydrogels. While the patterning of cell adhesion and phenotype has been well established in 2D models [28, 29], little work has been done assessing differences in cellular phenotype in patterned regions of 3D networks.

8.2 Experimental Design

The encapsulation protocols described below have been refined to maximize cytocompatibility through the use of simple hydrogel processing steps, and do not require any custom-built equipment. The process also allows for the synthesis of a large number of gels with relatively small batches of material (to conserve reagents) relative to other scaffold production techniques. In the following protocols, polymers containing multiple acrylates and thiol-containing peptides (either a pendant monocysteine or cross-linking bicysteine peptide) are used as representative network precursors. For instance, the cell adhesive pendant peptide GCGYGRGDSPG and proteolytically labile cross-linking peptide GCRDGPQG↓IWGQDRCG (arrow indicates site of matrix metalloprotease degradation) have been used in numerous studies [4, 8, 23]. It should also be noted, however, that any dithiol can be substituted as the cross-linker; dithiothreitol is a commonly used example. It is important to note that this model is not appropriate for all systems; for example, terminally functionalized linear polymers such as poly(ethylene glycol) diacrylate (PEGDA) require multifunctional cross-linkers for network formation via an addition mechanism. In general, the procedures given can be applied to a range of polymer systems that exhibit the appropriate functionality and reactivity. An illustrated schematic of the experimental protocol is shown in Figure 8.2.

8.3 Materials

The following materials are required for cell encapsulation and hydrogel fabrication, live/dead staining, and fixation of hydrogels for histological staining. Materials required for all other gel or encapsulated cell assessment techniques can be found in the references for each technique in Sections 8.4.4 and 8.4.5.

- 1-mL disposable syringes (BD Biosciences)
- 10-mL disposable syringes (BD Biosciences)
- 0.22-μm pore size nylon syringe filters (Fisher)
- Round glass cover slips (12-mm or 15-mm diameter, Bellco Glass)
- Fine tweezers or forceps

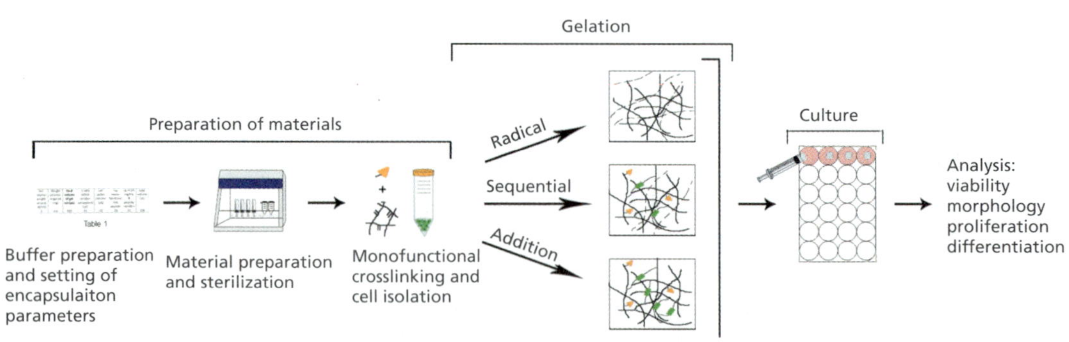

Figure 8.2 Flow diagram illustrating the steps for fabrication of a cell-encapsulated hydrogel. The labeled steps correspond directly to headings in Section 8.4.

- Wide orifice 200-μL pipette tips (Sigma)
- Triethanolamine (TEOA, Sigma)
- Phosphate-buffered saline (PBS, Invitrogen)
- Dimethyl sulfoxide (DMSO, Sigma)
- Irgacure 2959 (I2959) photoinitiator (Ciba)
- Light sources: 365-nm UV source for hydrogel polymerization (preferably equipped with a collimating lens for photopatterned gels; e.g., EXFO light guide system), and 254-nm germicidal source for sterilization (typical to any laminar flow cell culture hood)
- Functionalized polymer (e.g., acrylated HA, 4-arm PEG vinyl sulfone)
- Addition mechanism reagents (e.g., pendant monothiol or cross-linker dithiol peptides)
- Photomasks, printed on transparency film and with dimensions matching the hydrogel mold (4.5-mm diameter circles for the syringe tip molds described in the protocols below)
- Methacryloxyethyl thiocarbamoyl rhodamine B (MeRho, Polysciences)
- Cellular live/dead staining kit (Molecular Probes)
- Inverted microscope equipped with an epifluorescent lamp
- Bovine serum albumin (BSA, Sigma)
- Tween 20 (Tween, Sigma)
- Triton X-100 (Triton, Sigma)
- Formaldehyde (Sigma)

8.4 Methods

8.4.1 Preparation of materials

8.4.1.1 Preparation of buffers and stock solutions

1. A 0.5% w/v solution of I2959 photoinitiator dissolved in PBS (takes several days to dissolve) can be sterilized by syringe filtration, and stored long-term. A final concentration of 0.05 wt% I2959 (the stock solution is diluted ten-fold in the gelation) has been shown to provide optimum cytocompatibility [30, 31].
2. Addition and sequential cross-linking between peptide thiol and polymer vinyl groups is performed in a 0.3N TEOA-buffered saline. Prepare a solution of 0.2M TEOA in DI H_2O, adjust to pH 8.0 using 1N HCl, adjust to 0.3N via addition of NaCl, and sterilize by syringe filtration. Radical alone gels can be synthesized in sterile PBS.

8.4.1.2 Setting encapsulation parameters

It is suggested that addition and sequential gels be synthesized in sets of four or fewer for reasons given in the following protocols. The formulation for each gel set, an example of which is shown in Table 8.1 for four sequentially cross-linked 50-μL volume gels, can be easily created using a spreadsheet program:

Table 8.1 Example of Hydrogel Formulation Table

Gel Polymer Weight Percent (wt%)	Weight Polymer Required (mg)	Total Volume of Gel Set (mL)	0.5 wt% I2959 Solution Component (mL)	Cell Pellet Volume (mL)	mg Mono-functional (M) Peptide	mL of 20 mg/mL M Peptide Solution	mg Bifunctional (B) Peptide	mL of 60 mg/mL B Peptide Solution	Supplementary Volume (mL)
3	6.6	220	22	10	0.20	10	3	50	128

The mass of polymer can be calculated from the desired macromer concentration and total volume (it is suggested that extra precursor solution be prepared to account for some loss during transfer). For addition and sequential polymerizations, the mass of peptides required should then be calculated, based on a desired concentration in the gel. Finally, the remaining volume (used to dissolve the polymer), is calculated by subtracting the volume of each peptide solution, initiator solution, and cell pellets from the total volume. Depending on the objective of the specific experimental study, cells plated in 2D on tissue culture plastic, 100% radical, and 100% addition cross-linked hydrogels can each serve as control conditions.

8.4.1.3 Preparation and sterilization of materials

1. Place all materials in the biological safety cabinet for sterilization:
   - 1-mL syringes, with tips cut off using a 70% ethanol rinsed razor blade, and plunger adjusted to the desired gel volume (e.g., 50 μL). For radical encapsulations, syringes should be cut at a consistent height to prevent variability in the light intensity reaching the gel. For photopatterned gels, the molds should be cut as flat as possible to ensure uniform penetration of light through the mask and gel.
   - Eppendorf tubes (with tops open) containing polymer and peptides.
   - Round 12-mm or 15-mm cover slips (for sequential cross-linking).
   - Fine tweezers (for sequential cross-linking).
   - Transparency film photomasks (for patterned sequential cross-linking).
2. Sterilize materials with 254-nm germicidal light for 30 minutes.

8.4.2 Initiation of pendant addition reactions and preparation of cells for encapsulation

8.4.2.1 Initiation of pendant (e.g., adhesion site) reaction

1. Following sterilization, prepare solutions of the polymer (by adding the remaining volume of PBS for radically cross-linked gels or TEOA buffer for addition or sequentially cross-linked gels) and monofunctional peptide (by adding the volume of TEOA buffer required to achieve the prescribed concentration). Vortex to dissolve.
2. Add the required volume of the pendant peptide solution to the polymer solution, vortex to mix, and place in a 37°C incubator to react (if possible on a rotary stir plate). The required reaction time is typically < 20 minutes for appropriate choices of polymer and peptide functionalities (e.g., acrylates and thiols, as discussed briefly in Section 8.1.1).

8.4.2.2 Preparation of cells

1. While the pendant addition reaction is incubating, trypsinize and count cells. Based on each gel set volume and desired cell density, cells should be separated into

portions and centrifuged (e.g., 2.2 million cells should be centrifuged for a density of 10 million cells/mL in the example set). The choice of initial seeding density is balanced by biomimetic and practical considerations; while it is best to replicate the density found in vivo in the developing tissue of interest as closely as possible, certain quantitative characterization techniques such as PCR require significantly greater cell numbers than qualitative techniques such as staining.

8.4.3 Synthesis of hydrogels

The procedure(s) in the following sections should be repeated for each sample set following the centrifugation of cells.

8.4.3.1 Synthesis of radically cross-linked hydrogels

1. Add the photoinitiator component (10% v/v of 0.5% I2959/PBS, sterile) to the polymer solution and vortex to mix.
2. Resuspend the cell pellet in the polymer solution until the cells are well dispersed and aliquot into molds at the desired gel volume. This should be done rapidly to prevent settling of cells after aliquoting and before UV light exposure.
3. Expose the gels to UV light (typically, ~4 mW/cm^2 for 5–10 minutes) for network formation.
4. Following exposure, each gel can be plunged into a culture plate well containing the appropriate media.

8.4.3.2 Synthesis of addition or sequentially cross-linked hydrogels

1. If performing sequential cross-linking, add the photoinitiator component (10% v/v of 0.5% I2959/PBS, sterile) to the polymer solution and resuspend to mix.
2. Resuspend cell pellet in polymer solution until cells are well dispersed.
3. Using a wide orifice pipette tip, add the bifunctional cross-linker solution component of the gel to the cell-containing prepolymer solution, adjust the pipette volume to the desired gel volume, and aliquot into the sterile syringe tip molds. This step should be performed quickly, as the addition of the bifunctional cross-linker will initiate cross-linking and may rapidly increase the solution viscosity.
4. For sequential cross-linking, a sterile round cover slip should be placed on top of the syringe mold using tweezers immediately after aliquoting such that flush contact is made between each cover slip and gel. This step prevents oxygen exposure during radical cross-linking and ensures dual cross-linking throughout the entire hydrogel volume. For patterned sequential cross-linking, a photomask is substituted for the cover slip. (Note that there typically is some loss of UV light intensity through cover slips and transparency films; for UV sources with adjustable intensity, a radiometer can be used to determine the compensatory intensity increase needed to ensure the desired intensity reaches the gel.)
5. Allow the cross-linking to continue for 10–20 minutes (the optimal length of addition cross-linking for a given system can be determined using mechanical or chemical characterization as described later).

6. For sequential cross-linking, following incubation for addition cross-linking, expose the gels to UV light using the optimized parameters from radiometer calibration.

8.4.4 Characterization of hydrogels

The following techniques can be used to optimize gelation parameters (e.g., the intensity and length of exposure to UV light or length of addition cross-linking).

8.4.4.1 Mechanical properties (elastic modulus)

The elastic modulus of hydrogels is most typically measured via either compression (Young's modulus) or rheology (shear modulus), potentially depending upon what force the therapeutic target experiences in vivo. The elastic modulus of a gel is proportional to cross-link density, which correlates predictably with important hydrogel properties such as volumetric swelling ratio and swollen mesh size. The following methods can be used to assess the mechanical properties of hydrogels.

1. *Atomic force microscopy (AFM) (Young's modulus):* AFM measures the elasticity of a material by quantifying deflection of a cantilever tip that indents a very small portion of the gel at the surface [32, 33]. As such, it is a useful technique for measuring the elasticity of different regions of patterned gels. Since the technique deflects the gel-only microns in the z-direction, gel thickness effects are almost universally negligible for hydrogels synthesized using the protocols presented here.
2. *Parallel-plate compression testing (Young' modulus):* In typical compression testing of hydrogels, continuous stress or strain is applied to the gel, and the Young's modulus is calculated as the slope of the linear (elastic) region of the stress-strain curve (typically < 20% strain) [34, 35]. Creep stress and relaxation experiments have also been used to determine the equilibrium-confined compression aggregate modulus of hydrogels [36, 37].
3. *Parallel-plate rheology (shear modulus):* The shear modulus of hydrogels can be measured by oscillatory rheology using a frequency sweep and real-time measurements of the storage (elastic) and loss (viscous) moduli of the material, either during gelation (i.e., the hydrogel is formed directly on the instrument for optimal adhesion to the plates) or after swelling to the equilibrium [38, 39]. In the latter case, the elastic modulus should be constant across the frequency sweep; these values can be averaged to determine the modulus. In the former case, the gel point is determined when the storage modulus and loss modulus meet, and the elastic modulus can be read after its curve plateaus upon complete gelation.

8.4.4.2 Acellular validation of patterning

The following technique can be used to assess the resolution of the radical cross-linking pattern in acellular sequentially cross-linked hydrogels.

1. In setting encapsulation parameters (as shown in Table 8.1), add 5 μL of 0.2 mg/mL solution of methacryloxyethyl thiocarbamoyl rhodamine B (MeRho) in DMSO to give a final concentration of ~5 μM in the prepolymer solution.

2. Add the MeRho solution component to the prepolymer solution at the same time as the photoinitiator component (i.e., immediately prior to the addition of the bifunctional cross-linker).
3. Follow the remainder of the gelation protocol as described in Section 8.1.4.3. During the secondary cross-linking, MeRho binds to the hydrogel polymer only in UV-exposed regions (since the methacrylate group reacts very slowly during addition step, but rapidly during radical polymerization).
4. Wash hydrogels in PBS overnight, with additional washes the following day prior to imaging (next step). Thorough washing will allow unreacted MeRho to diffuse out of the gel.
5. Image the hydrogel using an epifluorescent microscope and TRITC (red) filter. Due to MeRho preferential binding to UV-exposed regions, unmasked regions of hydrogel will fluoresce brightly compared to mask-covered regions (Figure 8.3).
6. Draw lines across equivalent sections of mask and hydrogel pattern images using ImageJ (NIH) software, and record fluorescence intensity data for these lines. It is preferable to gather data from multiple crossimage lines for this step.
7. Set threshold values to define at what fluorescence level features begin and end, and calculate pixel width of features using this threshold value; width of mask features and gel features can be compared to determine pattern fidelity.

8.4.5 Characterization of cellular behavior in gels

Manufacturer's protocols included with assays for cell behavior are typically optimized for 2D culture. For effective translation to 3D, the methods typically require longer incubation times and/or increased reagent concentrations. For each following technique, references are provided in which the assay or stain being described was optimized for a 3D hydrogel system.

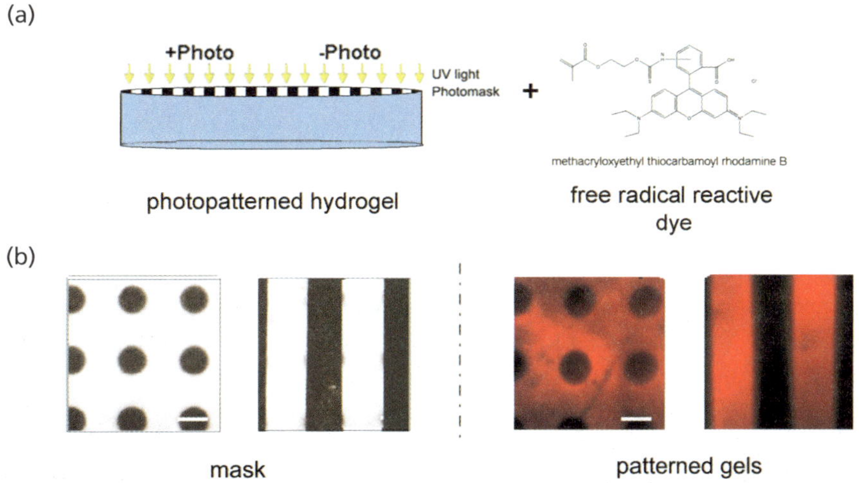

Figure 8.3 (a) Schematic for fluorescent imaging of hydrogel pattern. The fluorescent dye preferentially reacts into the network under transparent regions of the photomask. (b) Left: images of two different photomasks with hole and line features. Right: fluorescent images of hydrogels photopolymerized under masks at left. Scale bars = 100 μm.

8.4.5.1 Assessment of viability and proliferation

Qualitative assessment of cell viability is most easily performed using a commercially available live/dead staining kit (Figure 8.4). Gels are typically washed with PBS and incubated in the live/dead reagent solution. Though the exact mechanism and dye color can vary, the live probe typically emits fluorescence after cleavage by active esterases in live cells (e.g., Calcein-AM is converted to calcein, which fluoresces green after metabolism), while the dead probe enters through compromised regions of the cell membrane and fluoresces upon intercalation with DNA (e.g., ethidium homodimer). Gels are then washed again to remove excess dye and imaged with an epifluorescent microscope. An advantage of this approach is that it also provides an easy method for qualitatively assessing cell morphology.

Typically, cell viability assays do not measure viability directly, but instead measure proxies such as total metabolic activity or nucleic acid content. The PicoGreen assay measures total DNA content in the hydrogel. Assays measuring total metabolic activity in gels include the [3-(4,5-dimethylthiazol-2-yl)-2,5-diphenyl tetrazolium bromide] (MTT) or Alamar Blue assays. Assessment of viability using such techniques, however, is problematic because they are absolute and thus cannot distinguish between the contribution of cell viability and proliferation. Also, it is important to note that unencapsulated cells from the initial population may settle to the bottom of the culture well, adhere and proliferate, and confound gel viability studies. Thus, gels should be transferred to a fresh plate immediately before assays are performed. Also, it may be necessary to use a tissue grinder to better access all soluble dye components in the gels to obtain an accurate reading.

8.4.5.2 Visualization of cells in hydrogels using confocal microscopy

1. Fix gels by following or optimizing the protocol below, which has been developed in our lab for equilibrium swollen 3D hydrogels. Alternate fixation protocols are also available in [40–43].
   (a) Rinse constructs three times for 5 minutes with PBS.
   (b) Fix gels with incubation in 1 mL 4% formaldehyde for 30 minutes at room temperature.
   (c) Rinse constructs three times for 5 minutes with blocking solution containing 3% (w/v) BSA and 0.5% (w/v) Tween in PBS.

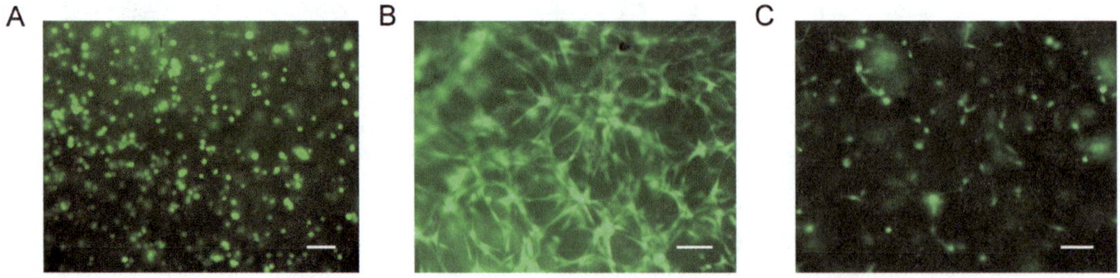

Figure 8.4 Images of calcein-stained human mesenchymal stem cells (hMSCs) encapsulated in hyaluronic acid based networks that were cross-linked (a)using a radical addition, (b) using cell adhesive and degradable oligopeptides, and (c) using a sequential (1:1 addition:radical) mechanism, respectively. Scale bar = 100 μm; all cultures were for 5 days.

(d) Permeabilize membrane with 0.25% (w/v) Triton X in blocking solution (for immunostaining, animal serum is also commonly added at this point to block nonspecific interactions).
(e) Rinse constructs three times with the blocking solution.
(f) Incubate in solution with staining reagent.

2. Following the generalized fixation protocol given above, the staining of hydrogels is accomplished by incubation with a reagent exhibiting affinity for the target of interest, either via direct binding or immunostaining. Common targets of staining for basic cellular visualization include but are not limited to (typical parameters for each technique are given in the subbullet):
   (a) Actin, via incubation in a solution of fluorescent phalloidin [40, 41]: 2 hours incubation in 0.66 μg/mL FITC-phalloidin in blocking solution.
   (b) Focal adhesions by immunostaining against vinculin [42, 43]. Vinculin: 10% (v/v) goat serum should be added during the permeabilization step—1 hour incubation in mouse monoclonal antivinculin IgG (diluted 1:250) in blocking solution, followed by 1 hour incubation in TRITC-conjugated donkey antimouse IgG.
   (c) Nuclei, via incubation in a solution of 4′,6-diamidino-2-phenylindole (DAPI) [41]—20 minutes in 0.4 μL/mL DAPI in PBS.
3. Following extensive final washing with PBS, gels can be imaged using either conventional microscopy with epifluorescence or confocal microscopy (most commonly confocal laser scanning microscopy, CLSM). This technique is especially useful for assessment of cellular migration and morphology due to its high resolution in the z-direction relative to conventional microscopy. Time-lapse photography can be used in conjunction with either bright field or confocal microscopy to provide high-resolution movies of temporal and spatial cell behavior [8, 44].

8.4.5.3 Quantitative assessment of cellular differentiation

Real-time PCR (RT-PCR) is a sensitive and accurate method for determining the gene expression of encapsulated cells. Because most reverse transcriptase protocols require 1 μg of RNA per sample, the initial seeding density of the hydrogels is important and often must be fairly high to ensure adequate RNA extraction for RT-PCR (e.g., 10 million cells/mL for 50-μL hydrogels). This minimum seeding density is influenced by numerous factors that affect total RNA per sample, including the hydrogel volume, type and batch of cells used, and type of media. Hydrogel culture is followed by RNA extraction, reverse transcriptase (RT), and RT-PCR. A protocol for RNA extraction, which primarily uses common laboratory reagents, has been optimized in our lab and is given below. A similar protocol is given here [45]. Protocols for RT and RT-PCR require more specialized reagents such as enzymes and buffers, can vary for 3D systems, and often use commercially available kits with modifications. Two examples for such protocols are given here [14, 45]. Primer/probe sets for genes that express many standard differentiation markers are available as "off-the-shelf" products from Applied Biosystems, Inc., but can also be customized. Typically, relative gene expression is calculated by the delta delta Ct method [46] using a housekeeping (i.e., constitutively expressed) gene as the internal control and a nonencapsulated cell portion from the gel synthesis procedure as an external control.

RNA Extraction protocol

1. Add 500-μL TRIZOL to one eppendorf per sample.
2. Transfer hydrogels to eppendorfs using a scoopula and add an additional 500-μL TRIZOL.
3. Use a pestle (plastic, cone-tipped tissue grinders) to homogenize the hydrogels until a clear solution is obtained. Clean or use a separate pestle for each sample.
4. Vortex each eppendorf for an additional 20 seconds to further homogenize the samples.
5. Incubate samples at room temperature for 5 minutes to permit complete dissociation of nucleoprotein complexes. Samples may be stored for at least 1 month at −70°C at this point.
6. Cool samples on ice for 20 minutes.
7. Add 200 μL (per mL TRIZOL) chloroform to samples and vortex until well mixed.
8. Incubate samples at room temperature for 5 minutes.
9. Centrifuge samples at 12,000 x g for 15 minutes.
10. Transfer the aqueous phase (i.e., the clear top layer) to a new eppendorf (avoiding interfacial region and lower red, phenol-chloroform phase). RNA remains in the clear aqueous phase; the polymer should remain in the red phase.
11. Add 500 μL IPA (−20°C) to each sample and invert by hand until haziness from separate phases disappears.
12. Incubate at room temperature for 10 minutes; turn on and warm a water bath to 65°C.
13. Centrifuge at 4°C for 10 minutes at 12,000 x g. The RNA precipitate forms a gel-like pellet at the bottom of the tube.
14. Aspirate supernatant (leave 50–100 μL) and rinse pellet with 1 mL cold (4°C) 75% ethanol and vortex. (RNA precipitate forms a more visible white pellet and may be stored for at least 1 week at −20°C in 75% ethanol.)
15. Centrifuge at 4°C for 10 minutes at 12,000 x g. Repeat steps 14–15.
16. Aspirate supernatant using gel-loading tips and air dry for 5 minutes at room temperature (65°C).
17. Dissolve the RNA pellet in 15-μL sterile H_2O to inactivate RNases.
18. Incubate sample in 65°C water bath for 10 minutes to denature the RNA pellet.
19. Read the concentration of the RNA (in 2 μL nanodrops preferred). Typical parameter values for nanodrop reader mRNA analysis are:
    (a) 260/280 ratio → RNA quality, should be between 1.9 and 2.1.
    (b) 260/230 ratio → level of protein contamination, per Applied Biosystems should be > 2.
20. Store sample at −70°C (up to one year).

8.4.5.4 Qualitative assessment of tissue composition—histology and immunostaining

Typically, staining of hydrogels for general composition (i.e., to visualize biochemically distinct regions such as cells versus connective tissue ECM) or for tissue-specific markers (i.e., as a proxy for encapsulated stem cell differentiation) involves dehydration, paraffin embedding, and sectioning of the construct. A protocol for this process that has been optimized in our lab for hydrogels is written next; another is given here [45].

Fixation and dehydration

1. Rinse specimen three times in PBS.
2. Fix for 5–30 minutes in 4% paraformaldehyde.
3. Rinse specimen three times in PBS.
4. Incubate sample in EtOH at 25°C for 1 hour at each of the following EtOH (v/v) concentrations in water (in order): 50%, 70%, 95%, 95%, 100%.
5. At this point, samples can be stored overnight at 25°C.

Standard procedures can be used for embedding and sectioning. Sectioning can be difficult with samples that contain a lot of polymer component, particularly if there is a mismatch in properties between the polymer and embedding media. Once sectioned, histological staining or immunostaining may be performed. If sufficient tissue is not produced in the constructs, section adherence to slides may be difficult. Alternatively, cryosectioning can be used, but paraffin has been feasible for gel systems used in our lab. Some typical regenerative targets and corresponding stains are mentioned below, with referenced studies in which the stain was performed on embedded and sectioned hydrogels.

1. *Cartilage*: Glycosaminoglycan (GAG) content—safranin O [45, 46], chondroitin sulfate [12, 47], Alcian blue (sulfated GAGs) [48, 49]; type II collagen [12, 50].
2. *Bone:* Von kossa (mineralization) [20, 22, 51]; osteocalcin [23, 51]; alkaline phosphatase [52].
3. *Vasculature:* Sarcomeric action (myofibrils) [29, 53]; PECAM1 (platelet endothelial cell adhesion molecule) [54].
4. *Nonspecific:* Hematoxylin and eosin [19, 45, 50]; type I collagen [50, 55]; Masson trichrome (connective tissue) [23, 56].

8.4.5.5 Assessment of cell behavior in spatially patterned hydrogels

The assessment of cell behavior in spatially patterned hydrogels requires some adjustment from the bulk hydrogel case. For any staining or qualitative methods, the procedures are identical, and differential cell behavior in adjacent regions of patterned gels can be confirmed directly through the appropriate visualization method (e.g., confocal microscopy for actin staining). The feasibility of using quantitative methods such as metabolic activity assays or RT-PCR to assess behavior in differential regions is limited. In this case, quantification is commonly performed indirectly with staining. For example, if assessing simultaneous differentiation of multiple lineages in a patterned hydrogel, staining for differentiation markers could be performed and relative differentiation determined by counting the number of cells exhibiting each marker.

8.5 Anticipated Results

Growing evidence in biomaterials research indicates that the physical and biochemical microenvironment of the cell (e.g., mechanical properties or adhesivity) directly instructs phenotype. As such, the predictive control of these properties in cell encapsulated hydrogels is of critical importance. Some universal trends in hydrogel mechanical and structural properties can be expected as a function of the ratio of radical to addition cross-linking. Radical cross-linking alone produces spatially constricted, bioinert and nondegradable cross links, resulting in a low network mesh size and swelling ratio, high cross-link density, and greater mechanical properties relative to addition cross-linked gels. Thus, increasing the ratio of addition to radical cross-linking should linearly decrease mechanical properties and cross-link density while increasing swelling and mesh size. The anticipated behavior of encapsulated cells as a function of cross-link composition is confounded by numerous other factors and is discussed in Section 8.1.7.

8.6 Discussion and Commentary

The protocols presented here afford the design and fabrication of hydrogel scaffolds for control of encapsulated cell behavior with a high degree of tunability of the bioactive, mechanical, and degradation properties of bulk and patterned hydrogels. For studies comparing cell behavior in addition versus radical gels, a major advantage to these 3D techniques is the ability to decouple adhesion and mechanics, most easily by adjusting the macromer concentration in addition gels to match those of radical gels. A side effect of such versatility is the difficulty in choosing parameters when working with a novel functionalized polymer. In this case, we have found that a useful strategy is to perform a pilot set of gelation experiments to define an approximate range of achievable hydrogel properties (e.g., mechanical and degradation characterization of 100% addition, 100% radical, and 50%/50% addition/radical hydrogels at several different macromer concentrations). When functionalizing the polymer with reactive groups, it is suggested that batch sizes be maximized in order to maximize the amount of macromer available for use after these initial characterization studies, since there may be batch-to-batch variations.

Troubleshooting Table

Problem	Explanation	Potential Solutions
Lack of gelation in radical system	Initiation parameters not sufficient	Increase initiator concentration, light intensity, or time of polymerization.
Difficulty dissolving polymer in remaining volume	Weight percent of initial polymer solution prohibitively high	Increase peptide solution concentration to increase remaining volume
Nonuniform cell distribution in remaining volumes	Cell pellet not adequately dispersed prior to gelation	Resuspend cells using a regular pipette tip (smaller bore than a wide cut), and then switch to a wide cup tip for the addition of the cross-linker solution.
Lack of patterning fidelity throughout the hydrogel	This is caused mainly by the diffraction of light outside the vertical channels of the pattern.	Reduce hydrogel thickness by lowering total volume, optimizing radical gelation parameters (lowest exposure time/intensity needed to retain complete cross-linking and cytocompatibility) and ensure syringe is flat in the tube holder.
Difficulty in performing shear or compressive modulus testing on addition gels	Surface topography of addition gels may not be smooth.	If necessary, perform cross-linking between slides.

8.7 Application Notes

A potentially valuable application for the techniques discussed here is the controlled differentiation of encapsulated stem cells toward tissue regeneration. As discussed, many of the factors influencing differentiation including mechanical properties, adhesivity, cell shape, and proteolytic degradability are tunable in hydrogels synthesized using the versatility in this procedure. The parameters that can be varied to tune hydrogel composition begin with the backbone composition, type of functional group and modification efficiency, and concentration of the macromer in the hydrogel. The composition of mono- or bifunctional chemical cross-linkers, the ratio of addition to radical cross-linking, and spatial patterning are further design parameters that expand the library of formulations. External variables such as cell seeding density, incubation with inductive medium, and dynamic cell culture (e.g., perfusion or mechanical loading) can be added to further control differentiation.

Spatial patterning of hydrogels offers some unique and exciting potential applications. Because cells modulate their phenotype based on material cues they "see" in 3D, the different regions of patterned gels may induce a distinct lineage commitment of encapsulated stem cells, possibly enabling the engineering of tissue interfaces (e.g., osteochondral composite tissue). Acellular spatially patterned hydrogels may also be valuable for implantation and regeneration of tissues with characteristically motile or sprouting cell phenotypes that lead to macroscopically anisotropic tissue such as vasculature or nervous tissue. The premise here is that native cells would penetrate bioactive, nonradically cross-linked regions of the hydrogels and deposit ECM in the dual cross-linked regions over time.

8.8 Summary Points

1. Addition, radical, and sequential cross-linking are a robust set of techniques to vary the microenvironments and behavior of encapsulated cells.
2. Spatial patterning of hydrogels can be performed to achieve zonal differential composition and cell behavior in a single gel.
3. The gelation procedure can be separated into three steps: material preparation, preparation of cells, and hydrogel network synthesis.
4. A wide variety of qualitative and quantitative characterization methods are available to assess properties of hydrogels and behavior of encapsulated cells.
5. As many of the characterization techniques used are written for 2D systems, some optimization for individual 3D systems likely will be required.
6. The design variables within the protocols can be combined with external techniques such as incubation with soluble growth factors or dynamic culture to enhance the desired phenotype.

References

[1] Engler, A., et al., "Matrix Elasticity Directs Stem Cell Lineage Specification," *Cell*, Vol. 126, No. 4, 2006, pp. 677–689.

[2] Chen, C., "Mechanotransduction—A Field Pulling Together?" *J. Cell. Sci.*, Vol. 121, No. 20 2008, pp. 3285–3292.

[3] Gumbiner, B., "Cell Adhesion: The Molecular Basis of Tissue Architecture and Morphogenesis," *Cell*, Vol. 84, No. 3, 1996, pp. 345–357.

[4] Khetan, S., J. Katz, and J. Burdick, "Sequential Crosslinking to Control Cellular Spreading in 3 Dimensional Hydrogels," *Soft Matter*, Vol. 5, 2008, pp. 1601–1606.

[5] Nguyen, K., and J. West, "Photopolymerizable Hydrogels for Tissue Engineering Applications," *Biomaterials*, Vol. 23, No. 22, 2002, pp. 4307–4314.

[6] Baroli, B., "Hydrogels for Tissue Engineering and Delivery of Tissue-Inducing Substances," *J. Pharm. Sci.*, Vol. 96, No. 9, 2007, pp. 2197–2223.

[7] Nicodemus, G., and S. Bryant, "Cell Encapsulation in Biodegradable Hydrogels for Tissue Engineering Applications," *Tissue Eng.*, Vol. 14, No. 2, 2008, pp. 149–165.

[8] Lutolf, M., et al., "Cell-Responsive Synthetic Hydrogels," *Adv. Mater.*, Vol. 15, No. 11, 2003, pp. 888–892.

[9] Kim, J., et al., "Synthesis and Characterization of Matrix Metalloprotease Sensitive-Low Molecular Weight Hyaluronic Acid Based Hydrogels," *J. Mater. Sci. Mater. Med.*, Vol. 9, No. 11, 2008, pp. 3311–3318.

[10] Vanderhooft, J., B. Mann, and G. Prestwich, "Synthesis and Characterization of Novel Thiol-Reactive Poly(Ethylene Glycol) Cross-Linkers for Extracellular-Matrix-Mimetic Biomaterials," *Biomacromolecules*, Vol. 8, No. 9, 2007, pp. 2883–2889.

[11] Ifkovits, J., and J. Burdick, "Review: Photopolymerizable and Degradable Biomaterials for Tissue Engineering Applications," *Tissue Eng.*, Vol. 13, No. 10, 2007, pp. 2369–2385.

[12] Chung, C., et al., "Effects of Auricular Chondrocyte Expansion on Neocartilage Formation in Photocrosslinked Hyaluronic Acid Networks," *Tissue Eng.*, Vol. 12, No. 9, 2006, pp. 2665–2773.

[13] Benoit, D., et al., "Small Functional Groups for Controlled Differentiation of Hydrogel-Encapsulated Human Mesenchymal Stem Cells," *Nat. Mater.*, Vol. 7, No. 10, 2008, pp. 816–823.

[14] Elisseeff, J., et al., "Cellular Photoencapsulation in Hydrogels," in G. V. Novakovic and R. I. Freshney, (eds.), *Culture of Cells for Tissue Engineering*, New York: Wiley-Liss, 2006.

[15] Li, Q., et al., "Photocrosslinkable Polysaccharides Based on Chondroitin Sulfate," *J. Biomed. Mater. Res. A*, Vol. 68, No. 1, 2004, pp. 28–33.

[16] Bryant, S., J. Arthur, and K. Anseth, "Incorporation of Tissue-Specific Molecules Alters Chondrocyte Metabolism and Gene Expression in Photocrosslinked Hydrogels," *Acta. Biomater.*, Vol. 1, No. 2, 2005, pp. 243–252.

[17] Yeh, J., et al., "Micromolding of Shape-Controlled, Harvestable Cell-Laden Hydrogels," *Biomaterials*, Vol. 27, No. 31, 2006, pp. 5391–5398.

[18] Masters, K., et al., "Crosslinked Hyaluronan Scaffolds as a Biologically Active Carrier for Valvular Interstitial Cells," *Biomaterials*, Vol. 26, No. 15, 2005, pp. 2517–2525.

[19] Almany, L., and D. Seliktar, "Biosynthetic Hydrogel Scaffolds Made from Fibrinogen and Polyethylene Glycol for 3D Cell Cultures," *Biomaterials*, Vol. 26, No. 15, 2005, pp. 2467–2477.

[20] Li, Q., et al., "Biodegradable and Photocrosslinkable Polyphosphoester Hydrogel," *Biomaterials*, Vol. 27, No. 7, 2006, pp. 1027–1034.

[21] Garagorri, N., et al., "Keratocyte Behavior in Three-Dimensional Photopolymerizable Poly(Ethylene Glycol) Hydrogels," *Acta. Biomater.*, Vol. 4, No. 5, 2008, pp. 1139–1147.

[22] Burdick, J., and K. Anseth, "Photoencapsulation of Osteoblasts in Injectable RGD-Modified PEG Hydrogels for Bone Tissue Engineering," *Biomaterials*, Vol. 23, No. 22, 2002, pp. 4315–4523.

[23] Kim, J., et al., "Bone Regeneration Using Hyaluronic Acid-Based Hydrogel with Bone Morphogenic Protein-2 and Human Mesenchymal Stem Cells," *Biomaterials*, Vol. 28, No. 10, 2007, pp. 1830–1837.

[24] Flynn, L., et al., "Adipose Tissue Engineering with Naturally Derived Scaffolds and Adipose-Derived Stem Cells," *Biomaterials*, Vol. 28, No. 26, 2007, pp. 3834–3842.

[25] Chung, I., et al., "Bioadhesive Hydrogel Microenvironments to Modulate Epithelial Morphogenesis," *Biomaterials*, Vol. 29, No. 17, 2008, pp. 2637–2645.

[26] Liu, Y., X. Shu, and G. Prestwich, "Osteochondral Defect Repair with Autologous Bone Marrow-Derived Mesenchymal Stem Cells in an Injectable, In Situ, Cross-Linked Synthetic Extracellular Matrix," *Tissue Eng.*, Vol. 12, No. 12, 2006, pp. 3405–3416.

[27] Zawko, S., et al., "Photopatterned Anisotropic Swelling of Dual-Crosslinked Hyaluronic Acid Hydrogels," *Acta Biomaterialia*, Vol. 5, No. 1, 2008, pp. 14–22.

[28] Chen, C., et al., "Micropatterned Surfaces for Control of Cell Shape, Position, and Function," *Biotechnol. Prog.*, Vol. 14, No. 3, 1998, pp. 356–363.

[29] Gauvreau, V., and G. Laroche, "Micropattern Printing of Adhesion, Spreading, and Migration Peptides on Poly(Tetrafluoroethylene) Films to Promote Endothelialization," *Bioconjug. Chem.*, Vol. 16, No. 5, 2005, pp. 1088–1097.

[30] Williams, C., et al., "Variable Cytocompatibility of Six Cell Lines with Photoinitiators Used for Polymerizing Hydrogels and Cell Encapsulation," *Biomaterials*, Vol. 26, No. 11, 2005, pp. 1211–1218.

[31] Bryant, S., C. Nuttelman, and K. Anseth, "Cytocompatibility of UV and Visible Light Photoinitiating Systems on Cultured NIH/3T3 Fibroblasts In Vitro," *J. Biomater. Sci. Polym. Ed.*, Vol. 11, No. 5, 2000, pp. 439–457.

[32] Lira, M., et al., "Comparative Study of Silicone-Hydrogel Contact Lenses Surfaces Before and After Wear Using Atomic Force Microscopy," *J. Biomed. Mater. Res. B Appl. Biomater.*, Vol. 85, No. 2, 2008, pp. 361–367.

[33] Huang, J., et al., "Research Article Synthesis and In Situ Atomic Force Microscopy Characterization of Temperature-Responsive Hydrogels Based on Poly(2-(Dimethylamino)Ethyl Methacrylate) Prepared by Atom Transfer Radical Polymerization," *Langmuir*, Vol. 23, No. 1, 2007, pp. 241–249.

[34] Park, S., C. Hung, and G. Ateshian, "Mechanical Response of Bovine Articular Cartilage Under Dynamic Unconfined Compression Loading at Physiological Stress Levels," *Osteoarthritis Cartilage*, Vol. 12, No. 1, 2004, pp. 65–73.

[35] Smeds, K., et al., "Photocrosslinkable Polysaccharides for In Situ Hydrogel Formation," *J. Biomed. Mater. Res.*, Vol. 54, No. 1, 2001, pp. 115–121.

[36] Chung, C., et al., "Differential Behavior of Auricular and Articular Chondrocytes in Hyaluronic Acid Hydrogels," *Tissue Eng.*, Vol. 14, No. 7, 2008, pp. 1121–1131.

[37] Moutos, F., L. Freed, and F. Guilak, "A Biomimetic Three-Dimensional Woven Composite Scaffold for Functional Tissue Engineering of Cartilage," *Nat. Mater.*, Vol. 6, No. 2, 2007, pp. 162–167.

[38] Nie, T., R. J. Akins, and K. Kiick, "Production of Heparin-Containing Hydrogels for Modulating Cell Responses," *Acta Biomater.*, Vol. 5, No. 3, 2009, pp. 865–875.

[39] Fatimi, A., et al., "The Rheological Properties of Silated Hydroxypropylmethylcellulose Tissue Engineering Matrices," *Biomaterials*, Vol. 29, No. 5, 2008, pp. 533–543.

[40] Lee, S., J. Moon, and J. West, "Three-Dimensional Micropatterning of Bioactive Hydrogels Via Two-Photon Laser Scanning Photolithography for Guided 3D Cell Migration," *Biomaterials*, Vol. 29, No. 20, 2008, pp. 2962–2968.

[41] Luo, Y., and M. Shoichet, "A Photolabile Hydrogel for Guided Three-Dimensional Cell Growth and Migration," *Nat. Mater.*, Vol. 3, No. 4, 2004, pp. 249–253.

[42] Peyton, S., et al., "The Use of Poly(Ethylene Glycol) Hydrogels to Investigate The Impact of ECM Chemistry and Mechanics on Smooth Muscle Cells," *Biomaterials*, Vol. 27, No. 28, 2006, pp. 4881–4893.

[43] Wacker, B., et al., "Endothelial Cell Migration on RGD-Peptide-Containing PEG Hydrogels in the Presence of Sphingosine 1-Phosphate," *Biophys. J.*, Vol. 94, No. 1, 2008, pp. 273–285.

[44] Kloxin, A., et al., "Photodegradable Hydrogels for Dynamic Tuning of Physical and Chemical Properties," *Science*, Vol. 324, No. 5923, 2009, pp. 59–63.

[45] Strehin, I., and J. Elisseeff, "Characterizing ECM Production by Cells Encapsulated in Hydrogels," *Methods Mol. Biol.*, Vol. No. 522, 2009, pp. 349–362.

[46] Burdick, J., et al., "Controlled Degradation and Mechanical Behavior of Photopolymerized Hyaluronic Acid Networks," *Biomacromolecules*, Vol. 6, No. 1, 2005, pp. 386–391.

[47] Sahoo, S., et al., "Hydrolytically Degradable Hyaluronic Acid Hydrogels with Controlled Temporal Structures," *Biomacromolecules*, Vol. 9, No. 4, 2008, pp. 1088–1092.

[48] Erickson, I., et al., "Differential Maturation and Structure-Function Relationships in Mesenchymal Stem Cell- and Chondrocyte-Seeded Hydrogels," *Tissue Eng. Part A*, Vol. 15, No. 5 2009, pp. 1041–1052.

[49] Cooper, J. J., et al., "Encapsulated Chondrocyte Response in a Pulsatile Flow Bioreactor," *Acta Biomater.*, Vol. 3, No. 1, 2007, pp. 13–21.

[50] Chung, C., et al., "Influence of Gel Properties on Neocartilage Formation by Auricular Chondrocytes Photoencapsulated in Hyaluronic Acid Networks," *J. Biomed. Mater. Res. A*, Vol. 77, No. 3, 2006, pp. 518–525.

[51] Na, K., et al., "Osteogenic Differentiation of Rabbit Mesenchymal Stem Cells in Thermo-Reversible Hydrogel Constructs Containing Hydroxyapatite and Bone Morphogenic Protein-2 (BMP-2)," *Biomaterials*, Vol. 28, No. 16, 2007, pp. 2631–2637.

[52] Fedorovich, N., et al., "The Effect of Photopolymerization on Stem Cells Embedded in Hydrogels," *Biomaterials*, Vol. 30, No. 3, 2009, pp. 344–353.

[53] Shapira-Schweitzer, K., et al., "A Photopolymerizable Hydrogel for 3D Culture of Human Embryonic Stem Cell-Derived Cardiomyocytes and Rat Neonatal Cardiac Cells," *J. Mol. Cell. Cardiol.*, Vol. 46, No. 2, 2009, pp. 213–224.

[54] Ferreira, L., et al., "Bioactive Hydrogel Scaffolds for Controllable Vascular Differentiation of Human Embryonic Stem Cells," *Biomaterials*, Vol. 28, No. 17, 2007, pp. 2706–2717.

[55] Hwang, N., et al., "Enhanced Chondrogenic Differentiation of Murine Embryonic Stem Cells in Hydrogels with Glucosamine," *Biomaterials*, Vol. 27, No. 36, 2006, pp. 6015–6023.

[56] Bryant, S., and K. Anseth, "The Effects of Scaffold Thickness on Tissue Engineered Cartilage in Photocrosslinked Poly(Ethylene Oxide) Hydrogels," *Biomaterials*, Vol. 22, No. 6, 2001, pp. 619–626.

CHAPTER

9

Micromolded Nonadhesive Hydrogels for the Self-Assembly of Scaffold-Free 3D Cellular Microtissues

Jacquelyn Youssef, Brian Bao, Toni-Marie Ferruccio, and Jeffrey R. Morgan

Department of Molecular Pharmacology, Physiology and Biotechnology, Center for Biomedical Engineering, Brown University, Providence, Rhode Island, Corresponding author: Jeffrey R. Morgan, address: Brown University, G-B 393, Biomed Center, 171 Meeting Street, Providence, RI 02912, phone: 401-863-9879, fax: 401-863-1753, e-mail: Jeffrey_Morgan@Brown.edu

Abstract

We present procedures for the fabrication and use of micromolded hydrogels for the self-assembly of three-dimensional (3D) multicellular microtissues. Computer-aided design, rapid prototyping, and replica molding are used to produce micromolds for the casting of hydrogels that are nonadhesive for cells and that guide the cells to form 3D microtissues. Cells seeded onto the surface of these micromolded nonadhesive hydrogels settle, aggregate, and self-assemble 3D microtissues whose size and shape are controlled by the design of the small recesses. In addition to forming thousands of spheroids of uniform size, the micromolds can direct the self-assembly of complex shapes such as honeycombs and can form microtissues with two or more different cell types. In addition to applications in tissue engineering, these scaffold-free microtissues can be used in drug discovery, toxicity testing, and stem cell and cancer research.

Key terms

aggregate
drug screening
microtissue
multicellular tumor spheroid
spheroid
three-dimensional (3D) cell culture
tissue engineering

9.1 Introduction

Three-dimensional (3D) cell culture models that more closely mimic in vivo tissue architecture and functions are growing in importance for study in the fields of developmental biology, cancer, drug discovery, regenerative medicine, and tissue engineering [1–3]. Most of these approaches combine cells with a scaffold (natural or synthetic) to achieve 3D cell culture and some have shown clinical promise as a substitute or replacement for diseased or injured tissues [4–6]. The scaffold is a large proportion of the mass of these structures and interactions of cells with the scaffold are a critical component. In many cases, cell-to-scaffold interactions are more important than cell-to-cell interactions. However, in most natural tissues, such as the liver, the opposite occurs. The scaffold or extracellular matrix (ECM) is a small proportion of the mass of the tissue, as cell density is high and cell-to-cell interactions predominate.

It has been known for some time that cells, in the absence of a scaffold, will undergo a process known as self-assembly [7]. In this process, monodispersed cells will spontaneously aggregate and form a 3D microtissue called a spheroid. It is thought that self-assembly mimics natural processes that occur during embryogenesis, morphogenesis, and organogenesis [7–9]. Many self-assembled spheroids mimic architectural and functional characteristics of their native tissue. Promising results include beating cardiomyocyte spheroids and liver-like hepatocyte spheroids [10–13] and vascularized smooth muscle cells and fibroblasts [14]. Human vascular endothelial cells (HUVECs) have been shown to vascularize fibroblast spheroids [13] and dorsal root ganglion cells have been shown to extend ganglion-like projections into embryonic fibroblast spheroids [15].

Through the years, two main methods have been used to study the self-assembly of spheroids from monodispersed cells, namely, spinner culture [24] and the hanging drop [18]. In the spinner culture method, monodispersed cells are pipetted into a spinner culture flask and prevented from attaching to a surface by constant mixing. During this time, cells collide with one another and form multicellular spheroids. The size of the spheroids is roughly controlled by the concentration of cells added, their relative adhesiveness, and the time in spinner culture. Spheroids of mixed cell populations have been produced in spinner culture and large numbers of spheroids can be easily harvested and so the method lends itself to scale up. Spinner culture, however, has several limitations. First, the self-assembly process occurs in an environment with significant shear forces and so may not be useful for cells that are less adhesive, sensitive to shear forces, slow to self-assemble, or prone to undergo apoptosis when detached. Due to constant mixing, it is impossible to obtain time lapse images to study the self-assembly process. The range of sizes of the spheroids produced by this method is not as uniform as other methods and due to the nature of the spinner flask, it is challenging to perform a mass balance and account for and/or document the self-assembly of all cells added. Medium changes and additions of drugs are easily performed, but seldom utilized. Few studies have used this method to examine the early kinetics and mechanisms of self-assembly. Most studies are end-point experiments that examine the final spheroid structure. Spinner culture produces only spheroids and so cannot be used to direct the self-assembly of cells into complex geometries.

In the hanging drop method, a small volume (~50 μL) of monodispersed cells is pipetted onto a surface, such as the lid of a tissue culture dish, and this surface is inverted so that the drop hangs under its own weight. The cells within this drop settle to the bottom of the drop, contact one another, and undergo self-assembly into a spheroid structure. The use of an automatic multichannel pipettor has enabled the production of a larger number of spheroids [2]. Spheroid size is readily controlled by the concentration of the cells in each drop and the range of distribution of sizes is shown to be uniform. Likewise, the cellular composition of the spheroid is easily controlled and spheroids of two or more cells can be generated and spheroids can be harvested for multiple purposes. Although widely used, the method has two significant limitations. First, the handling of hundreds of small drops can be challenging and simple acts routinely performed in tissue culture experiments, such as changing the medium, adding a drug or adding a second cell type, are nontrivial. Second, like spinner culture, the hanging drop method produces only spheroids and so cannot be used to direct the self-assembly of cells into complex geometries.

To address these limitations, we have developed a new method to self-assemble microtissues based on a micromolded nonadhesive hydrogel (e.g., agarose). Monodispersed cells are pipetted onto the hydrogel, the cells settle into the micromolded features, and because the agarose is nonadhesive for cell, cell-to-cell interactions predominate and cells spontaneously self-assemble into a multicellular aggregate (Figure 9.1). As our data show, micromolds of various geometries can be made and monodispersed cells in these molds will self-assemble a microtissue with a complex geometry (e.g., honeycomb) (Figure 9.2). The method relies on self-assembly, the same biological phenomenon that gives rise to spheroids in the spinner culture and the hanging drop. However, the micromolds, by virtue of their geometry, set the initial condi-

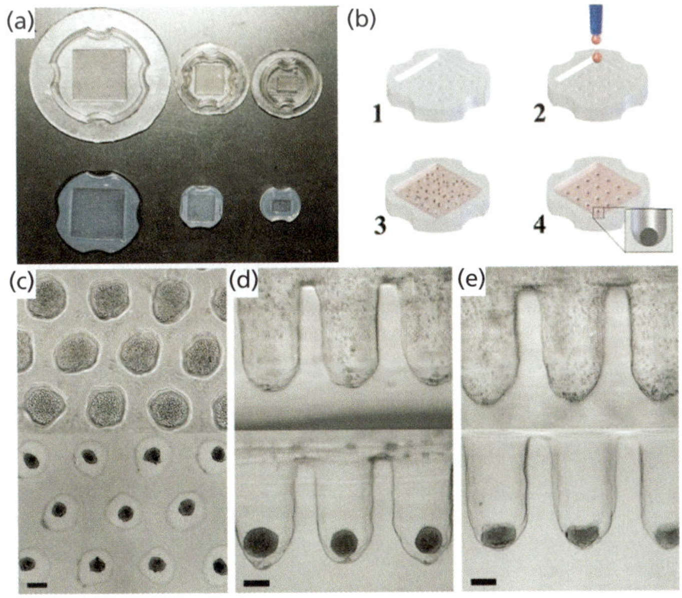

Figure 9.1 Micromolded nonadhesive hydrogels, the seeding process, and resulting microtissues. (a) The top row is the PDMS micromolded for the 6-, 12-, and 24-well plates, respectively. The bottom row is the resulting agarose micromolded hydrogels. (b) Schematic of cell seeding process. (1) The empty hydrogel. (2) A cell suspension is seeded into the hydrogel. (3) Cells begin to settle into the recesses of the hydrogel. (4) Cells aggregate and form microtissues. (c–e) Monodispersed cells being seeded into micromolded hydrogels and the resulting microtissues. (c) Conventional view of seeded cells and the resulting microtissues. Top panel shows side view images of monodispersed (d) NHFs and (e) H35s settling into the wells of the micromolded hydrogel. The bottom panel shows the resulting microtissues after 24 hours. Scale bars are 200 μm. ([18] © 2009 BioTechniques. Used by permission.)

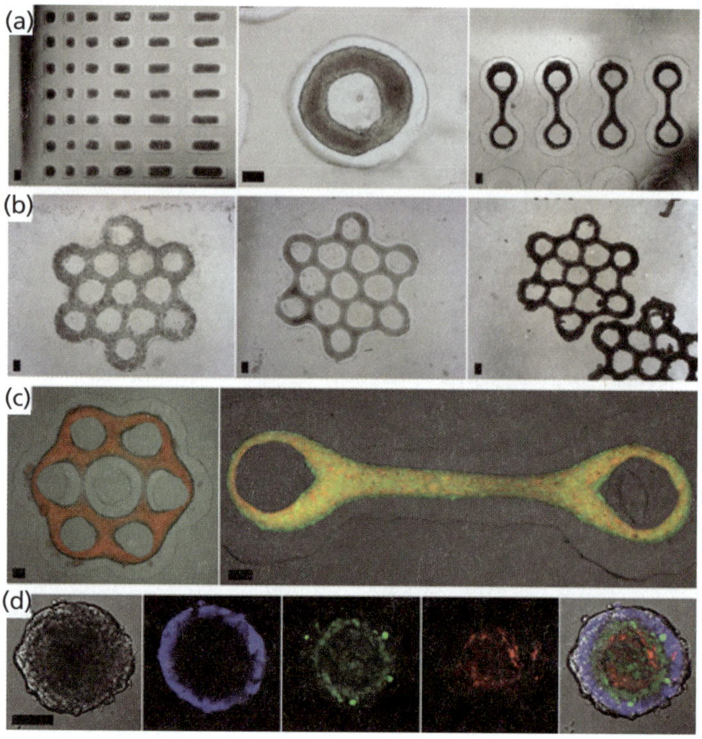

Figure 9.2 Micromolded nonadhesive hydrogels can be used to direct the assembly of complex and mixed cell type microtissues: (a) H35 rods (left), MCF-7 toroid (middle), H35 loop-ended dog bone (right). (b) MCF-7s seeded in honeycomb recesses (left) MCF-7 honeycomb compacts slightly 1 day after seeding (middle) MCF-7s maintain patent lumens of branched structure up to 3 days postremoval from gels(right). (c) Heterotypic honeycomb (left) and loop-ended dog bone (right) microtissues composed of NHFs and H35s (right). (d) Self-sorting of 2-day tritypic spheroid from left to right: differential interference contrast (DIC) microscopy; H35s; NHFs; human umbilical vein endothelial cells (HUVECs); and the composite image. Scale bars are 200 μm (a–c) or 100 μm (d). ([18] © 2009 BioTechniques. Used by permission.)

tions and configuration of cells from which self-assembly commences and also impose obstacles (e.g., nonadhesive agarose peg in a toroid) that also influence self-assembly. The outcome can be a structure far different from a simple spheroid structure. We refer to this process as directed self-assembly [16–24].

9.2 Experimental Design

The micromolded hydrogel was developed as a method to self-assemble cells in a simple yet effective way. We have designed these gels so that the process of self-assembly can be easily monitored and quantified using novel assays. This technology is distinct from other methods of self-assembly in that cells can be directed to self-assemble complex structures other than the spheroid. Complex shapes include lumen containing toroids, elongated rods, branched honeycomb structures with multiple lumens, and a constrained rod structures called the dog bone. All of these structures are free from any added extracellular material allowing for the concentrated study of cell-to-cell interactions.

9.3 Materials

- ThermoJet rapid prototyping machine (3D Systems Corporation)
- Vacuum chamber Model V0914A (Lindenberg/Blue)
- VWR 375 Hot plate/Stirrer (VWR)
- Dataplate Digital Hot Plate/Stirrer (PMC)
- Thermoforma Centrifuge 5682GFBR (ThermoForma)
- Dulbecco's modified Eagle's medium (DMEM) (Fisher Scientific)
- Fetal bovine serum (FBS) (Fisher Scientific)
- 1% penicillin/streptomycin (penn/strep) (Fisher Scientific)
- TRIS Buffer 0.5M, pH 7.4 (Fisher Scientific)
- 0.05% trypsin-EDTA (Fisher Scientific)
- Ammonium persulfate (APS) (Sigma)
- N,N,N'N'-Tetramethylethylenediamine (TEMED) (Sigma)
- Autoclave-sterilized powder Ultrapure Agarose (Invitrogen)
- Acrylamide/bis-acyrlamide 40% solution (Sigma)
- Phosphate buffered saline (PBS) (Invitrogen)
- CellTracker Green 5-chloromethylfluorescein diacetate (CMFDX) (Molecular Probes)
- CellTracker Red (CMPTX) (Molecular Probes)
- Dimethyl sulfoxide (DMSO) (Sigma)
- LIVE/DEAD Stain (Invitrogen)
- WST-1 Cell Proliferation Kit (Roche)
- Saline, 0.9% (w/v) NaCl
- Reprorubber (Flexbar Machine Corporation)
- Epoxy Parafilm Release Agent (Flexbar).
- Reprorubber Thin Pour 16116 (Flexbar)
- Sylgard 184 Polydimethylsiloxane (PDMS, Dow Corning Corporation)
- 70% Ethanol
- Micro cover glasses 24 × 50 mm No. 1 (VWR)
- 6-well tissue culture plates (Fisher Scientific)
- Sterile 50-ml centrifuge tubes (Fisher Scientific)
- Hemocytometer (Fisher Scientific)
- Autoclave sterilized spatulas
- Prism 3 mm (Thor labs)
- Glass Petri dish 100 cm (Fisher Scientific)
- 8-well 27.9 × 37.5 mm rectangular Petri dish (Nunc)
- Computer-assisted design software (CAD) (Solid Works Corporation)
- ImageJ Software (National Institute of Health, free software)
- MetaMorph Software (Molecular Devices)

9.4 Methods

9.4.1 Design and fabrication of micromolds

9.4.1.1 Wax micromold design and fabrication

Using computer-aided design (CAD) software, we have designed a number of micromolds with a variety of design features. The different designs are used to self-assemble a number of complex-shaped microtissues including spheroids, rods, toroids, honeycombs, and dog bones. A typical mold contains a rectangular box, which forms the cell seeding chamber, and extending from this box is an array of the micromolded features, which form the cell recesses. For the standard 6 well plate, the spheroid forming micromold recess feature is an 800-μm-tall cylindrical peg with a 600-μm hemispherical cap. For the side-view microscopy, the spheroid mold has the same 800-μm-tall cylindrical peg with a 600-μm hemispherical cap with only a single row of 21 features. CAD files are then printed into a wax micromold using a ThermoJet rapid prototyping machine.

9.4.1.2 Casting a Reprorubber negative replica of the wax mold

1. Remove any large debris from the wax mold and place in a 10-cm Petri dish with the features facing up.
2. Mix equal parts of the Reprorubber base and catalyst (approximately 4 ounces total). Mix well until the solution is green.
3. Pour the Reprorubber solution over the wax mold until the mold is completely covered.
4. Quickly degas the Reprorubber on the wax mold to remove any air bubbles from the small features. To degas, place the mold in a vacuum chamber and pull the vacuum until the bubbles rise out of the features. As the bubbles rise out of the features, open the valve to allow for venting. Take caution not to boil the Reprorubber.
5. Allow polymer to polymerize at room temperature for 5–10 minutes.
6. Carefully separate the wax mold from the Reprorubber micromold replica.
7. In a fume hood, spray the Reprorubber replica with an epoxy parafilm release agent ensuring that the features and sides of the replica are well coated. Allow the replica to dry in the fume hood for 10 minutes.

9.4.1.3 Casting the PDMS replica of a wax micromold

1. Mix a 10:1 (by weight) solution of 184 Sylgard PDMS base to curing agent. Be sure the solution is well mixed. Approximately 7 grams are needed for a single PDMS micromold.
2. Degas the PDMS until all the air bubbles are removed by pulling vacuum until the solution boils. As solution boils, open valve to allow for venting. Take caution to ensure that the PDMS solution does not boil over. Repeat pulling the vacuum and opening the valve until all the air bubbles are removed.
3. Place Reprorubber replica in a glass Petri dish and pour PDMS solution into Reprorubber replica so that all the features are covered in PDMS.

4. Degas the Reprorubber with PDMS by placing the molds in a vacuum chamber and pulling vacuum until the air bubbles rise out of the features. Open valve to allow for venting taking caution to prevent the solution from spilling over. Repeat pulling the vacuum and opening the valve until all the air bubbles are removed from the features.
5. Bake the PDMS at 95°C for 90 minutes and then gently remove the PDMS from the Reprorubber replica. Continue to bake the PDMS for 60 minutes at 95°C.
6. Sterilize the PDMS micromolds by autoclaving at 132°C for 30 minutes.
7. After use, the PDMS micromolds can be cleaned by washing the gels with soap and water, then air-drying the molds, and finally spraying the molds with 70% ethanol. Once the molds have dried, they can then be sterilized as described in step 6.

9.4.2 Casting of agarose micromolded hydrogels

1. Measure out 2g of Ultrapure agarose powder into a 150-ml autoclave safe glass bottle. Place a magnetic stir bar in the bottle with the agarose. Tighten the lid of the bottle so that it is just secured but still loose so that it is movable. To sterilize, autoclave the bottle with agarose at 132°C for 30 minutes on a dry cycle.
2. In a biosafety cabinent using an septic technique, prepare a 2% agarose solution by mixing 2g of the sterile Ultrapure agarose powder in 100-ml saline 0.9% (w/v) NaCl.
3. Using a hot plate with a stirring function; heat and stir the agarose solution on low heat until it is completely dissolved.
4. Pipette 1.0 ml of molten agarose solution into a sterile PDMS micromold.
5. Using a 10-ml pipette, quickly aspirate the air bubbles from the micromold features by drawing up molten agarose in the features and then replacing it. Other methods for removing air bubbles include using a sterile spatula and gently scraping the features until bubbles are removed or degassing the gel in a vacuum chamber until air bubbles come out of the features.
6. Replace any lost agarose, ensuring that the top surface is flat, neither convex nor concave.
7. Allow the agarose to set for 10 minutes.
8. Upon opacification of the agarose solution, gently separate the agarose gel from the PDMS micromold using a sterile spatula. Use caution to avoid damaging features or ripping the agarose hydrogel.
9. Transfer the agarose hydrogel to a 6-well tissue culture plate and equilibrate the gel overnight in 5 ml of the medium. Prior to seeding, make sure that the medium has been changed at least three times over the course of 12 hours to allow for proper gel equilibration.

9.4.3 Casting polyacrylamide micromolded hydrogels

1. Mix 1.75 ml of acrylamide/bis-acyrlamide 40% solution with 1.63 ml of DMEM, 1.63 ml of Tris buffer, and 25 μl of a 10% APS solution.
2. Degas the prepolymer by placing the solution in a vacuum chamber. Pull the vacuum until the solution boils. As the solution boils, open the valve to allow for

venting. Repeat pulling the vacuum and opening the valve until all the air bubbles are removed.

3. Add 50 μl of TEMED to initiate polymerization.
4. Add 400 μl of the polymer solution to the wax molds and place a glass cover slip over the top surface of the mold to create a flat surface.
5. After 10–15 minutes, remove the polyacrylamide hydrogel with a sterile spatula from the wax molds and transfer to a sterile tissue culture plate.
6. Rinse the gels twice with 4 ml of DMEM supplemented with 1% pen/strep leaving a few hours between rinses to allow the gels to equilibrate.
7. Aspirate off the medium and equilibrate the gels overnight at 37°C with 4 ml of the medium.

9.4.4 Formation of 3D microtissues

9.4.4.1 Agarose hydrogels

1. Remove the adherent cells with 0.05% trypsin-EDTA for 5 minutes. Quench trypsin by adding an equal volume of the culture medium with 10% FBS.
2. Transfer the cell suspension to a 50-ml centrifuge tube and centrifuge for 5 minutes at 800 rpm.
3. Aspirate the trypsin-containing supernatant, and resuspend the cells in the known volume of the culture medium.
4. Determine the total cell number using a hemocytometer. Centrifuge and resuspend cells in an appropriate volume to obtain the desired seeding density. Spheroids in the range of 150 to 250 μm in diameter contain between 400 and 1,500 cells/spheroid. Use Table 9.1 for approximate cell number values.
5. Pipette 200 μl of the cell suspension into seeding chamber of the gel.
6. Incubate the samples for 30 minutes and then carefully add 5 ml of culture medium via the media exchange port. Ensure that enough medium is added to cover the seeding chamber without washing out the cells.
7. Return the gels to the incubator at 37°C with the appropriate percentage of CO_2 specific to the cell type.

Table 9.1 Cell Number for Seeding 6-Well Spheroid Gels

Spheroid Diameter (mm)	Cells Per Gel (Cells/200 ml)	~Cells/ Spheroid
100	0.1 × 106	122
125	0.2 × 106	243
150	0.35 × 106	425
175	0.55 × 106	669
200	0.8 × 106	973
225	1.2 × 106	1,459
250	1.6 × 106	1,946
275	2.1 × 106	2,554
300	2.7 × 106	3,284

9.4.4.2 Polyacrylamide hydrogels

1. Trypsinize, count, and resuspend the cells to the desired cell concentration according to the standard protocol as described for the agarose hydrogel.
2. Prior to seeding, aspirate the medium and rinse the gels with 4 ml of the medium.
3. Seed 70 μl of the cell solution with the desired cell concentration into the seeding chamber. Use Table 9.1 for the approximate cell number values.
4. Allow the cells to settle to the bottom of the recess for 30 minutes at 37°C.
5. After 30 minutes, carefully pipette 3 ml of the medium into the well of the tissue culture plate and return the gels to incubator at 37°C with the appropriate percentage of CO_2 specific to the cell type.

9.4.5 Side-on viewing of self-assembly

9.4.5.1 Using right angle prisms

1. Place the side-view gels in a multiwell rectangular Petri dish with the thin wall of the gel positioned against a well wall that is shared with another well.
2. In the adjacent well, arrange a right angle prism so that its back face is snug against the wall shared with the side-view gel and with the hypotenuse of the prism facing upwards.
3. Position the plate so that the microscope objective is directly under the bottom face of the prism.
4. For epi-fluorescence, the excitation light will travel from the objective through the prism and be reflected into the sample. The emitted radiation will then return through the prism and into the objective.
5. For bright-field microscopy, bring an external light source and position the light source so that the light shines through the rear of the gel, through the sample, through the prism, and into the objective.

9.4.5.2 Using a modified microscope

We also view microtissues side-on using a modified traditional microscope. Currently, we are using a Mitutoyo FS-110. The microscope sits in a cradle that secures the microscope while it is positioned to lie on its back. The original stage has been replaced with one that translates and holds the samples perpendicular to both the original light source and objective. Using this modified microscope, we capture bright-field side view images of our microtissues.

9.4.6 Spheroid size quantification

1. Import side-view and conventional view images into Image J software.
2. After setting the appropriate size scale using the "Set scale" function, the diameter of a spheroid can be measured using the line tool, and the area can be measured with either the ellipse or the free-hand tool.
3. Multiple aggregates in the same field of view can be measured using the "Analyze particle" function.

4. To use this function, first threshold the image by going into Image → Adjust → Threshold.
5. A histogram will appear in which the levels of the image can be adjusted. Use the tabs to reduce noise while highlighting individual microtissues and then press "Apply."
6. The resulting image will be black and white. With this image still open, go to Image → Analyze Particles.
7. Set the upper and lower limit for the size of the microtissue and check off "Display results." Press "OK" and the dimensions of each microtissue will be displayed in a table.

9.4.7 Live cell fluorescent staining and determination of self-sorting patterns of cells

CellTracker (Invitrogen) is a membrane permeable dye that allows for the tracing and tracking of cells. The two most commonly used for staining microtissues are CellTracker Green CMFDA and CellTracker Red CMPTX.

9.4.7.1 Labeling cells with CellTracker stains

1. Thaw one 50-μg vial of either CellTracker Green or CellTracker Red stain for each T-175 flask.
2. To prevent photobleaching, work with the lights off in the tissue culture hood.
3. Resuspend the thawed CellTracker Green powder in 10.8 μl of DMSO.
4. Make a working solution of CellTracker Green by adding a reconstituted dye to 21.6 mL of the serum-free medium. Wrap the solution in foil to prevent photobleaching.
5. Resuspend the thawed CellTracker Red powder in 7.1 μl of DMSO.
6. Make a working solution of CellTracker Red by adding the reconstituted dye to 14.2 mL of the serum-free medium. Wrap the solution in foil to prevent photobleaching.
7. Incubate cells with a working solution of either CellTracker Green or CellTracker Red for 50 minutes at 37°C.
8. Aspirate off solution, tryspinize, harvest, and count cells as described above.
9. Combine the two cell populations in a 1:1 (red:green) ratio or other desired ratio.
10. Centrifuge the cells at 500 rpm for 6 minutes.
11. Seed hydrogels with appropriate seeding density according to Table 9.1, and incubate the cells for 24 hours at 37°C while self-assembly and self-sorting occurs.
12. Analyze the sorting patterns via epi-fluorescent and confocal microscopy.

9.4.8 WST-1 cell proliferation assay adapted for microtissues

1. Allow the spheroid microtissues to aggregate and assemble. (This length of time is cell type dependent.)
2. At desired time points, take one replicate of the hydrogel sample and aspirate the excess medium from the culture plate well.
3. In a centrifuge tube, mix a 10:1 solution of the medium and WST-1 reagent. Add 400 μl of this solution to the seeding chamber of each gel and incubate the hydrogel at 37°C for 4 hours.

4. Pipette 100 μl of the WST-1 containing medium from the seeding chamber of each gel and transfer to a 96-well plate.
5. Using a spectrophotometer, measure the optical density of the reagent/medium solution at an optical density of 440 nm minus 600 nm.
6. Repeat steps 2–5 for each replicate at the desired time point.
7. A standard curve can also be created by seeding the known cell numbers and measuring the absorbance at 440 nm minus 600 nm.
8. Plot the absorbance as a function of the cell number to create a standard curve. Using the standard curve, the proliferation of unknown samples can be determined.

9.4.9 Harvesting microtissues

9.4.9.1 By agitation (75–80% recovery)

1. Place 2.5 ml of the medium into a well of a sterile 6-well plate.
2. Remove the medium from the well holding the hydrogel and carefully remove the medium from the seeding chamber of the hydrogel itself.
3. Using a sterile spatula, remove the hydrogel and place into the new plate containing the medium. Invert the hydrogel over the well carefully, not creating an excess of bubbles.
4. Incubate for 5–10 minutes while gently shaking the plate and tapping the back of the hydrogel's seeding chamber with a spatula to release the microtissues.
5. View the plate under the microscope to ensure that microtissues have been released from the gel.
6. Repeat until all the microtissues are released. Remove the hydrogel with a spatula.

9.4.9.2 Centrifugation (90–99% recovery)

1. Place 2.5 ml of the medium into a well of a sterile 6-well plate.
2. Remove the medium from the well holding the hydrogel and carefully remove the medium from the seeding chamber of the hydrogel itself.
3. Remove the hydrogel with a sterile spatula, and invert the hydrogel in the new well. Be careful to not create air bubbles.
4. Place the 6-well plate in a swinging bucket rotor in a centrifuge and spin for 5 minutes at 500 rpm.
5. After centrifugation, view the hydrogel under the microscope to ensure that microtissues have been released.
6. Remove the empty hydrogel with a spatula.

9.4.10 LIVE/DEAD staining to determine microtissue viability

1. In a centrifuge tube prepare the LIVE/DEAD solution by adding 4-μl Ethidium homodimer-1, 1-μl calcein AM, and 2 ml of PBS that was warmed in a 37°C water bath.
2. Aspirate the medium from the well holding the hydrogel and gently tip the plate to carefully remove the excess medium from the seeding chamber of the gel.
3. Rinse the gel with 3 ml of warm PBS (37°C) and aspirate off the excess PBS.

4. Add 300 μl of the LIVE/DEAD solution to the seeding chamber of the hydrogel and incubate at room temperature for 30–45 minutes.
5. Image the samples within 45 minutes to ensure a bright signal.
6. To assess microtissue viability, MetaMorph image analysis software is used to calculate the live/dead ratio within a sample.
7. Use the Region Measurement free-hand tool to determine the average intensities of the green (live) or red (dead) pixels within a region of interest corresponding to the projected microtissue area.
8. The live/dead ratio for a single microtissue is the ratio of the average intensity of the green signal to the red signal. Average live/dead ratio ± standard deviation can be calculated for microtissues in a given sample.

9.4.11 Data analysis

Microtissues formed using the micromolded nonadhesive hydrogel technology can be analyzed using a wide variety of standard microscopy and biochemical techniques. Bright field and fluorescent images from the microscope can be quantified using standard image analysis software to measure the size and viability of the microtissues as well as the kinetics of their self-assembly and self-sorting. The easy formation of large numbers of microtissues of uniform size ensures that the microscopic measurements have a large sample size and are statistically significant. The metabolic activity and proliferation of microtissues can be analyzed by the addition of standard dyes, such as WST-1, which diffuse into the hydrogel and are metabolized by the microtissues. These metabolic products equilibrate with the medium surrounding the hydrogel and so medium can be harvested and metabolites quantified using standard multiwell plate readers that measure absorbance or fluorescence. Since large numbers of microtissues are easily formed, microtissues can be harvested from the micromolds and subjected to analyses widely used in molecular biology including Western blots, RT-PCR, and immunostaining.

9.5 Anticipated Results

Using the nonadhesive micromolded hydrogel gel, cells can be directed to self-assemble microtissues with a number of shapes and sizes. With these procedures, the microtissue size should be reproducible and uniform, and self-assembly and self-sorting behavior should be easy to monitor. We anticipate that this technology will be compatible with a number of cell types that readily form cell-to-cell adhesions. To date, over 20 different adherent cell lines from a variety of tissues (liver, skin, bone, cartilage, brain) have been shown to self- assemble 3D microtissues using this technology. Depending on the cell type, different factors including cell number, medium components, gas levels, and incubation time should be carefully considered to match the requirements of each cell type.

9.6 Discussion and Commentary

The nonadhesive micromolded hydrogel is a straightforward approach to direct the self-assembly of cells into 3D microtissues. This new method presents a number of benefits in comparison to the past methods of self-assembly. Unlike other methods of self-assembly, which are laborious and/or have low throughput, this method is quite simple in that with a single pipetting step, cells can be assembled into over 800 microtissues [16]. From past studies, we have determined that by simply changing the seeding density we can control microtissue size and by using different recess features we can direct the cells to aggregate into a number of complex shapes [16–18]. We have also shown that these microtissues can be harvested [17], fused to create larger tissues [23], encapsulated [22], and monitored for metabolic activity [18]. In addition, this method is well suited for using multiple cell types, creating heterotypic microtissues, which is of key importance as tissues are often a collection of multiple cell types.

We have also established that the nonadhesive micromolded hydrogel is a great tool for assaying the process and contributors of self-assembly. Using the hydrogel, we have developed a rod contraction assay, which is very useful for comparing the self-assembly rate of cell types. In particular, we have compared the rate of self-assembly for two very different cell types: normal human fibroblast (NHFs) and H35, a rat hepatocyte cell line [17].We have determined that NHFs assemble and contract from an elongated rod structure into a spheroid within 12 hours, while H35s contract but maintain an elongated rod structure for days [17]. Using the rod contraction assay, we have examined the role of rho kinase (ROCK) mediated contraction in self-assembly and self-sorting [17]. Previously, it was thought that both self-sorting and self-assembly were directed solely by surface proteins, specifically cadherins [9, 18]. However, by treating NHFs with a ROCK inhibitor, Y-27632, the rate of self-assembly was slowed significantly and self-sorting was also altered indicating that ROCK-mediated contraction has an important role in self-assembly [17]. We have also used complex-shaped geometries such as the dog bone to reveal the dynamic process in fibroblasts of extending and contracting dendritic processes, a phenomenon that had not been observed in self-assembled microtissues.

Relevant to self-sorting and tissue engineering, we have used the technology to fuse spheroids into larger microtissues and have shown that cell position can be directed contrary to intrinsic sorting behavior. By seeding a combination of monodispersed cells and spheroids precultured for a variety of times, a number of heterotypic fused microtissue structures were developed, each with a distinct reproducible sorting pattern [23]. This finding is significant as the ability to control cell position is important to engineering epithelialized and vascularized tissue structures.

Troubleshooting Table

Problem	Explanation	Potential Solutions
PDMS does not release from the Reprorubber replica.	Reprorubber replica was not sufficiently sprayed with release agent.	When spraying replica with the release agent, ensure that the agent has covered all surfaces by running your gloved finger around all the crevices and edges of the replica. Multiple sprays may also be employed to ensure sufficient coverage.
Agarose gel breaks upon release from the PDMS micromold.	Agarose gel was not separated from the PDMS micromold slowly enough or the setting time for agarose was too long.	Use a sterile spatula to first separate each corner of the agarose, allowing air to enter underneath. Then use the spatula to slowly separate each corner of the seeding chamber, prior to complete separation from the PDMS micromold. As well, if the agarose is allowed to gel too long, it becomes very brittle make sure to remove the gel once it has become opaque.
Small features in the agarose break upon release from the PDMS micromold.	Inappropriate time for agarose solidification.	Wait for the agarose to become opaque, signifying that the agarose has solidified and adequately molded the small features.
Polyacrylamide gel breaks.	Gel was not separated from wax micromold gently enough or the polymerization time was too long.	With a sterile spatula gently separate the walls of the gel from the wax mold. Then, starting at one of the short walls, gently slide the spatula under the gel, popping it out from the wax mold. If the gel still breaks, decrease the polymerization time.
Small aggregates/low cell seeding number.	Cells did not stay in the gel after seeding due to a crack in the gel or the cells were washed out when the medium was added.	Take care when removing gels from the PDMS, ensuring that the gel does not have cracks. To check for cracks, pipette a small volume of medium into the seeding chamber prior to seeding and check if the medium remains in the chamber. When adding the medium, make sure that the medium is being added slowly into the well of the culture plate and that it is not being added directly over the seeding chamber, which could wash out the cells.
Features were not formed in agarose or polyacrylamide gel.	Air bubbles were in the features at the time of gel formation.	For agarose gels, use one of the three methods to ensure that bubbles are removed from the features. For polyacrylamide, a degassing step can be added after the polymer has been added to the wax mold.
Microtissues are not removed during harvesting.	Aggregates may be physically stuck due to their size or an air bubble may be between the inverted gel and the medium.	If the aggregate is too large, it will become physically trapped by the walls of the well. Make sure at the time of the seeding that the number of cells seeded will not be too large considering the time for proliferation and the culture time prior to harvesting. Adjust the seeding number or the time before the harvest to ensure that the aggregate is within the size constraints of the well. If an air bubble is between the gel and the medium, gently prop up the inverted gel, allowing the medium to fill space, and release. Repeat until the air bubble is removed.

9.7 Application Notes

Beyond applications in self-assembly and tissue engineering, we anticipate that the micromolded hydrogel technology will be useful for applications in toxicology and drug discovery. The ease with which large numbers of microtissues can be formed and the ability to analyze microtissues by standard microscopy lend themselves well to automation and applications in high-content screening. Because the microtissues are 3D (a significant step closer to the in vivo environment) and can be formed with human cells, the technology may be useful for in vitro toxicology assays. Also, because the microtissues maximize cell-to-cell interactions (homotypic and heterotypic cell interactions), the technology may be useful for identifying new drug targets that are the manifestation of the contact and communication between two cells types such as the neuromuscular junction.

9.8 Summary Points

1. We have developed a novel method to direct the self-assembly of cells into 3D microtissues. This method presents many benefits including ease of use, flexibility of design, and high throughput. Unique to the micromolded hydrogel is the ability to self-assemble complex-shaped microtissues.
2. Micromolded hydrogels allow for the ease of monitoring microtissue self-assembly and function using a variety of microscopy techniques. The gel also allows for microtissue harvesting, fusion, and encapsulation.
3. Micromolded hydrogels can be used for a number of research applications including tissue engineering, developmental biology, cancer research, and stem cell research as well as determining the role of specific proteins and protein systems in cell-to-cell adhesion. As well, the platform is compatible for applications in drug discovery and toxicity testing.
4. We and others have shown that a number of cell types from a variety of tissues and organs including skin, liver, heart, ovary, breast, and brain can be self-assembled into 3D microtissues using the micromolded hydrogels. New and untested cell types require some optimization in terms of micromold design, cell number, medium components, and time for self-assembly.

Acknowledgments

This work was funded, in part, by the NIH (R01EB008664-01A1) and the MRSEC Program of the National Science Foundation under award DMR-0520651.

References

[1] Abbott, A., "Cell Culture: Biology's New Dimension," *Nature*, Vol. 424, 2003, pp. 870–872.

[2] Kelm, J. M., and M. Fussenegger, "Microscale Tissue Engineering Using Gravity-Enforced Cell Assembly," *Trends in Biotechnology*, Vol. 22, 2004, pp. 195–202.

[3] Enmon, R. M., Jr., et al., "Dynamics of Spheroid Self-Assembly in Liquid-Overlay Culture of DU 145 Human Prostate Cancer Cells," *Biotechnology and Bioengineering*, Vol. 72, 2001, pp. 579–591.

[4] Langer, R., and J. P. Vacanti, "Tissue Engineering," *Science*, Vol. 260, No. 5110, 2003, pp. 920–926.

[5] Griffith, L. G., and G. Naughton, "Tissue Engineering—Current Challenges and Expanding Opportunities," *Science*, Vol. 295, No. 5557, 2002, pp. 1009–1014.

[6] Ingber, D. E., and M. Levin, "What Lies at the Interface of Regenerative Medicine and Developmental Biology?" *Development*, Vol. 134, No. 14, 2007, pp. 2541–2547.

[7] Moscona A., and H. Moscona, "The Dissociation and Aggregation of Cells from Organ Rudiments of the Early Chick Embryo," *J. Anat.*, Vol. 86, No. 287, 1952.

[8] Foty, R. A., et al., "Surface Tensions of Embryonic Tissues Predict Their Mutual Envelopment Behavior," *Development*, Vol. 122, 1996, pp. 1611–1620.

[9] Duguay, D., R. A. Foty, and M. S. Steinberg, "Cadherin-Mediated Cell Adhesion and Tissue Segregation: Qualitative and Quantitative Determinants," *Developmental Biology*, Vol. 253, 2003, pp. 309–323.

[10] Kelm, J. M., and M. Fussenegger, "Microscale Tissue Engineering Using Gravity-Enforced Cell Assembly," *Trends in Biotech.*, Vol. 22, No. 195, 2004.

[11] Fukuda, J., S. Yusuke, and K. Nakazawa, "Novel Hepatocyte Culture System Developed Using Microfabrication and Collagen/Polyethylene Glycol Microcontact Printing," *Biomaterials*, Vol. 1, 2005.

[12] Fukuda, J., and K. Nakazawa, "Orderly Arrangement of Hepatocyte Spheroids on a Microfabricated Chip," *Tissue Eng.*, Vol. 11, No. 1254, 2005.

[13] Kunz-Schughart, L. A., et al., "Potential of Fibroblasts to Regulate the Formation of Three-Dimensional Vessel-Like Structures from Endothelial Cells In Vitro," *Am. J. Physiol. Cell Physiol.*, Vol. 290, 1385.

[14] Rouwkema, J., J. de Boer, and C. A. Van Blitterswijk, "Endothelial Cells Assemble into a 3-Dimensional Prevascular Network in a Bone Tissue Engineering Construct," *Tissue Eng.*, 12, 2006, pp. 2685–2693.

[15] Kelm, J. M., et al., "Self-Assembly of Sensory Neurons into Ganglia-Like Micro-Tissues," *J. of Biotech.*, Vol. 121, No. 86, 2005.

[16] Napolitano, A. P., et al., "Dynamics of the Self-Assembly of Complex Cellular Aggregates on Micro-Molded Nonadhesive Hydrogels," *Tissue Eng.*, Vol. 13, No. 8, 2007, pp. 2087–2094.

[17] Dean, D. M., et al., "Rods, Tori and Honeycombs. The Directed Self-Assembly of Microtissues with Prescribed Microscale Geometries," *FASEB J.*, Vol. 21, 2007, pp. 4005–4012.

[18] Napolitano, A. P., et al., "Scaffold-Free 3-Dimensional Cell Culture Utilizing Micro-Molded Nonadhesive Hydrogels," *BioTechniques*, Vol. 43, 2007, pp. 494–500.

[19] Rago, A. P., A. P. Napolitano, and J. R. Morgan, "Miniaturization of an Anoikis Assay Using Nonadhesive Micromolded Hydrogels," *Cytotechnology*, Vol. 56, 2008, pp. 81–90.

[20] Barbone, D., et al., "mTOR Contributes to the Acquired Multicellular Apoptotic Resistance of Human Malignant Mesothelioma Spheroids," *J. Biol. Chem.*, Vol. 283, 2008, pp. 13021–13030.

[21] Dean, D. M., and J. R. Morgan, "Cytoskeletal-Mediated Tension Modulates the Directed Self-Assembly of Microtissues," *Tissue Eng.*, Vol. 14, 2008, pp. 1989–1997.

[22] Rago, A. P., P. Chai, and J. R. Morgan, "Encapsulated Arrays of Self-Assembled Micro-Tissues: An Alternative to Spherical Microcapsules," *Tissue Eng.*, Vol. 15, 2009, pp. 387–395.

[23] Rago, A. P., D. M. Dean, and J. R. Morgan, "Controlling Cell Position in Complex Heterotypic 3D Microtissues by Tissue Fusion," *Biotech. and Bioeng.*, Vol. 102, 2009, pp. 1231–1241.

[24] Dean, D. M., and J. R. Morgan, "Fibroblast Elongation and Dendritic Extensions in Constrained Versus Unconstrained Microtissues," *Cell Motility and the Cytoskeleton*, Vol. 66, 2009, pp. 129–141.

CHAPTER

10

On-Demand 3D Freeform Fabrication of Tissue Structures Using Bioprinting

Seung-Schik Yoo,[1] Wonhye Lee,[2] and Je-Kyun Park[2]

[1]Department of Radiology, Brigham and Women's Hospital, Harvard Medical School, Boston, MA
[2]Department of Bio and Brain Engineering, College of Life Science and Bioengineering, KAIST, Daejeon, Republic of Korea, Corresponding author: Seung-Schik Yoo, address: Department of Radiology, Brigham and Women's Hospital, Harvard Medical School, Boston, MA 02115, phone: 617-525-3308, e-mail: yoo@bwh.harvard.edu

Abstract

We present procedures for constructing multilayered cell-hydrogel composites through on-demand three-dimensional (3D) freeform fabrication (FF) based on bioprinting. A robotic 3D biological printer was developed to dispense various liquid materials including hydrogel precursors and cell-containing media in user-defined patterns. A low pneumatic pressure was applied to the fluid path to dispense the droplets of materials through miniature microvalves. A novel cross-linking technique was applied to the printed hydrogel layer to cross-link the hydrogel scaffold in a layer-by-layer fashion, rendering the construction of engineered 3D tissue with flexibility in on-demand generation of user-definable macroscopic tissue architecture. We administered the method in various tissue engineering applications, including multilayered printing of human skin cells directly onto a nonplanar poly(dimethylsiloxane) (PDMS) substrate as well as a 3D patterning of rat embryonic neural cells in a collagen scaffold. We introduce the key technical elements and methods to enable on-demand production of the engineered 3D tissue.

Key terms

3D freeform fabrication
bioprinting
cell printing
collagen hydrogel
hydrogel printing
tissue engineering

10.1 Introduction

The discipline of tissue engineering aims to create artificially engineered tissue products made of naturally driven or synthetic biomaterials with a strategic placement of cells exhibiting a normal functional potency to replace damaged or defective tissues. Various tissue engineering techniques can be used to fabricate 3D cellular environments that mimic the natural physiological/geometrical conditions of major organ systems [1]. The construction of such a cellular assembly will also serve as a useful biomedical research tool to help understand the pathology of specific diseases and thus may result in many potential clinical applications such as drug-screening and testing platforms, control of stem cell differentiation and proliferation, and, ultimately, the regeneration of human organs [2].

By constructing an artificial tissue from an assembly of cells and biomaterials, tissue engineering techniques can offer 3D cellular environments that mimic the natural physiological/geometrical architecture of a biological tissue. Traditionally, the cells of interest are embedded in or attached to biocompatible materials that serve as temporary scaffolds that support their integration into the existing physiological environment. Solid scaffolds with built-in porosity have been assembled in 3D to provide the cells with adequate perfusion as well as surface attachment [3]. However, culturing cells on or within porous solid 3D scaffolds often does not provide the appropriate tissue architecture, especially in mimicking soft tissues, thus making them unsuitable for engineering complex and complete biological tissues of interest.

Synthetic and naturally driven hydrogels have gained popularity as candidate scaffold materials for nonskeletal tissue engineering due to their ability to facilitate the transport of oxygen through passive diffusion and to integrate readily into the surrounding extracellular matrix (ECM). Controllable dissociation/biodegradation of hydrogels in physiological environments also makes hydrogels useful materials in tissue engineering [4]. With these advantages over solid scaffold materials, hydrogels have been used to provide the necessary 3D cell culture environments for chondrocytes and hepatocytes [5].

The 3D cellular structure is crucial for the recreation of the cell-to-cell or cell-to-ECM environment necessary for normal tissue/organ function and development. Stratified layers of skin, lobular structures found in liver/endocrine organs, and neural tissue architecture in brain cortices are a few examples of such structures. With the advancement of microfabrication technology and microfluidics, mammalian cells can be patterned and cultured in 3D. In these methods, the spatial distribution of cells and cellular environment are patterned in 2D and extended to construct a 3D structure in a layer-by-layer fashion [4]. For example, photo-patterning of a cell-containing hydrogel [6] was proposed to pattern and stamp hydrogels using ultraviolet (UV) light, which activates the curing agents of a polymer solution containing the cells within. However, the method is limited by the optical "smears" between layers and the potential harmful effects of UV light on cells. Fabrication of microfluidic channels, strategically laid to pattern the different cell layers inside of the channel, was suggested to construct tubular structures such as biomimetic blood vessels [7]. Although the soft lithographic approach can reliably generate the biological patterns with cell-level accuracy, it needs sophisticated production and coalignment of individual lithographic masks for the production of a multilayered cell structure, rendering the high-throughput, rapid construction of a tissue with heterogeneous cells difficult to achieve.

A new breed of techniques has emerged in the past few years to enable the direct injection/printing of cells along with a hydrogel-based scaffold material in an attempt to construct tissues and organs in 3D [8]. Freeform fabrication (FF), also known as rapid prototyping, has been applied to assemble user-defined 3D structures layer by layer. Computer-aided design (CAD) software is typically used for transforming the cross-sectional plane of a 3D object into individual 2D layers. FF technology has emerged as a new means to create an engineered tissue whereby cells and other tissue constructs are dispensed (as liquid droplets) and patterned onto the desired spatial locations without the use of lithographic approaches [9].

To construct multilayered cell-hydrogel composites in 3D, the hydrogel precursors, dispensed in the liquid phase, must be cross-linked to form a hydrogel layer before printing subsequent layers. One of the hurdles preventing the multilayered construction of a hydrogel-cell composite is that printed hydrogel precursors (before gelation) are prone to being distorted during the application of the cross-linking material [10]. The dispensing of hydrogel precursors and cross-linking agents onto the same location does not generate the desired printing pattern since two liquid drops, when placed in close proximity, immediately merge together due to the surface tension. This tends to distort the intended morphology of the tissue constructs severely. The problem worsens when droplets exceeding 100 μm in diameter are used for patterning.

Boland et al. [8] printed the cross-linker (aqueous calcium chloride) pattern onto the uncross-linked hydrogel precursor (alginic acid), thus achieving patterns with a droplet-size resolution (on the order of 50 μm). More recently, Chang et al. [11] proposed the extrusion of a viscous alginate hydrogel precursor as a continuous strand onto a bed of aqueous calcium chloride to form a 3D micro-organ. The schematics of the procedure are illustrated in Figure 10.1. First, the target stage is lowered and submerged into the container with hydrogel precursor in an aqueous solution, which coats the surface. The stage is then elevated back to the surface and the cross-linking material (for the hydrogel precursor) is printed on the target to form the planar hydrogel layer. Cells can be printed on the gel surface and the stage is submerged back to the hydrogel precursor solution to prepare the second layer. The process is repeated to enable multilayered construction.

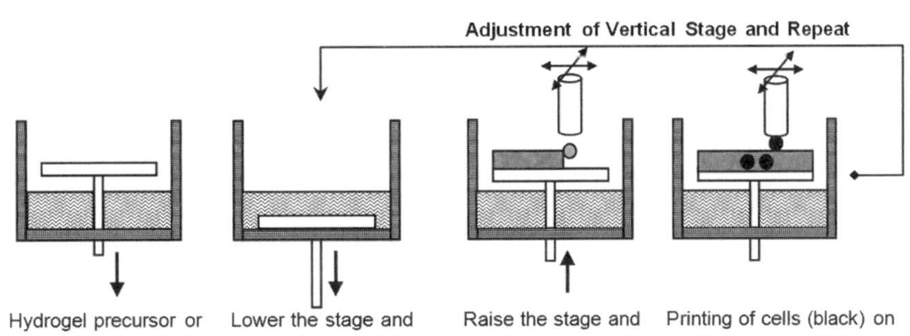

Figure 10.1 The conventional approach. First, the target stage is lowered into the container that has hydrogel precursor in aqueous solution, submerged into the uncross-linked hydrogel, coating the surface. After the coating, the stage is elevated back to the surface and cross-linking material (for the hydrogel precursor) is printed on the target to form the planar hydrogel layer. Cells can be printed onto the gel surface and the stage is submerged back into the hydrogel precursor solution bed to prepare the second layer. The process is repeated to enable a multilayered construction. Alternatively, the stage can be submerged into the cross-linking solution and the hydrogel precursor can be printed instead.

Alternatively, the target stage can be submerged into the cross-linking solution and the hydrogel precursor can be printed instead. This method carries the risk of washing off the printed product during the "dipping" process. In addition, they require a separate container (illustrated in Figure 10.1) to prepare a leveled surface of hydrogel or cross-linking materials.

To overcome the limitations of this approach, we developed a novel method [10] to enable the construction of multilayered 3D hydrogel composites. The overall schematics of the process are illustrated in Figure 10.2. The substrate surface (either a Petri dish or a PDMS) is first coated with a cross-linking agent using nebulization via an ultrasonic transducer. During this process, the application of ultrafine mists with droplets less than 2 μm in diameter is crucial to cross-link the hydrogel precursors without macroscopically distorting the morphology. The uncross-linked hydrogel precursor layer is then printed on the coated surface and cross-linked to form a gel. The droplets of cell suspension in culture media are then dispensed on the partially cross-linked hydrogel layer to be lodged inside. A cross-linking solution in a nebulized form is applied to cross-link the remainder of the hydrogel layer. The cross-linker coating on the top surface serves as the cross-linking material for the next layer to be printed. The process is repeated to construct multiple layers of cell/hydrogel composites in 3D. It is important to note that this technique allows for printing the tissue layers directly onto nonplanar surfaces without the need for a separate container to house cross-linking materials (see Figure 10.1 for the conventional approach).

10.2 Experimental Design

The experimental methods for the construction of multilayered on-demand 3D printing of skin cells (human fibroblasts and keratinocytes) and neural cells (rat embryonic neurons and astrocytes) in collagen hydrogel scaffold are introduced. The custom-built 3D biological printer (called a U-printer) provided a crucial element to enable the construction of the 3D cell hydrogel composites. The detailed specifications of the biological printer are described elsewhere [10]. A brief summary of the operating principle is given in Section 10.3. The 3D bioprinter prints droplets of various liquid materials, including hydrogel precursors and cell-containing media, in user-defined coordinates. The high cell viability was demonstrated due to a low dispensing pressure (less than 15 psi; typical

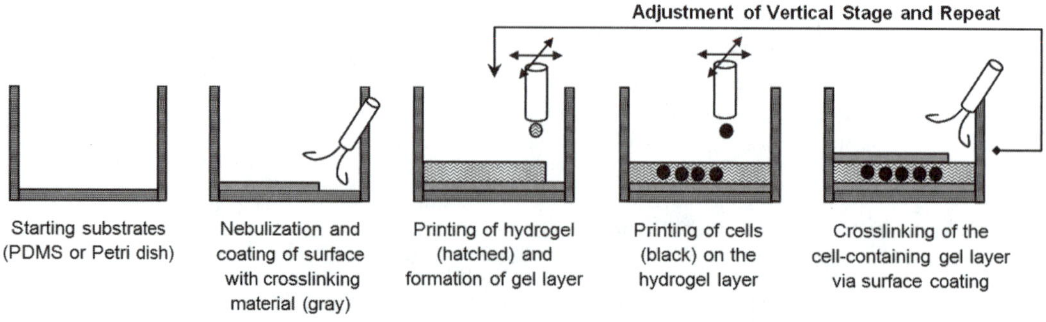

Figure 10.2 The schematic of the multilayered composition of hydrogels and cells by administering nebulized cross-linking agent on the printed hydrogel precursors.

operating range 1–7 psi) and the use of miniature electromechanical valves for fluid gating. A novel gelation technique based on the coating of a nebulized cross-linker was applied to enable the layer-by-layer construction of the cell-containing hydrogel scaffold. Here we introduce the technique to construct collagen-based 3D engineered tissue consisting of human skin cells (fibroblasts and keratinocytes) and embryonic day 18 rat-derived neural cells.

10.3 Materials

10.3.1 Reagents

- Rat tail type I collagen (BD Biosciences, 354236) stored in 4°C
- 1× Phosphate buffered saline (PBS) (GIBCO, 10010) (in 4°C to dilute collagen precursor with pH change)
- 0.02N acetic acid (CH_3COOH) in 4°C to dilute the collagen precursor without a pH change
- Sodium bicarbonate ($NaHCO_3$, Arm & Hammer Baking Soda)
- Distilled water (GIBCO, 15230)
- 100% Ethanol
- Live/Dead Viability/Cytotoxicity Kit (Invitrogen, L3224)

10.3.1.1 Fibroblast culture

- Human dermal fibroblasts-adult (frozen vial, ScienCell, 2320)
- Fibroblast medium 500 mL (ScienCell, 2301)
- Fetal bovine serum (FBS) 10 mL (ScienCell, 0010)
- Fibroblast growth supplement 5 mL (ScienCell, 2352)
- Penicillin/streptomycin (ScienCell, 0503)
- 1× Dulbecco's phosphate buffered saline (DPBS) (ScienCell, 0303)
- 0.05% Trypsin-EDTA 1× (GIBCO, 25300)

10.3.1.2 Keratinocyte culture

- Human epidermal keratinocytes-adult (frozen vial, ScienCell, 2110)
- Keratinocyte medium 500 mL (ScienCell, 2101)
- Keratinocyte growth supplement 5 mL (ScienCell, 2152)
- Penicillin/streptomycin (ScienCell, 0503)
- 1× DPBS (ScienCell, 0303)
- 0.05% Trypsin-EDTA 1× (GIBCO, 25300)

10.3.1.3 Neuron culture

- Combined hippocampus, cortex, and ventricular zone from embryonic day 18 rat (BrainBits)

- Neurobasal medium (-) L-glutamine (GIBCO, 21103)
- B27 supplement (GIBCO, 17504)
- L-glutamine 200 mM (100×) (GIBCO, 25030)
- Glutamate, caged (SIGMA, G3291-10MG)

10.3.1.4 Astrocyte culture

- Astrocytes from cortex, embryonic day 18 rat (BrainBits)
- Neurobasal medium (-) L-glutamine (GIBCO, 21103)
- B27 supplement (GIBCO, 17504)
- L-glutamine 200 mM (100×) (GIBCO, 25030)
- Horse serum (GIBCO, 16050)

10.3.1.5 Immunostaining of cells

- 1× PBS (GIBCO, 10010)
- 2–4% formaldehyde in PBS for cell fixation
- Blocking buffer: To prepare 25 mL, add 1.25 mL (5% (v/v)) of normal serum from the same species as the secondary antibody in 23.75 mL of 1× PBS with 75-μl Triton X-100 (100%)
- Antibody dilution buffer: To prepare 40 mL, add 0.4g bovine serum albumin (BSA) to 1× PBS and mix well and then add 120 μl of Triton X-100 (100%)
- Immunostaining of fibroblasts and keratinocytes: Pan-keratin (C11) mouse monoclonal antibody (Cell Signaling Technology, 4545), β-tubulin (9F3) rabbit monoclonal antibody (Cell Signaling Technology, 4523), and fluorescence-labeled secondary antibodies
- Immunostaining of neurons and astrocytes: MAP-2 (H-300) rabbit polyclonal antibody (Santa Cruz, SC 20172), GFAP (GA-5) mouse monoclonal antibody (Santa Cruz, SC 58766), and fluorescence-labeled secondary antibodies

10.3.2 Facilities/equipment

- Ultrasonic transducer (SU-1051, Sunpentown, City of Industry, California) or equivalent equipment which can generate the fine mists (diameter less than 10 microns) of aqueous solutions
- Custom-built 3D biological printer; schematics and plan are available (contact Seung-Schik Yoo for more information)
- Humidity control (higher than room humidity is preferred) to decrease the chance of drying the printed substrates; 100% humidity is preferred, but >30% humidity can be used

10.3.3 Overview of the robotic 3D bioprinter

The robotic 3D bioprinter consisted of a four-channel dispenser array, syringe reservoirs/tubing, a planar (2D) robotic stage which mounted the dispenser array, and a vertical robotic stage (defined as the Z-axis in Figure 10.3) on which the substrates were located. The horizontal coordinates (defined as X and Y in Figure 10.3) of the dispenser array and the location of the vertical stage were computer-controlled. The location of the vertical stage was adjusted to maintain the distance between the dispenser and the target substrate (i.e., tissue culture dish). The robotic stage (Newmark Systems, California) had a 5-μm bidirectional spatial reproducibility with a 0.4-μm movement resolution. The fluidic pathways through the dispenser array and syringes (10-mL capacity,

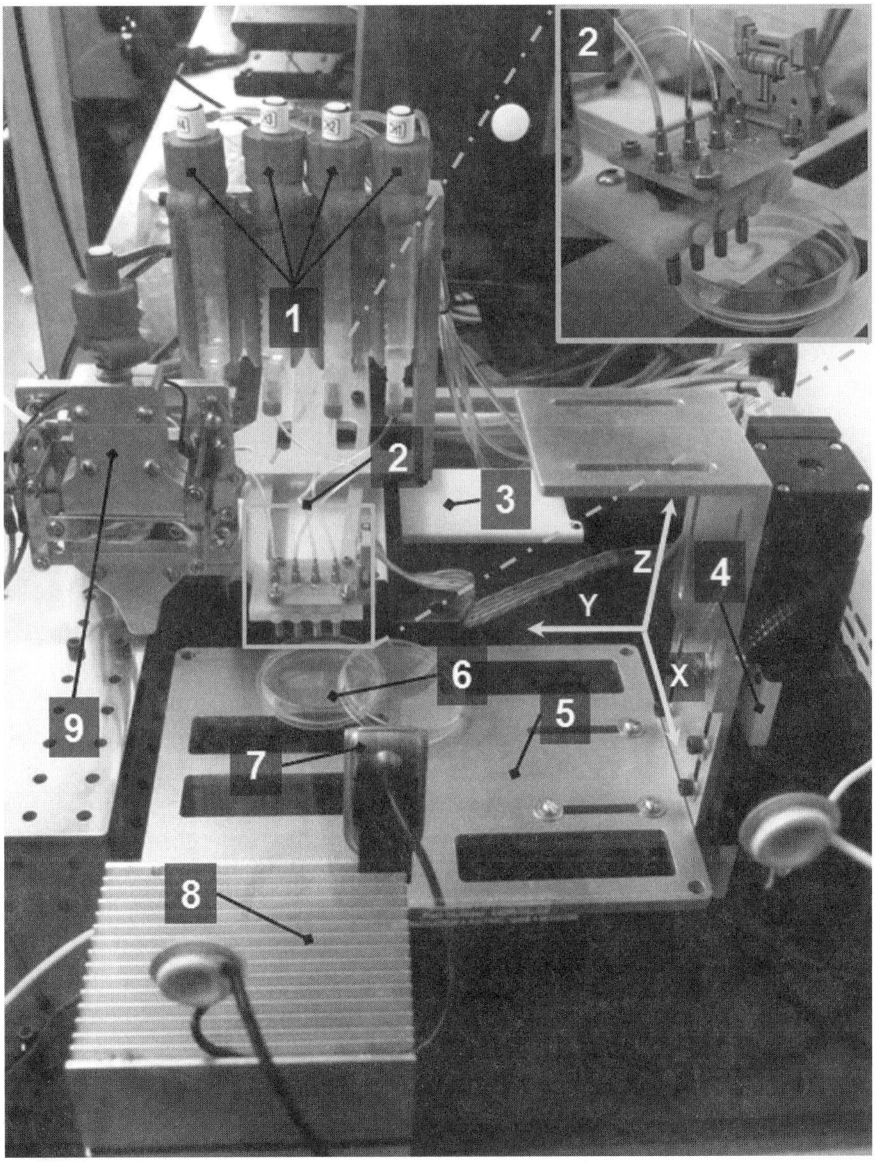

Figure 10.3 Side view of the 3D bioprinter platform shown with: (1) a four-channel syringe array as cartridges for cells and hydrogel precursors; (2) a four-channel dispenser array; (3) X-Y axes control; (4) Z-axis control; (5) the vertical stage; (6) the target substrate; (7) a video camera for the monitoring of 3D printing process; (8) a vertical stage heater/cooler; and (9) independent heating/cooling unit for a dispenser. Inset: a close-up view of the four-channel dispenser array.

serving as reservoirs for printing materials, analogous to a printer cartridge) were pneumatically pressurized and controlled (0–15 psi) independently using a set of four pressure regulators (ITV-2010; SMC, Japan). The fluid pathway was gated using electro-mechanical valves with a nozzle diameter of 150 μm (SMLD, Fritz Gyger AG, Thun-Gwatt, Switzerland) by adjusting the timing and the width of the transistor-transistor logic (TTL) signal (200–750 μs) applied to the valves. Prior to printing, the applied pressure and nozzle gating duration of the printed materials were adjusted to measure/calibrate the dispensed droplet volume. The 3D bioprinter itself was placed in a laminar flow hood. By changing the pressure level and valve on/off gating time on the microdispenser of the printer, the volume of dispensed droplets was able to be controlled with a high viability of the dispensed cells equivalent to conventionally plated cells. The printer can dispense fluidic material reliably with viscosities up to 20 cP. However, materials with high viscosities (up to 80 cP) can be printed if one does not require a controlled dispensing of small droplets (nominally on the order of 200 μm in diameter).

10.3.4 Software for the 3D bioprinter operations

In-house software was developed (MATLAB, Mathworks, Natick, Massachusetts, and Visual Basic, Microsoft, Redmond, Washington) to generate printing coordinates and to control the three-axis robot stage movement for dispensing location and dispenser nozzle gating.

The developed MATLAB software was used to generate the dispensing spatial coordinates from raw input images that can be prepared as bitmap images (*bmp extension file) using most of the standard photographic image software. One should pay attention to the image resolution and size to ensure that the pixel resolution exceeds the printing resolution. The raw images were prepared from a slice-by-slice profile, representing a desired 3D structure. The 3D computer-aided design (CAD) files or 3D radiological images from MRI or CT scans can be sources of the 3D structure information.

The dispensing coordinates were then spatially sampled from the 2D sectional images. The distance between each dispensing locations (printing resolution) was user-definable (in a resolution of 5 μm, limited to the robot stage resolution). The sampled printing coordinates were routed to the path planner algorithm (either through the vector or a coordinate-by-coordinate mode), which prescribed the printing sequence. This process is similar to the printing routine for many types of commercial plotters. The spatial gradient of dispensing density as well as the clustering of dispensing sequence (to save printing time) can be implemented, with a 3D preview function to help the user to plan or monitor the 3D printing process. To operate the robotic 3D bioprinter, in-house software (coded with Visual Basic) was used to generate the robot control code based on the sequence and spatial coordinates of printing.

The droplet volume can be changed independently across all four channels of dispensers by controlling the pneumatic pressure to the fluid paths or by controlling the gating duration of the valve-based dispenser. Other ECM materials or cytokines prepared as or dissolved in liquid can be dispensed and integrated into previously printed composites during sequential dispensing.

The procedure pertaining to the preparation of the printer is outlined next.

10.3.5 Sterilization of the fluidic pathways in the 3D bioprinter for biomaterial printing

1. Sterilize the syringes and fluidic pathways by printing droplets of 70% alcohol with a pressure of 15 psi, a valve gating time of 750 μs, and a gating frequency of 5 Hz for 10–15 minutes.
2. After sterilization, wash the fluidic pathways, including the syringes, by printing droplets of endotoxin-free, sterilized distilled water with a pressure of 15 psi, a valve gating time of 750 μs, and a gating frequency of 5 Hz for 10–15 minutes.
3. Dry the fluidic pathways via a high efficiency particulate air (HEPA) filtered air with a pressure of 15 psi, a valve gating time of 750 μs, and a gating frequency of 5 Hz for 10–15 minutes.
4. Ensure that the fluidic path does not contain residual alcohol or other nonwater liquid since they may inadvertently cross-link the hydrogel precursor during printing and clog the microvalve.

10.3.6 Loading of materials to the printer

1. Place liquid materials such as cell-containing media or an uncross-linked hydrogel precursor in the 10-mL disposable syringes installed in the 3D bioprinter. Prepare cell-containing media at a concentration of lower than 5×10^6 cells/mL to prevent cells from aggregating and clogging the fluidic pathway or dispenser.
2. Cells prepared in higher concentrations or small volumes (up to 100 μl) can be directly loaded to the fluid paths prior to printing via aspiration. To do so, detach the tubing from the syringe and split the fluid path using the Y connector (Upchurch, P-512). Reroute the other end of the tubing to a 1-mL syringe that will be used to aspirate the small quantity of fluid of interest. The fluid paths are manually rerouted by shutoff valves (Upchurch, P-782) to the Y-connector. Use at least 10 cm of tubing between the Y connector and the microvalve to allow enough volume to accommodate the aspired fluid.
3. Detach the tubing from the microvalve and gently aspire the fluid by retracting the plunger of the 1-mL syringe. Make sure to close the path to the 10-mL syringe. After loading the fluid into the tubing, reconnect the tube to the microvalve. Then reroute the normal dispensing path using the shutoff valves.

10.3.7 Control of droplet dispensing

1. Fasten the cap of the syringes and pressurize (0–15 psi) the liquid material loaded in the syringe. Each syringe is independently fed from the pressurized air tank (as a main pressure source), while the pressure to each syringe is controlled by a digital pressure regulator (ITV-2010; SMC, Japan). Please avoid the use of high pressure (greater than 30 psi) for the main pressure source and make sure that there are no air leaks in the tubings before use. If possible, apply the HEPA filter to the main pressure source before feeding it to the pressure regulator.
2. Find the working pressure range for stable droplet dispensing of the material by dispensing droplets at variable microvalve gating time up to 750 μs. The gating

duration can be monitored by a standard oscilloscope (>10-MHz sampling is preferred).

3. At the same time, adjust the pressure range based on the readings from the pressure regulator.
4. To get a desired droplet volume, image and measure the ejected droplets using a high-speed CCD camera or examine the dispensed droplet size using a microscope.

10.3.8 Cleaning of the printing path and microvalve after use

1. Remove the remaining materials in the fluidic pathway by flushing. Do not let the materials dry in the fluidic pathway. Flush the fluidic pathway with distilled water first at a pressure of 15 psi, a valve gating time of 750 μs, and a gating frequency of 5 Hz for 10 minutes.
2. Repeat the steps as in Section 10.3.5.
3. In case there is clogging present, immediately stop the printing and relieve the pressure by closing the applied pressure valve; detach the tubing from the microvalve. Connect a new clean tube to the microvalve connected to the 10-mL syringe and gently aspirate distilled water (make sure to apply a back pressure of less than 25 psi) while operating microvalve on/off gating at 1–2 Hz using a 500-μs valve opening duration. This allows the aspiration of clean water with the clogged materials away from the valve.
4. Continue this process until no clogging is detected. Flush the valve with 100% ethanol if necessary.

10.4 Methods

10.4.1 Optimization of the printing resolution for a cell-laden single-layer hydrogel scaffold

1. Sterilize the fluidic pathways of the 3D bioprinter (see Section 10.3.5).
2. Prepare printing patterns for single-layer hydrogel and cells with proper printing resolutions. To print a layer of hydrogel, we printed an $N \times N$ array of hydrogel droplets on a 10×10 mm^2 area. N was decided by the printing resolution. For example, we used the printing resolution of 600 μm for the printing of 1.12 mg/mL and 2.05 mg/mL type I collagen precursor (pH 4.5, rat tail origin), and therefore the N for the layer of 10×10 mm^2 area was 16. For cell printing, the cell concentration of cell-containing media needs to be planned in advance to obtain the desired cell seeding density after printing. In our previous studies utilizing skin cells and neural cells, 1×10^6 cells/mL to 3×10^6 cells/mL were used with the printing resolutions of 300 μm and 150 μm, respectively. Do not print too many droplets of cell-containing media into the printed hydrogel precursor, which may prevent the cross-linking of the hydrogel precursor in the next step. One should find the optimal conditions of the cell concentration and the printing resolution of cell-containing media for specific cell patterning.
3. Prepare the liquid hydrogel precursor and cell-containing media, and place those into separate syringes.

4. Find the conditions of pressure and the valve gating time for the prepared liquid hydrogel precursor and the cell-containing media (see Section 10.3.8). For example, we used pressures of 1.8 psi and 2 psi with a valve gating time of 600 μs for the printing of 1.12 mg/mL and 2.05 mg/mL type I collagen precursor (pH 4.5, rat tail origin), respectively. For cell-containing media with concentrations of 1×10^6 cells/mL to 3×10^6 cells/mL, a pressure of 1.2 psi and a valve gating time of 500 μs were used for printing.
5. Prepare a target substrate (a tissue culture dish) and coat the surface uniformly with an aerosol of a nebulized cross-linking agent for 5–15 seconds, while avoiding the formation of condensation. For a collagen hydrogel precursor, we used a 0.8M sodium bicarbonate ($NaHCO_3$) solution in distilled water as a cross-linking agent.
6. Print a layer of hydrogel using a prepared printing pattern on the target substrate.
7. Print the cell-containing media using the prepared printing pattern onto the printed uncross-linked single-layer hydrogel.
8. Cross-link the layer of hydrogel by coating it with a nebulized cross-linking agent for 5–15 seconds. Do not drench the surface with the cross-linking agent. Wait 1–3 minutes without touching the tissue culture dish for the stable immobilization of cells inside the hydrogel scaffold during the gelation before the move. For collagen hydrogel, the waiting time is necessary for the cross-linking of collagen precursor.
9. Move the tissue culture dish containing the cell-laden scaffold to the incubator and incubate for 10–15 minutes.
10. Inspect the morphology of printed hydrogel patterns using bright field microscopy. If the surface of the printed hydrogel layer is not uniform, change the inter-dispensing distance (printing resolution) and repeat steps 2–9. Avoid a high printing resolution of the hydrogel to prevent the formation of an excessively thick hydrogel layer. If the printed layer appears to be fluidic/mobile, the hydrogel precursor in the layer may not have been sufficiently cross-linked in steps 7–9.
11. Add a warm cell culture medium to the tissue culture dish and culture in an incubator.
12. Change the culture medium following the cell vendor's protocol and monitor the cell growth.

10.4.2 Multilayer cell-laden hydrogel scaffold

1. Print a single-layer cell-laden hydrogel scaffold as in steps 1–7 in Section 10.4.1.
2. Cross-link the layer of the cell-laden hydrogel layer by coating the surface with the nebulized cross-linking agent for 5–15 seconds and wait 1–2 minutes for the hydrogel gelation. Do not drench the scaffold surface with the cross-linking agent.
3. Print the next layer of the hydrogel using the prepared printing pattern on the printed cell-laden hydrogel scaffold. Then print the cell-containing media using the prepared printing pattern to embed cells in the printed/uncross-linked hydrogel layer.
4. Cross-link the cell embedded uncross-linked hydrogel layer by coating the surface with the nebulized cross-linking agent for 5–15 seconds and wait 1–2 minutes for

hydrogel gelation. Avoid excessive coating (visual inspection of condensation and droplet formation) of the cross-linking agent. Excessive coating will prevent the gelation of the next layer and the stable construction of the multilayered structure, and it may distort the morphology of the constructed cell-hydrogel composites.

5. Repeat steps 3–4 to construct the desired multiple layers of the cell-laden hydrogel scaffold.
6. Wait 5–10 minutes without touching the tissue culture dish for the stable immobilization of cells inside the hydrogel scaffold during cross-linking.
7. Move the tissue culture dish containing the cell-laden scaffold to the incubator and incubate for 15 minutes.
8. Add a warm cell culture medium to the tissue culture dish to submerge the printed cell-laden scaffold and culture.
9. Change the culture medium following the cell vendor's protocol and monitor the cell growth.

10.4.3 Cell-laden hydrogel scaffold on a nonplanar surface

1. Prepare the desired nonplanar surface using PDMS and sterilize it using 70% ethanol.
2. Get the slice-by-slice information of the 3D structure for the nonplanar surface. Arrange and sort the slices from bottom to top.
3. Coat the nonplanar surface with an aerosol of a nebulized cross-linking agent for 5–15 seconds. Do not drench the surface with the cross-linking agent.
4. Print a layer of the hydrogel by sequentially printing the sorted slices from the bottom to top. After printing the entire sequence for a hydrogel layer, wait 1–2 minutes.
5. Print the cell-containing media into the printed, uncross-linked hydrogel layer using the desired patterns.
6. Cross-link the layer of hydrogel by coating the hydrogel with a nebulized cross-linking agent for 5–15 seconds. Wait 1–2 minutes for hydrogel cross-linking with cell immobilization.
7. Do not drench the scaffold surface with the cross-linking agent.
8. Repeat steps 4–6 to construct the desired multilayered cell-laden hydrogel composites on the nonplanar area. One may need to increase the waiting time for the cross-linking of a printed hydrogel layer when the number of layers is increased, especially when the nonplanar surface has a steep gradient. Depending on the cross-linking speed of the specific hydrogel, the intermediate waiting time may need to be increased for the creation of a stable multilayered hydrogel scaffold.
9. Wait 5–10 minutes without touching the PDMS mold containing the cell-hydrogel composite for the stable cell immobilization.
10. Move the PDMS mold containing the printed cell-laden composites to an incubator and incubate for 15 minutes.
11. Add a warm cell culture medium to the well of PDMS mold to submerge the printed cell-laden scaffold and culture.
12. Change the culture medium following the cell vendor's protocol and monitor the cell growth.

10.4.4 Staining and imaging

10.4.4.1 Live/dead viability/cytotoxicity staining

1. Prepared live/dead viability/cytotoxicity staining solution of 5 μl of calcein AM and 20 μl of ethidium homodimer-1 in 10 mL of warm (37.5°C) DPBS in the dark.
2. The cell-laden hydrogel scaffold samples were rinsed with DPBS on a laboratory rocker (~3 Hz) at room temperature.
3. The rinsed cell-laden hydrogel scaffold sample was submerged and incubated for 40 minutes in the staining solution on the laboratory rocker (~3 Hz) at room temperature in the dark.
4. Inspect the fluorescent intensity of the stained sample using fluorescent microscopy.
5. Remove the staining solution and briefly rinse the cell-laden hydrogel scaffold samples in DPBS to remove the background fluorescent signals at room temperature in the dark.
6. Observe the stained cells in hydrogel scaffold using a fluorescent microscope.

10.4.4.2 Fixation and immunostaining

1. Aspirate the culture media and briefly rinse the cell-laden scaffold in PBS.
2. Aspirate the PBS and submerge the cell-laden scaffold to a depth of 2–3 mm with 2–4% formaldehyde in PBS.
3. Allow the cells in the hydrogel scaffold to fix for 15 minutes at room temperature on a laboratory rocker (~3 Hz).
4. Aspirate the fixative and rinse three times in PBS for 5 minutes each on a laboratory rocker (~3 Hz).
5. Block the cell-laden scaffold in a blocking buffer for 60 minutes on a laboratory rocker (~3 Hz).
6. While blocking, prepare the primary antibody by diluting as indicated on the vendor's datasheet in the antibody dilution buffer (see Section 10.3.1).
7. Aspirate the blocking solution and apply the diluted primary antibody.
8. Incubate overnight at 4°C on a laboratory rocker (~3 Hz).
9. Rinse three times in PBS for 5 minutes each at room temperature on a laboratory rocker (~3 Hz).
10. Incubate the cell-laden scaffold in fluorescence-conjugated secondary antibodies at their appropriate dilutions in an antibody dilution buffer for 1–2 hours at room temperature in the dark on a laboratory rocker (~3 Hz).
11. Rinse in PBS as in step 9 in the dark.
12. Examine the stained sample immediately using the fluorescent microscope.

10.4.4.3 Estimation of the thickness of a printed hydrogel scaffold

1. Using a bright field microscope, observe and find the depths of focus on the top and bottom of the printed hydrogel scaffold. If it is difficult to find the focuses, then locate cells that can be fluorescently stained or equivalent fluorescent particles at the bottom and top of the scaffold during the construction, and find the depth of the focuses under the fluorescent microscope.

2. Using the different depths of focus between the top and bottom, get the thickness of the hydrogel scaffold. From the thickness of the scaffold, the thickness of a single hydrogel layer can be estimated.

10.5 Anticipated Results, Data Acquisition, and Interpretation

Utilizing these procedures, the on-demand cell-laden hydrogel scaffold can be constructed in a layer-by-layer fashion. The construction method of a multilayer cell-laden hydrogel scaffold can be employed on most chemically cross-linkable or pH-sensitive hydrogels on the conditions that the hydrogel precursors are printable and/or the cross-linking materials can be nebulized for coating on the printed hydrogel surface.

We anticipate that the presented method will provide the needed flexibility in the manufacturing process of user-defined artificial tissues, which enables the examinations of both cell-to-cell and cell-to-extracellular matrix (ECM) interactions with on-demand cell positioning and patterning in 3D locations. For instance, in our previous study, the human skin cells of fibroblasts (FB) and keratinocytes (KC) were printed on-demand for in vivo like locations, while a 3D collagen scaffold was constructed with a type I collagen layer by layer (Figure 10.4). The skin mimetic composites were successfully structured on both planar and nonplanar target substrates [10]. Through 3D bioprinting of neurons and astrocytes, 2D and 3D patterning and coculture of the neuronal cells in collagen scaffold were also demonstrated [12] (Figure 10.5).

With the semitransparency and high porosity and diffusivity of hydrogels used for scaffold construction, the cells embedded in the 3D scaffold can be studied and investigated using conventional fluorescent staining methods. For example, histological assays using immunostaining, interactions of cell-cell or cell-ECM, or cell-based drug toxicity assays all can be visualized in real, biomimetic 3D environments with well-developed staining methods.

For the successful visualization and interpretation of the assays in the cell-laden hydrogel scaffold, the 3D image acquisition of the scaffold is crucial. For 3D imaging, fluorescent microscopy with a motorized stage or motorized confocal microscope is indispensable. We used the z-stacking methods for 3D inspections. Montage methods were additionally conducted when a wide area inspection in 3D was necessary (Figure 10.5) [12]. Software-based volumetric 3D image reconstruction and visualization of a resliced plane of the 3D rendering are required for interpretation.

10.6 Discussion and Commentary

The presented method based on direct cell printing enables the on-demand rapid production of 3D multicellular composites. The use of electromechanical valves for dispensing the hydrogel allowed for the adjustment of dispensing volumes. The low pneumatic pressure (< 5 psi) and passive gating of the fluid path were also conducive to high cell viability if the cells need to be embedded simultaneously. Although the method described herein demonstrates the use of pH-sensitive collagen, a wide spectrum of hydrogel materials can be adopted for printing. For example, the independently temper-

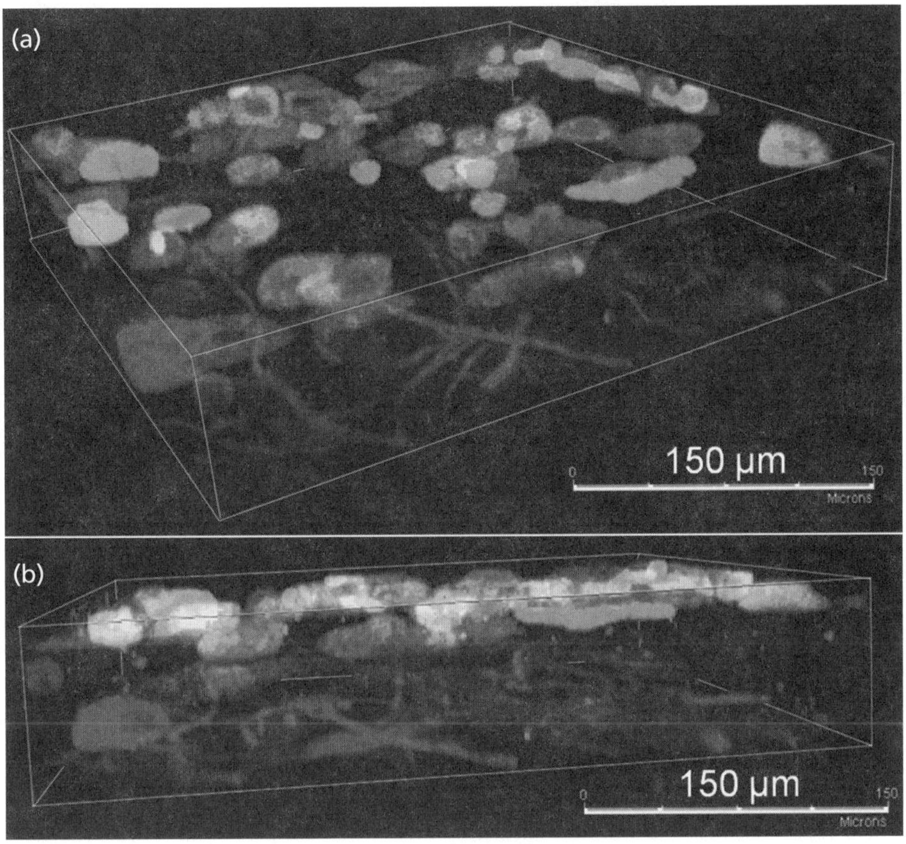

Figure 10.4 Immunostaining images after multilayered printing and culture of human skin FB and KC on a tissue culture dish. (a) Volume-rendered 3D images of a multilayered printing of FB and KC and its side view of (b) distinctive layers of keratin-containing KC layer (only the upper layer) and β-tubulin-containing KC and FB (both upper and lower layers). (*After:* [10].)

ature-controlled dispenser (Figure 10.3 [9]) can be used to print temperature-sensitive materials such as gelatin and thermoreversible gels [13]. In this case, the separate administration of the cross-linker is not necessary. Enzymatically cross-linked gels (e.g., fibrinogen and thrombin to form a fibrin gel) as well as chemically cross-linked gels (e.g., calcium chloride and alginate) can also be used. It is important, however, to note that the viscosity of the materials (in aqueous form) should be low enough to be dispensed using the microvalves.

In terms of the mechanical properties of the printed hydrogel, we have constructed up to 17 layers of a collagen hydrogel with a thickness exceeding 1 mm without structural cracks or collapse. However, it is reasonable to predict that the construction of thicker hydrogel materials will eventually require either submerging the printed layers in media or adding mechanical supports within the scaffolds.

While it is true that the printing resolution featured in this chapter is much lower than that available through the soft lithography methods, the use of a computer-guided robotic printer allowed a significant improvement in the flexibility of creating multilayered fluidic hydrogel scaffolds. Since the printing resolution, viscosity (it would merge the dispensed droplets, thus changing the intended morphology), and printed droplet volume may influence the printed morphology, more study is needed to characterize

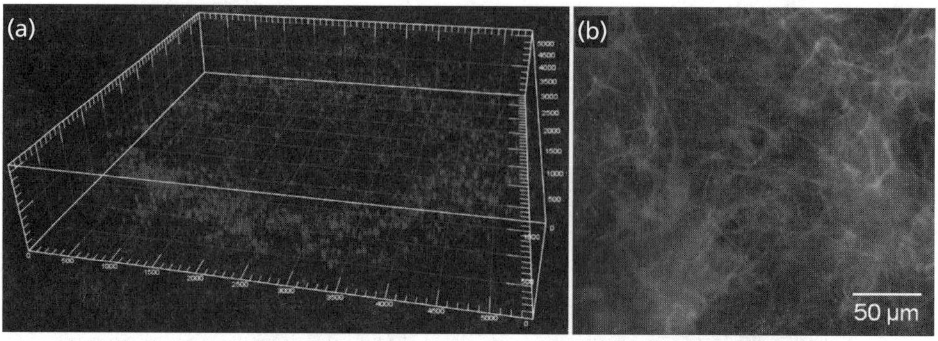

Figure 10.5 Immunostaining of printed neural cells. (a) Multilayer patterning of three neuron rings within eight layers of collagen. Each layer of the printed neuron rings was distinct from each other. (b) Coculture of printed neurons and astrocytes in a single-layer collagen scaffold (*After:* [12].)

the mechanical/geometric properties and shapes in relation to the droplet volume. Such characterization is commonly employed for calibrating dispensers used in commercial ink-jet printers. The use of different dispensers with the capability to print picoliter-range droplets will potentially generate the 3D tissue structure with higher spatial resolution. The current in-house software allows for the adjustment of the geometry of the dispenser units as well as the printing resolution with an accuracy of 7 μm.

The volume of the printed droplets was adjusted independently across all four channels of dispensers by controlling the pneumatic pressure (0–15 psi) to the fluid paths or the gating duration of the valve (nozzle diameter of 150 μm). Since the valve (with a dispensing nozzle diameter of 150 μm) and controlling mechanism allow for dispensing viscous liquid materials (up to 200 cP) along with an independent temperature control, a wide range of hydrogel materials (gelatin, collagen, Matrigel, agarose, and fibrin) have been successfully printed and cross-linked. We have printed more than 30 human and animal cell lines (e.g., chondrocytes, PC6, AML12, C166, HL1, HeLa, neural precursor cells, mesenchymal stem cells, and mouse embryonic stem cells) and tested the cell viability after printing using a commercially available live/dead assay kit (Invitrogen, MA). There was no significant difference in viability (all > 95%) compared to manually plated cells, suggesting that our cell printing technique can be generally applied to most of cell types.

Based on our novel bioprinting method enabling the high-throughput construction of hydrogel-based multicellular biomimetic tissues in a layer-by-layer fashion, the described method can be applied to create multicellular organs with embedded fluidic channels in a bioreactor, that is, organ-on-a-chip. With the integration and design of a bioreactor that promotes the culture and growth of an engineered tissue, a stand-alone mini artificial organ system can be realized. The creation of a miniature multicellular structure resembling a healthy/diseased human organ system will present a unique opportunity to establish the undesired side effects of therapeutic medications and to construct toxicity profiles against various types of chemical stressors. In addition, these mini organs can be manufactured to include different cell lines with various pathological phenotypes (such as cancer cells); therefore, these disease-specific tissues and organs will also provide an in vitro testing bed for drug testing/screening of newly-developed pharmaceutical agents.

Apart from the value of the basic understanding of toxicological responses of printed organs, the developed techniques and hardware will have an extended impact on stem cell research and regenerative medicine. The proliferation and differentiation of stem cells are known to be dependent on the surrounding microcellular environment, as well as on cell-to-cell interactions. One example of these dependencies can be found from the effect of feeder cells for the lineage induction of embryonic stem cell lines [14]. On-demand 3D bioprinting techniques can strategically place stem cells in a user-definable cellular environment with the aim of a targeted differentiation of desired cell lines for potential application in regenerative medicine. For example, based on the ability to differentiate mesenchymal stem cells (MSCs) to osteoblasts in collagen scaffolds, patient-specific 3D bone grafts can be designed and printed using bone marrow–derived MSCs. During this process, cytokines such as growth factors can be printed in a fibrin gel matrix, which allows for the time release of factors to promote bone growth and integration with existing bone structure.

The 3D bioprinter can also pattern different types of cells in sophisticated spatial geometries with gradients of cell density. This ability will provide a unique opportunity for studying physiological mechanisms such as cell signaling properties in vitro. An example of such a study includes the placement of neural cells onto an array of electrodes to study neural network processing. The processes of neural growth and development, such as neuronal proliferation and migration, can be studied in a more controlled environment, all in a 3D space.

Troubleshooting Table

Problem	Explanation	Potential Solutions
Cells alive but do not proliferate	Collagen matrix too dense	Dilute the collagen precursor to the extent that the integrity of the structure is preserved after printing.
Collagen scaffold detached from the culture dish during culture period	Surface characteristics of the culture dish or excessive amount of cross-linking material	Coat the dish surface with collagen to create a film of dried collagen gel in the sterile condition or reduce the amount of nebulized cross-linking material.
Collagen scaffolds do not gelate upon cross-linking	Faulty collagen	Test the material without printing and measure the pH of the hydrogel precursor using a pH strip. Get a new vial of collagen with a different lot number from the vendor.
Dispensing location altered during printing	Aggregation of dispensing material on the tip of the microvalve	Gently wipe the tip of the microvalve nozzle with sterile tissue paper.
Satellite droplet printing	Unoptimized dispensing parameter	Increase the valve opening duration or pneumatic pressure to the appropriate printing channel.
Cells aggregate within the dispensing syringe	Cell aggregation	Gently agitate the syringe or resuspend the cells.
Cells stained nonuniformly	Not enough staining time	Increase the staining time with the use of a rocker to an extended time.
Reduction in cell viability	Some cell types are sensitive to the duration of suspension and potential contaminants in the printing path.	Limit the experimental time per given cell types. Make sure that all the printing paths are free of contaminants. Replace the tubing if necessary.

10.7 Application Notes

One of the important and immediate applications of the proposed technique is the on-demand construction of fluidic channels within hydrogel scaffolds. One of the challenges in tissue engineering is to provide adequate supplies of oxygen and nutrients to cells within the engineered tissue construct. Soft lithographic techniques have allowed the generation of hydrogel scaffolds containing a network of fluidic channels, but at the cost of complicated and often time-consuming manufacturing steps. We recently reported [13] that the technique introduced in this chapter can be used for the construct hydrogel scaffolds containing fluidic channels. The collagen hydrogel precursor is printed and subsequently cross-linked through a coating with a nebulized sodium bicarbonate solution. The heated gelatin solution is printed between the collagen layers, which serves as a sacrificial element for the fluidic channels. The process is repeated in a layer-by-layer fashion to form a composite, 3D hydrogel block. The entire collagen-gelatin block is heated to 37°C, which allows the gelatin to be selectively liquefied and drained, generating a hollow channel within the collagen scaffold. This ability may promote the vascularization of tissue constructs by printing angiogenic factors or vascular endothelial cells in the inner layer of these fluidic channels.

The technique can be also applied to generate an artificial tissue-engineered product containing water-soluble growth factors or an embedded extracellular matrix (ECM) for the support of the cell function. Since the hydrogel cannot retain the water-soluble factors, the introduction of material which bound to the factors is necessary during the 3D tissue printing. For example, we have demonstrated that the vascular endothelial growth factor (VEGF) can be mixed with fibrinogen and subsequently printed along with thrombin to construct a collagen block containing C17.2 neural cells. The VEGF-containing fibrin gel released the growth factor over an extended period (more than 3 days), promoting cell proliferation and chemotaxis toward the printed fibrin gel. To demonstrate the flexibility of the developed system for inducing selective cell-to-cell interactions, rat hippocampal cells and oligodendrocytes can be patterned in 3D, and the effects of concentration gradients of neural cytokines such as nerve growth factor (NGF) and basic fibroblast growth factor (bFGF) on the printed neural cells can be studied.

10.8 Summary Points

1. We have developed on-demand biological printer based on 3D freeform fabrication techniques. The administration of a nebulized cross-linker on the target surface provided the gelation necessary for the multilayered construction of the hydrogel-cell composites. This fabrication procedure also enables the printing of the hydrogel structure on nonplanar surfaces, which may facilitate the integration of the bioreactor made of, for example, PDMS.
2. The volume of the printed droplets was adjusted independently across all four channels of dispensers by controlling the pneumatic pressure to the fluid paths or the gating duration of the valve. Due to the flexible design of the apparatus and the low mechanical pressure needed to print the cells, a wide range of hydrogel materials have been successfully printed and cross-linked while most of cell lines have been successfully printed without the reduction in viability.

3. A degree of optimization for the printing parameters is necessary for the type of cells and hydrogel scaffold material used since the density of the hydrogel tends to affect the cell growth and mechanical properties of the printed 3D tissue. The droplet size of the printed material needed to be characterized prior to the printing.
4. The tissue printing can be used for printing stem cells to induce specific proliferation and differentiation patterns of the cells to be used in the context of regenerative medicine by providing a controllable means of cell-to-cell and cell-to-environment interactions.
5. The full potential of the proposed method needs to be expanded to address printing of variable cell concentrations and multiple hydrogel materials along with the addition of ECM materials. We continue to enhance this system to increase the number of printed channels while maintaining the high-throughput characteristics of the system.

Acknowledgments

We appreciated the editorial support of Mr. Samuel Polio. We also thank the Chung Moon Soul Center for BioInformation and BioElectronics, KAIST.

References

[1] Griffith, L. G., and G. Naughton, "Tissue Engineering—Current Challenges and Expanding Opportunities," *Science*. Vol. 295, No. 5557, 2002, pp. 1009–1014.

[2] Whitesides, G. M., et al., "Soft Lithography in Biology and Biochemistry," *Annu. Rev. Biomed. Eng.*, Vol. 3, No. 1, 2001, pp. 335–373.

[3] Hutmacher, D. W., M. Sittinger, and M. V. Risbud, "Scaffold-Based Tissue Engineering: Rationale for Computer-Aided Design and Solid Free-Form Fabrication Systems," *Trends Biotechnol.*, Vol. 22, No. 7, 2004, pp. 354–362.

[4] Khademhosseini, A., et al., "Microscale Technologies for Tissue Engineering and Biology," *Proc. Natl. Acad. Sci. USA*, Vol. 103, No. 8, 2006, pp. 2480–2487.

[5] Underhill, G. H., et al., "Assessment of Hepatocellular Function Within PEG Hydrogels," *Biomaterials*. Vol. 28, No. 2, 2007, pp. 256–270.

[6] Liu Tsang, V., et al., "Fabrication of 3D Hepatic Tissues by Additive Photopatterning of Cellular Hydrogels," *FASEB J.* Vol. 21, No. 3, 2007, pp. 790–801.

[7] Tan, W., and T. A. Desai, "Layer-by-Layer Microfluidics for Biomimetic Three-Dimensional Structures," *Biomaterials*, Vol. 25, No. 7-8, 2004, pp. 1355–1364.

[8] Boland, T., et al., "Application of Inkjet Printing to Tissue Engineering," *Biotechnol. J.*, Vol. 1, No. 9, 2006, pp. 910–917.

[9] Mironov, V., C. Drake, and X. Wen, "Research Project: Charleston Bioengineered Kidney Project," *Biotechnol. J.*, Vol. 1, No. 9, 2006, pp. 903–905.

[10] Lee, W., et al., "Multi-Layered Culture of Human Skin Fibroblasts and Keratinocytes Through Three-Dimensional Freeform Fabrication," *Biomaterials*, Vol. 30, No. 8, 2009, pp. 1587–1595.

[11] Chang, R., J. Nam, and W. Sun, "Direct Cell Writing of 3D Microorgan for In Vitro Pharmacokinetic Model," *Tissue Eng. Part C Methods*, Vol. 14, No. 2, 2008, pp. 157–166.

[12] Lee, W., et al., "Three-Dimensional Bioprinting of Rat Embryonic Neural Cells," *Neuroreport*, Vol. 20, No. 8, 2009, pp. 798–803.

[13] Lee, W., et al., "On-Demand Three-Dimensional Freeform Fabrication of Multi-Layered Hydrogel Scaffold with Fluidic Channels," *Biotechnol. Bioeng.*, Vol. 105, No. 6, 2010, pp. 1178–1186.

[14] Bongso, A., and S. Tan, "Human Blastocyst Culture and Derivation of Embryonic Stem Cell Lines," *Stem Cell Rev.*, Vol. 1, No. 2, 2005, pp. 87–98.

CHAPTER

11

Three-Dimensional Neuronal Cultures

Michelle C. LaPlaca, Varadraj N. Vernekar, James T. Shoemaker, and D. Kacy Cullen

Wallace H. Coulter Department of Biomedical Engineering, Parker H. Petit Institute for Bioengineering and Bioscience, Laboratory for Neuroengineering, Georgia Institute of Technology, Corresponding author: Michelle C. LaPlaca, address: Neural Injury Biomechanics and Repair Group, Laboratory of Neuroengineering, Georgia Institute of Technology, Georgia Tech/Emory Coulter Department of Biomedical Engineering, 313 Ferst Drive, Atlanta, GA 30332-0535, phone: 404-385-0629, fax: 404-385-5044, e-mail: michelle.laplaca@bme.gatech.edu

Abstract

In vitro models utilizing neural cells in three-dimensional (3D) cultures may be a more accurate representation of the in vivo environment than two-dimensional (2D) cultures while maintaining many of the benefits. We have developed a 3D neural cell culture system using primary rat cortical neurons embedded throughout Matrigel, a protein-based thermoreversible hydrogel scaffold. Here we present the methodology for reproducing these cultures, as well as selected characterization and analysis techniques. Specifically, we examined viability as a function of cell density and morphology of neurons in both 2D and 3D configurations. We review and discuss the criteria for cell source, cell viability, scaffold selection, and application-specific considerations. The 3D neural models may more accurately represent in vivo neural responses and permit the development of enabling technologies for neurobiological and tissue engineering applications. The engineering of novel culture models is critical for in vitro advances in neuroscience and neural engineering, providing custom and modular design capabilities.

Key terms
cell culture
neuron
neurobiology
scaffold
three-dimensional

11.1 Introduction

11.1.1 2D versus 3D culture models

In vitro models are invaluable tools for studying cell behavior in a highly controlled setting. However, the interpretation of cellular responses in traditional planar, two-dimensional (2D) models may be confounded by atypical cell-cell/cell-matrix interactions and cellular morphology. Three-dimensional (3D) culture models, in which cells are grown within a scaffold such that the thickness is at least 10 cell diameters, maintain many positive aspects of in vitro cultures (e.g., real-time imaging, simplicity), but mimic the cytoarchitecture of in situ tissue to a higher degree than cells grown on nonphysiologic hard surfaces. A 3D environment provides a high surface area for growth and migration, which can be tuned to support other cell behaviors, such as differentiation or maturation. The scaffold may act to protect cells from environmental disturbances, such as media changes, and can be designed for physiological structural stability. Scaffolds can also be designed for optimal permeability (per network configuration, pore, or mesh size) for both nutrient and waste diffusion.

Fundamental differences exist between cells cultured in a monolayer versus 3D configurations in terms of access to soluble factors and the distribution and types of cell-cell and cell-matrix interactions [1–5], which may be constrained in planar cultures (see Table 11.1). Cells stay more spherical when embedded within a scaffold than 2D cultures and, in the case of neurons and other process-extending cells, outgrowth can occur in all directions. In vivo–like cell-cell interactions may lead to increased cellular survival and more realistic gene expression and cellular behavior. For example, it has been shown that dopaminergic neurons harvested from embryonic brain are viable longer when grown in 3D than in monolayer cultures [6]. The 3D cultures have been shown to result in longer neurite outgrowth, higher levels of survival, and different patterns of differentiation as compared to 2D monolayers [7–11]. When comparing 2D versus 3D embryonic mesencephalon tissue, more cell death occurred in dissociated monolayer cultures, while tissue explants and 3D cultures in collagen gels survived to a much greater extent [12]. Hippocampal neurons grown on a 3D aragonite matrix also survived to a greater extent than 2D counterparts, and formed higher-density networks [13]. We

Table 11.1 A Summary of the Comparisons Between 2D and 3D Cultures in Terms of Culture Configuration, Functional Measures, and Applicability to Modeling In Vivo Physiology

2D Versus 3D Cell Culture	Advantages	Limitations
2D Cultures	Environmental control and cell observation, measurement, and manipulation are easier than 3D A rich body of literature exists, to which outcome measures can be compared	2D systems may be inherently unable to depict traits exhibited by in vivo systems, (e.g., altered gene expression and growth characteristics due to a deficiency in cell-cell and cell-matrix interactions) Less compatibility with in vivo systems Increased drug sensitivity Cells have a majority of their surface exposed
3D Cultures	Cells are in proximity with other cells on all sides Neurites are able to extend in all directions More accurate representation of in vivo cytoarchitecture Survival and other cell behavior more in vivo–like	Diffusional transport limitations: O_2 and other essential nutrients may not reach all of the cells; accumulation of toxic waste products within scaffold space Culture-dependent alterations in gene expression, cell proliferation, viability, productivity and product quality due to nutrient deprivation

have also shown differences in the response of 2D versus 3D neural cultures to mechanical injury, in which 3D cultures sustained more cell death than 2D cultures subjected to the same strain and strain rate [14].

11.1.2 Cell type and culture configurations

Different types of 3D cultures can be created, including reaggregate or sphere cultures, rotary bioreactor cultures with cell aggregates or microcarriers, hydrogel/scaffold cultures, and organotypic slice cultures. These vary in terms of cell dispersion and preservation of tissue function and organization. Organotypic cultures are slices of tissue with the architecture maintained, thus preserving networks in the cut plane, whereas the former categories generally utilize dissociated cells, which reorganize according to cell type, media conditions, adhesiveness to a substrate or surrounding cells. Reaggregate cultures can be made by rotation-induced reassociation [9] or by providing conditions that promote sphere formation [15]. Although there is some difficulty in controlling extracellular components and the cellular distribution of reaggregate cultures, these can be excellent models to study cell-cell interactions. Cell models have been developed in which neurons are plated above a matrix material [16–18], which recapitulates aspects of 3D morphology; however, cell-cell and cell-matrix interactions are spatially limited. Cells that are grown throughout a 3D scaffold or matrix produce perhaps the most controllable 3D culture models, since cell type(s) can be chosen, as can the extracellular composition [19–22].

11.2 Experimental Design

The overall objective of this study was to establish and characterize primary cortical neurons cultured in a 3D configuration using a Matrigel matrix. We used both multiwell plates (typically 24-well) and custom-made PDMS chambers mounted on to glass cover slips. We varied the cell density to optimize viability for the chambers and culture thickness described later. It is advisable to repeat this characterization before using these cultures. Parallel methods for 2D cultures are presented in some sections for comparison to 3D cultures as needed. As discussed, this system is flexible and can be used to incorporate other features, such as multiple cell types.

11.3 Materials

11.3.1 Harvest

- Time-pregnant (embryonic day 18 (E18)) Sasco Sprague-Dawley rats (Charles River)
- Surgical tools
- Autoclave
- Laminar flow hood
- 4–6 100-mm Petri dishes
- Sterile Hanks Balanced Salt Solution (HBSS, Gibco)
- Ice

- 50-mL centrifuge tube
- Fume hood
- Isoflurane
- Anesthetization chamber
- Guillotine
- Sterile dissection hood
- 70% ethanol
- 15-mL centrifuge tube
- 2-mL L-15 supplemented with 2% B-27
- Aluminum foil

11.3.2 Dissociation

- Cortical hemispheres
- 5-mL trypsin (0.25% + 1mM EDTA) (Invitrogen) and 400-μL deoxyribonuclease I (DNase, 1.5 mg/mL, Sigma)
- 37°C water bath
- Ice
- Ca^{2+}- and Mg^{2+}-free Hanks Balanced Salt Solution (CMF-HBSS)
- 50-mL centrifuge tube
- Plugged Pasteur pipette or serological pipette
- DMEM/F12 (Invitrogen) + 10% fetal bovine serum (FBS, Invitrogen)
- Neuronal medium: 100-mL neurobasal medium + 2 mL B-27 + 250-μL Glutamax (0.5-mM final Glutamax concentration)
- 200–400-μL DNase
- Vortex
- Flame-narrowed Pasteur pipette
- Centrifuge
- 190-μL HBSS
- 200-μL trypan blue
- Hemocytometer

11.3.3 Plating

- Neuronal medium: 100-mL neurobasal medium + 2-mL B-27 + 250-μL Glutamax
- Poly-D-Lysine (PDL, stock solution 1 mg/mL, dilute to working concentration of 0.05 mg/mL in deionized water (di-H_2O) prior to use (1:20 dilution))
- Autoclave
- 70% EtOH
- UV
- Incubator (37°C, 5% CO_2, 95% RH)
- Laminar flow hood
- Protein precoat (e.g., laminin, fibronectin, collagen, Matrigel)

- Feeding media
- DNase (7.5 μg/mL) in HBSS
- HBSS

11.3.4 Assessment

- Viability/cytotoxicity
- Immunocytochemistry
- Microscope
- Hemocytometer

11.4 Methods

11.4.1 Harvest

11.4.1.1 Notes

1. Time-pregnant (embryonic day 18 (E18)) Sasco Sprague-Dawley rats (Charles River).
2. This procedure may also be used for a harvest from E17 rat pups.
3. All surgical tools should be sterilized by an autoclave prior to dissection.
4. Dissection is performed within a horizontal laminar flow hood.
5. Prior to dissection, fill 4–6 100-mm Petri dishes with 15 mL each of sterile Hanks Balanced Salt Solution (HBSS, Gibco) and place on ice
6. If cortices will be stored rather than dissociated immediately, then prior to dissection, fill a 50-mL centrifuge tube with 25 mL of sterile HBSS, and place on ice (for rinse steps). If cortices will be dissociated immediately following harvest, see Section 11.4.2.1.

11.4.1.2 Procedure

1. In a closed chamber with a hose inlet, anesthetize the dam using 3–5% isoflurane in oxygen for approximately 5 minutes, until unconscious and unresponsive to tail pinch.
2. Rapidly decapitate using a guillotine.
3. Transfer the carcass to a sterile dissection hood.
4. Lay the carcass ventral side up and rinse the abdomen thoroughly with 70% ethanol.
5. Cut beginning at the lower abdomen extending rostrally to expose the uterus.
6. Remove the uterus and place in a Petri dish with ice-cold HBSS.
7. Remove each fetus from the amniotic sacs and transfer to a new Petri dish containing ice-cold HBSS.
8. Decapitate each fetus and remove brains by cutting and peeling back the top portion of the skull.
9. Transfer brains to a new Petri dish containing ice-cold HBSS.
10. Cortical isolation:
    a. Remove the hindbrain and perform a midsaggital cut.
    b. Remove the midbrains and place hemispheres with lateral surfaces facing down.

c. Remove the olfactory bulbs and turn over hemispheres such that the medial surface faces down.
d. Detach the meninges and again turn the hemispheres over such that the lateral surface faces down.
e. Remove the cortical region from the remaining midbrain and cut the hippocampal region from the cortex (hippocampal regions may also be saved, dissociated, and cultured).
f. Transfer the cortical regions to a 15-mL centrifuge tube (4–6 cortical hemispheres per tube) and place on ice.

11. Immediately proceed with the dissociation procedure or follow the storage procedure outlined in the next step.
12. Storage procedure:
    a. Rinse twice with cold HBSS (removing small debris)
    b. Add 2-mL L-15 supplemented with 2% B-27.
    c. Wrap the tube in aluminum foil and place the tube on its side at 4°C, ensuring that all cortices are submerged.
    d. For optimal viability, dissociate within 2 days (>90% cells viable).

11.4.2 Dissociation

11.4.2.1 Notes

1. This procedure is typically for 2–3 brains (4–6 cortical hemispheres); the expected yield is 3–5 million cells/cortical hemisphere.
2. Prior to dissociation, transfer 5-mL trypsin (0.25% + 1mM EDTA) (Invitrogen) and 400-μL deoxyribonuclease I (DNase, 1.5 mg/mL, Sigma) to a 37°C water bath.
3. Keep the tissue/cells on ice throughout the procedure (except the trypsin step) and perform the rinses with ice-cold Ca^{2+}- and Mg^{2+}-free Hanks Balanced Salt Solution (CMF-HBSS).
4. Prior to dissociation, fill a 50-mL centrifuge tube with 25 mL of sterile CMF-HBSS and place on ice (for rinse steps, it may be same tube prepared prior to dissection).
5. Rinses may be performed using a plugged Pasteur pipette or serological pipette
6. Prepare DMEM/F12 (Invitrogen) + 10% fetal bovine serum (FBS, Invitrogen) and place on ice (to deactivate trypsin)
7. Prepare the neuronal medium: 100-mL neurobasal medium + 2-mL B-27 + 250-μL Glutamax (0.5-mM final Glutamax concentration) and place it on ice.

11.4.2.2 Procedure

1. Acquire the cortical (or hippocampal) region from E18 rat fetuses (cortices will be in HBSS or L-15 + B-27; see Section 11.4.1).
2. Rinse twice with CMF-HBSS (remove small debris).
3. Add 5-mL trypsin (0.25% + 1mM EDTA) prewarmed to 37°C, manually agitate tube once to mix, and place the tube in a water bath:
    a. At 5–7 minutes, manually agitate the tube to mix and check clumping.
    b. Check periodically; stop trypsinization if the tissue is one large clump.

c. Stop at ~10 minutes (time can be up to 15 minutes, depending on the trypsin strength):
   - Remove the trypsin, being careful not to disturb the tissue.
   - Rinse with cold DMEM/F12 + 10% FBS and gently wash twice with CMF-HBSS.
   - Add 1.8-mL CMF-HBSS + 200–400-μL DNase (final concentration 0.15–0.30 mg/mL).
   - Vortex for 30 seconds and/or triturate 5–10 times with a flame-narrowed Pasteur pipette to break up tissue clumps (any clumps remaining after 10 triturations may be removed and discarded).
   - Centrifuge cells at 200 rcf for 3 minutes.
   - Aspirate supernatant and resuspend the pellet in 2 mL of the neuronal medium (to redissociate cells, use a serological pipette, a flame-narrowed Pasteur pipette, or revortex).
   - Dilute the cells to the desired density.

4. Ensure that the cell solution is well mixed (gently triturate 3–5 times) and remove a small sample to dilute and count. Typically use a 1:40 dilution consisting of 10-μL cell solution + 190-μL HBSS and 200-μL trypan blue (let the diluted cell solution sit for 30 seconds prior to the trypan blue addition).
5. Ensure that the diluted cell solution is well mixed (gently triturate) and transfer 10 μL to each chamber of a hemocytometer.
6. Count the cells on the hemocytometer to determine the total cell number and percent viability via a trypan blue exclusion.
7. The total cell yield should be 3–5 million cells/cortical hemisphere. Do not proceed if the yield is substantially less than this amount.
8. If the neuronal viability is less than 90%, then do not proceed.
9. Dilute with the neuronal medium to desired density: sample 2D cell density: 4×10^5 cells/mL, and sample 3D cell density: 7.5×10^6 cells/mL.

11.4.3 Plating

11.4.3.1 Solutions

1. Neuronal medium: 100-mL neurobasal medium + 2-mL B-27 + 250-μL Glutamax (0.5 mM final Glutamax concentration).
2. Poly-D-Lysine (PDL, stock solution 1 mg/mL, dilute to working concentration of 0.05 mg/mL in di-H_2O prior to use (1:20 dilution)).

11.4.3.2 Surface prep (specific to plating surface)

1. Sterilize (e.g., autoclave, 70% EtOH, UV, flame (glass only)).
2. PDL treatment (0.05 mg/mL):
   a. Add 250 μL/cm^2 and place in incubator (37°C, 5%CO_2, 95%RH) for 4–12 hours.
   b. Aspirate PDL, gently rinse once with sterile di-H_2O, and let the excess evaporate by leaving the lid open under a laminar flow hood for ~2 minutes.
   c. Optional protein precoat (e.g., Ln, Fn, Cn, Matrigel): 0.5 mg/mL, 250 μL/cm^2, and place in an incubator (37°C, 5% CO_2, 95% RH) for 4–12 hours.

11.4.3.3 Procedure

1. Add cells:
   a. 2D final density: 50,000–125,000 cells/cm^2, volume = 250 μL/cm^2.
   b. 3D final density: 3.75–5.00 × 10^6 cells/cm^3, add appropriate volume for desired thickness, final Matrigel concentration = 7.5 mg/mL.
2. Place the cultures in the incubator (37°C, 5% CO_2, 95% RH).
3. Feed/change the media:
   a. 2D: change the media at 24 hours postplating and feed every 3–4 days thereafter by replacing 50% media.
   b. 3D: add the feeding media 30 minutes postplate and feed at 24 hours and every other day thereafter by replacing 50% media.
4. Remove DNA fragments (2D only, optional):
   a. At 24 hours postplate, aspirate the medium and treat with DNase (7.5 μg/mL) in HBSS for 5 minutes.
   b. Aspirate DNase and rinse twice with HBSS.
   c. Add the neuronal medium and return the cultures to incubator.

11.4.4 General assessment: staining, imaging, and data acquisition

11.4.4.1 Notes

1. Cultures should exhibit minimal clustering, meaning that there should be some small multicell clusters, but most neurons should not be in direct soma-soma contact.
2. Cultures may be assayed at different time points based on experimental objectives; however, more neuronal maturation is observed post–first week in culture.
3. Viability should be done with the entire culture and imaged and quantified using a confocal microscope.
4. Immunostaining can be performed with the whole 3D culture, assuming that culture density allows antibody penetration. Thick (1–2 mm) cultures can be fresh-sectioned using a vibrotome.
5. Otherwise, cryofix and section the culture on a cryostat or a microtome at a 30–40-μm thickness.
6. Besides viability and phenotypic analysis, electrical activity or other outcome measures may be considered (e.g., metabolic state, network properties, and gene and protein expression over time).

11.4.4.2 Procedures and criteria

1. Cell viability: >90% (assessed by viability/cytotoxicity assay):
   a. Incubate with a 4-μM ethidium homodimer-1 (EthD-1) and 2 μM calcein AM (Molecular Probes) at 37°C for 30 minutes.
   b. Rinse with 0.1M Dulbecco's phosphate-buffered saline (DPBS, Invitrogen).
   c. The percentage of viable cells is calculated by counting the number of live cells (fluorescing green by AM cleavage) and the number of cells with compromised membranes (nuclei fluorescing red by EthD-1).

   d. In 3D neuronal cultures, the viability was assessed at cell densities of 1,250; 2,500; 3,750; 5,000; 6,250; and 7,500 cells/mm^3 at 7 DIV (n = 6, 10, 10, 10, 6, 6, respectively).
   e. In neuronal cultures at a density of 3,750 cells/mm^3, viability was assessed at 7–8, 13–14, and 21 DIV (n = 5, 6, 4, respectively) and compared to viability in 2D cultures (n = 5, 6, 5, respectively) (data not shown).
2. Cell type: >95% neuronal (assessed by immunocytochemistry) (data not shown):
   a. Fix cells or sections in 3.7% formaldehyde (Fisher, Fairlawn, New Jersey) for 30 minutes, rinse in PBS, and permeabilize using 0.3% Triton X100 (Kodak, Rochester, New York) + 4% goat serum (Invitrogen) for 20 minutes.
   b. Add the primary antibodies (in PBS + 4% serum) at 18–24°C for 4 hours.
   c. After rinsing, add the appropriate secondary fluorophore-conjugated antibodies (FITC or TRITC-conjugated IgG, Jackson Immuno Research, West Grove, Pennsylvania, or Alexa 488 or 546-conjugated IgG, Molecular Probes) (in PBS + 4% serum) at 18–24°C for 2 hours.
   d. Primary antibodies that can be used are as follows:
      - Glial fibrillary acidic protein (GFAP) (AB5804, 1:400; MAB360, 1:400, Chemicon, Temecula, California), for contaminating astrocytes.
      - Tau-5 (MS247P, 1:200, NeoMarkers, Fremont, California), a microtubule-associated protein expressed predominantly in neurons.
      - Synapsin I (A6442, 1:200, Molecular Probes), a synaptic vesicle protein localized in presynaptic specializations.
      - Counterstain with Hoechst 33258 (1:1000, Molecular Probes).
3. Cell density: perform cell counts in 3–5 random microscopic fields of view and divide by the total volume of field of view. Verify the correspondence with the initial plating density.
4. Electrical activity:
   a. A 3D MEA biochip (Ayanda Biosystems, Lausanne, Switzerland) with an 8 × 8 matrix of microelectrode hillocks can be used to assess extracellular field recording parameters such as the spike rate and burst rate [23]. In our hands, we observed that the spike rate as well as the burst rates increased rapidly in the first week in culture, leveling off during the second week, suggesting an adaptation or saturation. This was followed by a gradual and slight drop in the third week suggesting pruning and/or culture degradation. This activity was responsive to agents known to interfere with synaptic transmission, confirming a biological response (data not shown).
   b. A patch clamp can also be used to assess the electrical properties of 3D neuronal cultures either when cells are cultured atop a 3D matrix [17, 24] or by penetrating the 3D culture [25]. Note that more synapsin positive cells are present with neurons are cocultured with astrocytes, and thus, electrical activity may be quite different between mono- and multitypic cultures (data not shown).
5. Cell morphology and cell distribution with scanning electron microscopy:
   a. Low-voltage, high-resolution scanning electron microscopy (LVHR-SEM) was used to qualitatively assess cell and culture morphology.
   b. Cultures were plated on pretreated silicon wafers and fixed using 2.5% EM-grade glutaraldehyde in 0.1M cacodylate buffer (pH 7.4) at 4°C for 24 hours.

c. Cultures were washed in di-H_2O and then postfixed with 1% OsO_4 in 0.1M cacodylate buffer (pH 7.4) for 1 hour and then rinsed.

d. A graded series of ethanol (30, 50, 70, 3 × 100%, 15 minutes each) was used to substitute culture fluids prior to wrapping individual gels in parafilm.

e. Samples were loaded into a Polaron E-3000 critical point dryer (CPD) and an exchange with CO_2 was made while monitoring the exhaust gas rate. The CPD was thermally regulated to the critical temperature and pressure and, following the phase transition, the CO_2 gas was released at a constant flow rate. Prior to LVHR-SEM, all specimens were sputter-coated with 3 nm of chromium.

11.4.5 Data analysis

Outcome measures were analyzed using quantitative microscopy to verify viability and phenotype and to examine morphology. After viability and immunocytochemistry assays, cells were viewed using fluorescent microscopy techniques on an epifluorescent microscope (Eclipse TE300, Nikon, Melville, New York) or a confocal laser scanning microscope (LSM 510, Zeiss, Oberkochen, Germany). For epifluorescent microscopy, images were digitally captured (DKC5T5/DMC, Sony, Tokyo, Japan) and analyzed using Image-Pro Plus (Media Cybernetics, Silver Spring, Maryland). Confocal images were acquired across the full thickness of the cultures and were analyzed using the LSM Image Browser (Zeiss). Three to five randomly selected regions per culture were digitally captured and counted for statistical analysis of viability. Data are presented as mean ± standard deviation. All confocal photomicrographs from 3D cultures are 100-μm-thick reconstructions (from 500–750-μm-thick cultures). A general linear model ANOVA was performed followed by Tukey's pairwise comparisons (p-value < 0.05 was considered significant).

11.5 Anticipated Results and Discussion

11.5.1 Characterization of cell morphology and viability in 3D neuronal cultures

By following these procedures, it is possible to generate 3D primary neuronal cultures that are viable for several weeks and maintain typical neuronal morphology and function. SEM was used to qualitatively assess cell and culture morphology in 2D and 3D neuronal cultures (Figure 11.1). Cells cultured on tissue culture plastic remained relatively flattened as compared to 3D neuronal cultures, presumably due to the properties of Matrigel, allowing for rounded cells with a more elaborate process extension. In order to determine the optimal cell density for neuronal viability in 3D culture, neurons were plated at various densities. Cell viability followed a parabolic relationship with cell density, with an optimum viability of ~90% at 3,750 cells/mm^3 (Figure 11.2). Throughout various 3D platings, it was observed that cell culture chambers of smaller cross-sectional area (~0.3 cm^2) did not support viable cells at the culture thicknesses utilized in this study (data not shown). This observation suggests an interaction between culture thickness and the cross-sectional area for diffusion that exists independent of cell density.

As highlighted in this chapter, 3D neural cultures can be created with primary neurons and a Matrigel matrix. It is anticipated that the needs of many applications can be

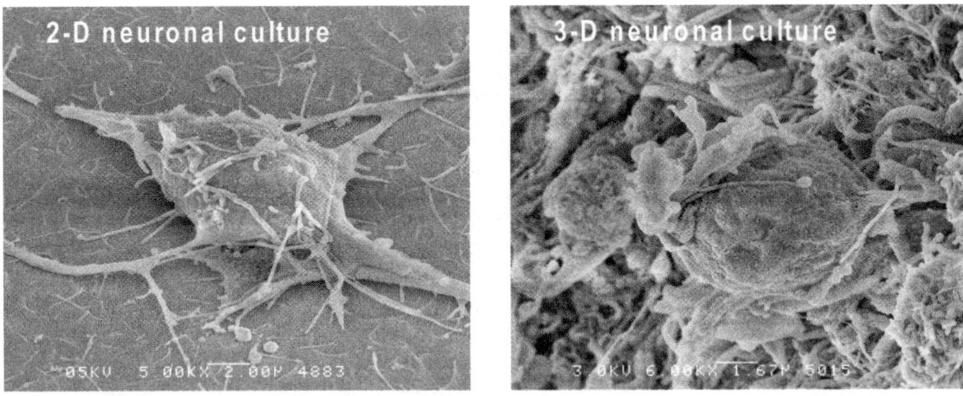

Figure 11.1 Electronmicrographs of neuronal cultures in 2D (left) and 3D (right). Neurons in 2D have a flattened morphology, while neurons cultured in a 3D matrix of Matrigel present a rounded morphology with matrix interactions possible in all spatial dimensions. (The authors thank Dr. Robert P. Apkarian, the director of the Integrated Microscopy and Microanalytical Facility at Emory University, for his assistance in electron microscopy.)

met with these procedures, but specific scenarios may require different protocols. There are several potential aspects of the methodology that are prone to variability and worth some discussion. Troubleshooting suggestions are offered below to stimulate innovative solutions to common as well as potential problems. For example, one must optimize the cell density and overall culture shape according to the application, keeping in mind that shape and size of the culture will likely change the surface area-to-volume ratio, and therefore some intralaboratory troubleshooting, outside of that described here, may be necessary. This general methodology provides an experimental framework on which to build, including varying the cell type, adding additional cell types, modifying or changing the scaffold, or interfacing with other systems, such as electrodes, fluidic support, or other cell systems.

11.5.2 Cell considerations

The 3D cultures allow tissue-like, multidimensional cell-cell/cell-matrix contacts. Slices and other explants are valuable for some applications, but 3D cultures allow the construction of a defined system with respect to cell type, cell ratios, and orientation (whether random for a more uniform response, or patterned in some way, allowing for a designed culture architecture). Cells from transgenic animals can also be introduced, allowing the probing of mechanisms or identification of a cell subpopulation. Extracellular proteins and other constituents can be added to bind to or enter cells. Synthetic components like electrodes or artificial microvessels can be easily introduced, as the cultures can be "cast" around micromachined devices. The choice of cell type is important and the advantages and disadvantages for adult versus fetal cells, primary cells versus cell lines, and human versus animal should be considered. The selection of media formulation is equally important; serum-containing media are not as well characterized as serum-free defined media, yet contain many essential components. Conditioned media are an option for some culture conditions as well, yet consistency in composition should be verified. In choosing and optimizing a protein-based scaffold, appropriate adhesion receptors should be assessed. Also, will the chosen cell type pro-

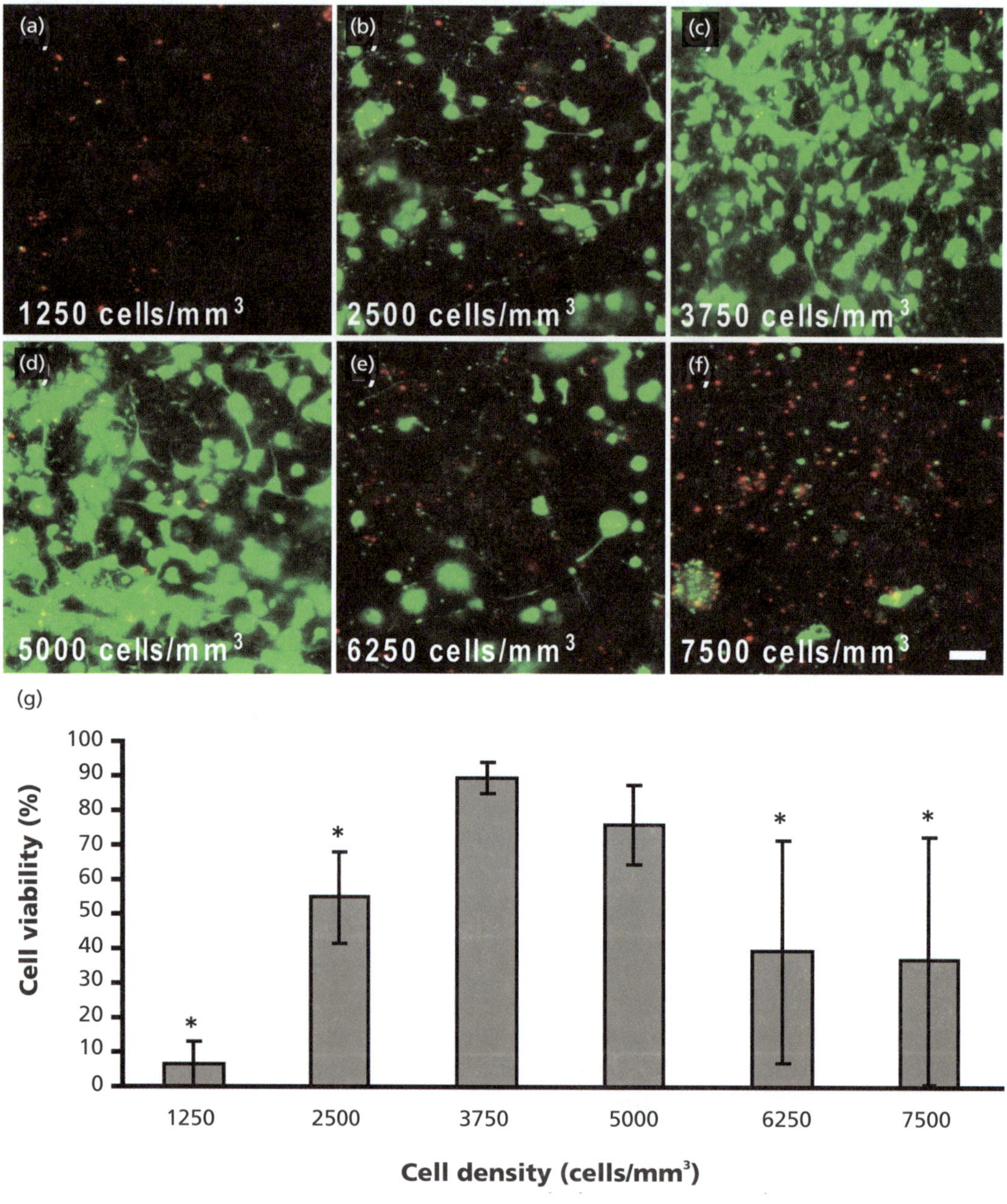

Figure 11.2 Neuronal survival was assessed as a function of 3D cell density. (a–f) Fluorescent confocal reconstructions of representative neuronal cultures plated at various cell densities. At 7 DIV, cells were stained to discriminate live cells (green) and the nuclei of dead cells (red). Scale bar = 50 μm. (g) The percentage of viable cells in 3D neuronal cultures at 7 DIV as a function of cell density (cells per mm^3). In this culture model, cell density was found to be a significant factor in neuronal survival. *Groups varied significantly from the peak cell viability attained at a cell density of 3,750 cells/mm^3 ($p < 0.05$).

duce, secrete, and adhere to endogenously made adhesive proteins? What is the minimum and maximum time in culture required for a particular application? Cell-produced enzymes and adhesive proteins may alter a biological scaffold, perhaps replacing it in some cases. The addition of other cell types is another important consideration. The addition of astrocytes, microglia, and endothelial cells may all change the response, yet are ultimately necessary if trying to mimic brain tissue. Optimal cell type ratios should be experimentally determined, with clear outcome criteria established.

The harvesting of cells or tissue regions from whole tissue inherently involves some injury in the process of slicing or dissociation. While this is often seen as a limitation of in vitro systems, it is important to choose cells that maintain a high viability during harvest (otherwise there is a risk of selecting populations other than those desired) and to have the ability to measure recovery from the potential trauma of such manipulation. This being said, cells should be treated as fragile and care should be taken to be consistent and avoid unnecessary handling.

As mentioned earlier, cell density is critical to culture behavior. The human cortex has approximately 10^5 neurons/mm^3, with thousands of synapses, both locally and over long distances. This is in contrast to culture conditions, especially 2D cultures, in which most synapses are with neighboring cells. In addition, most of the central nervous system is composed of interneurons with thousands of synapses to other neurons. Some of these neurons as well as the projection neurons synapse with distant neurons, further supporting the need for 3D culture conditions, where the average neuron-to-neuron distance is much greater than 2D cultures, in which neurons are constrained to synapse with neighboring cells. Several methods for increasing cell density to approach that of the brain have been explored. Of note, layered 3D neuronal networks using silica beads allow elaborate networks to form, the density of which is dependent on bead size [26]. In our laboratory, we have designed a convective microperfusion chamber to permit survival of high density cultures [27, 28].

11.5.3 Scaffold considerations

The neural cell culture models described here have been developed using the Matrigel matrix, a reconstituted basement membrane that is biologically active for neural cells (e.g., collagen, laminin) [29] and cytokine-related interactions [30] and has been shown to promote neurite outgrowth [31, 32]. Matrigel is prone to degradation, however, especially in the presence of astrocytes; therefore, enzyme-specific inhibitors are a possible addition to the culture medium. Possible scaffold materials (both protein-based and synthetic) are presented in Table 11.2. The choice of scaffold is quite important and may affect gene expression [33] and other functions. There are several criteria that should be met for 3D culture scaffold choice (see also [34]).

Scaffolds for 3D cultures must have a strong but porous structure to which the cells can adhere, but also must be able to extend processes (neurons) and migrate (microglia), as well as allow for the adequate diffusion/perfusion of medium components. The scaffold should have a defined composition such that the cells are the only black box in the system. Ideally, the scaffold should have adjustable mechanical properties (e.g., via concentration adjustment) such that the properties of neural tissue can be approximated. If the desire is to recreate the ECM as realistically as possible, then the defined composition should include components that are prevalent in the specific ECM (e.g., hyaluronic acid, HSPGs, collagens). The ECM of the brain contains few collagen/fibrillar components, so we must question making a biomimetic brain using traditional culture scaffolds like collagen I. Given the gelation and mechanical properties of collagen I, however, it may

Table 11.2 A Selection of Materials That Have Merit for Consideration as Scaffolds for 3D Cultures

Scaffold	Source	Description	Composition	Gelling Method	Pros	Cons
Matrigel	BD 354263	ECM from Murine EHS tumor cells	Laminin, collagen IV, HSPG, entactin/nidogen	Thermal	Primary cells survive well in it	Cost; incompletely defined composition
PuraMatrix	BD 354250	Synthetic peptide nanofiber scaffold	RADA16	Ionic strength	Very high water content; no factors added; can be modified to include binding motifs	Low pH; gelling method limits functionality; modified forms would be costly to produce
ECM gel	Sigma E1270	ECM from Murine EHS tumor cells (effectively the same as standard Matrigel)	Laminin, collagen IV, HSPG, entactin	Thermal	Primary cells survive well in it	Cost; incompletely defined composition
MaxGel	Sigma E0282	In vitro–produced nondenatured human ECM	Collagens, laminin, fibronectin, tenascin, elastin, PGs, and GAGs	Thermal	Nondenatured proteins more in vivo–like	No 3D application documented
HydroMatrix	Sigma A6982	Synthetic peptide nanofiber scaffold	Not specified	Thermal or ionic strength	Same as PuraMatrix	Same as PuraMatrix
Extracel	Glycosan	Chemically defined ECM	Hyaluronan and gelatin (thiol-modified)	Thiol-reactive crosslinker (PEGDA)	Defined composition	Not tested with primary neural cultures
Extracel-HP	Glycosan	Chemically defined ECM modified to allow for slow-release of factors	Hyaluronan, HA, heparin, and gelatin (thiol-modified)	Thiol-reactive crosslinker (PEGDA)	Defined composition; thiolated heparin which ionically bind growth factors	Not tested with primary neural cultures
Extracel-SS	Glycosan	Chemically defined ECM modified to allow for easy cellular retrieval	Hyaluronan and gelatin (thiol-modified)	PEGSSDA (reducible PEGDA)	Defined composition; hydrogel can be dissolved by treatment with mild reducing agent	Not tested with primary neural cultures

Other materials are also presented in the text. Application-specific criteria should be applied, including cell type, cell surface adhesion receptors, stability and degradation potential, porosity, and cytocompatibility.

be considered as a structural component (natural or denatured), used in combination with Matrigel [35] or other proteins or peptides. Related to this issue of protein scaffold choice, the cell adhesion surface receptors for any particular cell type should play a prominent role in scaffold selection. The issue of using synthetic versus natural components for a 3D culture scaffold is important and the possibility of developing bioartificial, or combination, scaffolds may be attractive in some instances. *N*-(2-hydroxypropyl) methacrylamide polymer HPMA + collagen I hydrogels, for example, have been shown to have potential as a 3D neural scaffold [22]. Other synthetic scaffold materials include poly(ethylene oxide) (PEO), poly(glycolic acid) (PGA), poly(L-lactic acid) (PLLA), polycaprolactone, polyester urethane, methylcellulose, poly(acrylonitrile) (PAN), poly(vinyl chloride) (PAN/PVC), and polysulfone (PS). The cytocompatibility of the material and the breakdown products should be carefully assessed (see [36, 37] for more on cytocompatiblity assays). Biological scaffolds include

Matrigel, as well as chitosan [38], collagens, fibronectin, laminin, fibrin, hyaluronic acid derivatives, and decellularized tissue (see Table 11.2).

The *porosity* is critical to cell performance within a 3D culture. The scaffold should be permeable to low molecular weight molecules, gases, and nutrients, and avoid waste buildup or trapping. Sufficient pore volume should exist to permit cell-cell interactions and migration, as well as neurite extension. In addition, the surface area must permit cell attachment and physiological spreading. Scaffolds should balance ligand density with stiffness and pore size, a relationship that may vary from material to material. For example, a decrease in pore size was observed in agarose gels when coupled to laminin peptides [39].

The *stiffness* and *pore size* of a scaffold are related and this relationship will differ from system to system. Distance between cross-links in the polymer chains will positively correlate with the pore size of the hydrogel. For example, in agarose gels, the average pore size was found to decrease exponentially as the concentration (i.e., the stiffness) increased [40]. The elastic modulus of poly(2-hydroxyethyl methacrylate (pHEMA) hydrogels was not, however, affected by increased porosity until pores became interconnected [41]. This *tortuosity*, or path windiness among the pores, will also play an important role in cell behavior, as neurites extend and synapses form. The *charge* of the gel will also affect cell function and the porosity. For example, a positive charge was shown to facilitate neurite outgrowth, while a negative charge inhibits outgrowth [40].

There are many methods for measuring porosity and other scaffold properties. The permeability coefficient can be used to estimate pore size. A slice of the gel with a known thickness is placed in a water column and is subject to a known hydraulic pressure [7]. The water collection over the unit time is used to measure porosity. Porosity may also be examined using scanning or transmission electron microscopy, but the preparation procedure may affect pore size, thus introducing an artifact into the system. Electron microscopy under physiological conditions or in combination with other methods should always be considered. In addition, hydrogels may swell while under culture conditions. Therefore, the characterization of any hydrogel should include the measurement of fluid uptake and formulation adjustment, as this may affect *osmolarity* of the extracellular fluid. The *stability* of a scaffold is vital to consistent culture conditions, whether for short-term cultures or cultures designed to support cells for weeks or months. Scaffolds can be affected by enzymatic degradation or mere culture erosion over time. This can be used as an advantage, however, as neurite outgrowth of photoencapsulated cells within polyethylene glycol has been shown to be controllable by varying the degradation rate [42].

11.5.3.1 Gelation method

The method for gelation is an important design feature, especially for those cultures in which cells are entrapped or "cast" at the same time as scaffold gelation. Many different methods are possible, perhaps with temperature phase transition being the most common (see Table 11.2). Extreme heat or cold, however, should be avoided, as proteolytic processes and immediate early genes may be activated and the transient insult may affect cell behavior. A change in pH transition, ionic strength, and photo cross-linking procedures are also common in the literature and may be considered for particular applications. Caution must be used when considering any gelation methods in terms of potential toxicity from unpolymerized monomers, change in osmotic pressure during polymerization, heat production, or free radical production.

11.6 Application Notes and Commentary

One of the major challenges in neuroscience is to translate basic findings in neurobiology to real clinical solutions. Robust 3D culture models that can be reproduced will help to accelerate neuroresearch in general and neuropharmaceutical progress in particular. While culture models are not a replacement for animal or human research, they have long been engrained in the beginnings of basic neuroscience research and yet are archaic in many respects. For example, we often model adult disease processes using fetal cells; we model complex neurobiological processes using neuron-only cultures; and we apply drugs without considering systemic effects. While much is to be learned using established fetal cultures (and cell lines), there is a tremendous need to increase complexity in a rational, systematic way, without compromising feasibility and reproducibility. The challenges are to choose the most appropriate building blocks to create complex 3D neural cultures, and to define and measure physiological homeostasis and functional fluctuations. These challenges stem from specific needs: current in vitro systems are limited and many processes and mechanisms cannot be isolated in vivo, given the complexity. Realistic neural tissue equivalents are expected to be invaluable tools for neuroscience and neurotherapeutics. For example, successful 3D neural platforms can be adopted for assessing disease mechanisms via microsampling and micro-based assays, optimizing drug delivery to the brain, and preclinical testing for mono- and combination therapies in a semi-high-throughput fashion.

11.7 Summary Points

1. Electron microscopy revealed distinct morphological differences between planar cultures, which present a flat morphology, compared to cells distributed throughout a matrix, which present a bulbous morphology with cell-matrix contact in all dimensions.
2. Viability in 3D neuronal cultures was highly dependent on cell density (with optimal viability at 3,750 cells/mm^3 for 500-μm-thick cultures) up to 21 days in vitro (DIV).
3. Functional measures, such as intracellular and extracellular electrophysiology can be performed on 3D cultures.
4. Phenotypic markers can be assessed as a function of time in culture to monitor maturity and other changes.
5. The cell type presented here is primary fetal rat cortical cells. Other cell types or additional cell types can be incorporated into the cultures as needed, but density and ratio must be optimized for viability and function.
6. The scaffold used in these methods is Matrigel. While it has many advantages and most cell types encountered by our laboratory thrive in it, it is prudent to consider alternatives as cultures become more sophisticated.
7. The 3D neural culture models potentially provide enhanced physiological relevance over 2D planar cultures and will be valuable in the mechanistic study of cell growth,

cell-cell/cell-matrix interactions, as well as the responses to chemical or mechanical perturbations.

Acknowledgments

This work was supported in part by the NIH, NSF, and the Whitaker Foundation.

References

[1] Hoffman, R. M., "To Do Tissue Culture in Two or Three Dimensions? That Is the Question," *Stem Cells*, Vol. 11, 1993, pp. 105–111.

[2] Cukierman, E., et al., "Taking Cell-Matrix Adhesions to the Third Dimension," *Science*, Vol. 294, No. 5547, 2001, pp. 1708–1712.

[3] Cukierman, E., R. Pankov, and K. M. Yamada, "Cell Interactions with Three-Dimensional Matrices," *Curr. Opin. Cell. Biol.*, Vol. 14, No. 5, 2002, pp. 633–639.

[4] Schmeichel, K. L., and M. J. Bissell, "Modeling Tissue-Specific Signaling and Organ Function in Three Dimensions," *J. Cell Sci.*, Vol. 116, Pt. 12, 2003, pp. 2377–2388.

[5] Yamada, K. M., R. Pankov, and E. Cukierman, "Dimensions and Dynamics in Integrin Function," *Braz. J. Med. Biol. Res.*, Vol. 36, No. 8, 2003, pp. 959–966.

[6] Fawcett, J. W., R. A. Barker, and S. B. Dunnett, "Dopaminergic Neuronal Survival and the Effects of bFGF in Explant, Three Dimensional and Monolayer Cultures of Embryonic Rat Ventral Mesencephalon," *Experimental Brain Research*, Vol. 106, 1995, pp. 275–282.

[7] Bellamkonda, R., et al., "Hydrogel-Based Three-Dimensional Matrix for Neural Cells," *Journal of Biomedical Materials Research*, Vol. 29, 1995, pp. 663–671.

[8] Blackshaw, S. E., et al., "Promotion of Regeneration and Axon Growth Following Injury in an Invertebrate Nervous System by the Use of Three-Dimensional Collagen Gels," *Proceedings of the Royal Society London*, Vol. 264, 1997, pp. 657–661.

[9] Choi, H. K., L. Won, and A. Heller, "Dopaminergic Neurons Grown in Three-Dimensional Reaggregate Culture for Periods of Up to One Year," *Journal of Neuroscience Methods*, Vol. 46, 1993, pp. 233–244.

[10] Horie, H., and Y. Akahori, "Three-Dimensional Cell Aggregation Enhances Growth-Promoting Activity of NGF in Adult DRG," *Neuroreport*, Vol. 6, 1994, pp. 37–40.

[11] Pardo, B. and P. Honegger, "Differentiation of Rat Striatal Embryonic Stem Cells In Vitro: Monolayer Culture Vs. Three-Dimensional Coculture with Differentiated Brain Cells," *Journal of Neuroscience Research*, Vol. 59, 2000, pp. 504–512.

[12] O'Connor, S. M., et al., "Primary Neural Precursor Cell Expansion, Differentiation and Cytosolic Ca(2+) Response in Three-Dimensional Collagen Gel," *J. Neurosci. Methods*, Vol. 102, No. 2, 2000, pp. 187–195.

[13] Peretz, H., et al., "Superior Survival and Durability of Neurons and Astrocytes on 3-Dimensional Aragonite Biomatrices," *Tissue Eng.*, Vol. 13, No. 3, 2007, pp. 461–472.

[14] Cullen, D. K., and M. C. LaPlaca, "Neuronal Response to High Rate Shear Deformation Depends on Heterogeneity of the Local Strain Field," *J. Neurotrauma*, Vol. 23, No. 9, 2006, pp. 1304–1319.

[15] Hulspas, R., et al., "In Vitro Cell Density-Dependent Clonal Growth of EGF-Responsive Murine Neural Progenitor Cells Under Serum-Free Conditions," *Exp. Neurol.*, Vol. 148, No. 1, 1997, pp. 147–156.

[16] Coates, P. W., et al., "Utilization of Three-Dimensional Culture for Early Morphometric and Electrophysiological Analyses of Solitary Cerebellar Neurons," *Dev. Neurosci.*, Vol. 14, No. 1, 1992, pp. 35–43.

[17] Coates, P. W., and R. D. Nathan, "Feasibility of Electrical Recordings from Unconnected Vertebrate CNS Neurons Cultured in a Three-Dimensional Extracellular Matrix," *J. Neurosci. Methods*, Vol. 20, No. 3, 1987, pp. 203–210.

[18] O'Shaughnessy, T. J., H. J. Lin, and W. Ma, "Functional Synapse Formation Among Rat Cortical Neurons Grown on Three-Dimensional Collagen Gels," *Neurosci. Lett.*, Vol. 340, No. 3, 2003, pp. 169–172.

[19] Cullen, D. K., M. C. Lessing, and M. C. LaPlaca, "Collagen-Dependent Neurite Outgrowth and Response to Dynamic Deformation in Three-Dimensional Neuronal Cultures," *Ann. Biomed. Eng.*, Vol. 35, No. 5, 2007, pp. 835–846.

[20] O'Connor, S. M., et al., "Immobilization of Neural Cells in Three-Dimensional Matrices for Biosensor Applications," *Biosens. Bioelectron.*, Vol. 14, No. 10-11, 2000, pp. 871–881.

[21] O'Connor, S. M., et al., "Survival and Neurite Outgrowth of Rat Cortical Neurons in Three-Dimensional Agarose and Collagen Gel Matrices," *Neurosci. Lett.*, Vol. 304, No. 3, 2001, pp. 189–193.

[22] Woerly, S., G. W. Plant, and A. R. Harvey, "Neural Tissue Engineering: From Polymer to Biohybrid Organs," *Biomaterials*, Vol. 17, No. 3, 1996, pp. 301–310.

[23] Heuschkel, M. O., et al., "Development of 3-D Multi-Electrode Arrays for Use with Acute Tissue Slices," in *Advances in Network Electrophysiology Using Multi-Electrode Arrays*, M. Taketani and M. Baudry, (eds.), New York: Springer Science+Business Media, 2006, pp. 69–111.

[24] Ma, W., et al., "CNS Stem and Progenitor Cell Differentiation into Functional Neuronal Circuits in Three-Dimensional Collagen Gels," *Exp. Neurol.*, Vol. 190, No. 2, 2004, pp. 276–288.

[25] Irons, H. R., et al., "Three-Dimensional Neural Constructs: A Novel Platform for Neurophysiological Investigation," *J. Neural Eng.*, Vol. 5, No. 3, 2008, pp. 333–341.

[26] Pautot, S., C. Wyart, and E. Y. Isacoff, "Colloid-Guided Assembly of Oriented 3D Neuronal Networks," *Nat. Methods*, Vol. 5, No. 8, 2008, pp. 735–740.

[27] Cullen, D. K., et al., "Microfluidic Engineered High Cell Density Three-Dimensional Neural Cultures," *J. Neural Eng.*, Vol. 4, No. 2, 2007, pp. 159–172.

[28] Vukasinovic, J., et al., "A Microperfused Incubator for Tissue Mimetic 3D Cultures," *Biomedical Microdevices*, June 27, 2009.

[29] Kleinman, H. K., et al., "Basement Membrane Complexes with Biological Activity," *Biochemistry*, Vol. 25, No. 2, 1986, pp. 312–318.

[30] Vukicevic, S., et al., "Identification of Multiple Active Growth Factors in Basement Membrane Matrigel Suggests Caution in Interpretation of Cellular Activity Related to Extracellular Matrix Components," *Exp. Cell Res.*, Vol. 202, No. 1, 1992, pp. 1–8.

[31] Wells, M. R., et al., "Gel Matrix Vehicles for Growth Factor Application in Nerve Gap Injuries Repaired with Tubes: A Comparison of Biomatrix, Collagen, and Methylcellulose," *Exp. Neurol.*, Vol. 146, No. 2, 1997, pp. 395–402.

[32] Madison, R., et al., "Increased Rate of Peripheral Nerve Regeneration Using Bioresorbable Nerve Guides and a Laminin-Containing Gel," *Exp. Neurol.*, Vol. 88, No. 3, 1985, pp. 767–772.

[33] Li, G. N., et al., "Genomic and Morphological Changes of Neuroblastoma Cells in Response to Three-Dimensional Matrices," *Tissue Eng.*, Vol. 13, No. 5, 2007, pp. 1035–1047.

[34] Drury, J. L., and D. J. Mooney, "Hydrogels for Tissue Engineering: Scaffold Design Variables and Applications," *Biomaterials*, Vol. 24, No. 24, 2003, pp. 4337–4351.

[35] Dewitt, D. D., et al., "Collagen I-Matrigel Scaffolds for Enhanced Schwann Cell Survival and Control of Three-Dimensional Cell Morphology," *Tissue Eng. Part A*, Vol. 15, No. 10, 2009, pp. 2785–2793.

[36] Brown, S., "Cell-Culture Test Methods," *ASTM Special Technical Publication*, Vol. 810, 1983.

[37] Lontz, J., M. Nadijcka, and R. Holmes, "Assessment of Biocompatibility of Orofacial Materials and Devices by Culturing with Human Excised Donor Tissues," *ASTM Special Technical Publication Cell-Culture Test Methods*, 1983, pp. 77–87.

[38] Crompton, K. E., et al., "Polylysine-Functionalised Thermoresponsive Chitosan Hydrogel for Neural Tissue Engineering," *Biomaterials*, Vol. 28, No. 3, 2007, pp. 441–449.

[39] Borkenhagen, M., et al., "Three-Dimensional Extracellular Matrix Engineering in the Nervous System," *J. Biomed. Mater. Res.*, Vol. 40, No. 3, 1998, pp. 392–400.

[40] Dillon, G. P., et al., "The Influence of Physical Structure and Charge on Neurite Extension in a 3D Hydrogel Scaffold," *J. Biomater. Sci. Polym. Ed.*, Vol. 9, No. 10, 1998, pp. 1049–1069.

[41] Liu, Q., et al., "Preparation of Macroporous Poly(2-Hydroxyethyl Methacrylate) Hydrogels by Enhanced Phase Separation," *Biomaterials*, Vol. 21, No. 21, 2000, pp. 2163–2169.

[42] Mahoney, M. J., and K. S. Anseth, "Three-Dimensional Growth and Function of Neural Tissue in Degradable Polyethylene Glycol Hydrogels," *Biomaterials*, Vol. 27, No. 10, 2006, pp. 2265–2274.

CHAPTER

12

Engineering Cartilage Tissue with Zonal Properties

June E. Jeon,[1] Jos Malda,[1,2] Karsten Schrobback,[1] Daisy Irawan,[1] Koichi Masuda,[3] Robert L. Sah,[4] Dietmar W. Hutmacher,[1] and Travis J. Klein[1]

[1]Institute of Health and Biomedical Innovation, Queensland University of Technology, Brisbane, Australia, [2]Department of Orthopaedics, University Medical Center Utrecht, the Netherlands, [3]Department of Orthopaedic Surgery, University of California, San Diego, CA, [4]Department of Bioengineering, University of California, San Diego, CA, corresponding author: Travis J. Klein, address: Institute of Health and Biomedical Innovation, Queensland University of Technology, 60 Musk Avenue, Kelvin Grove, QLD 4059 Australia, phone: +61 7 3138 6142 ,fax: +61 7 3138 6030, e-mail: T2.klein@qut.edu.au

Abstract

Normal articular cartilage has a functionally important zonal structure, with biochemical and biomechanical variations with depth into the tissue. Cartilage tissue engineering approaches to replace and regenerate damaged articular cartilage have generally not been designed to achieve this level of organization and have had limited clinical success. Methods have been recently developed to form cartilaginous tissue with biomimetic organization and properties. Vital to the success of these techniques is the ability to isolate cells from different cartilage zones, encapsulate them in an appropriate arrangement, monitor them in vitro and in vivo, and assess the biochemical and biomechanical characteristics of the construct. This chapter details the key methods for the production and analysis of zonal cartilaginous tissue.

Key terms

cartilage
cell printing
hydrogel
regenerative medicine
tissue engineering

12.1 Introduction

Articular cartilage is a load-bearing tissue that covers the ends of diarthrodial joints. Even in a harsh mechanical environment, articular cartilage demonstrates excellent resiliency despite its aneural and avascular nature [1]. However, once damaged, cartilage does not display an inherent ability to heal itself. When left untreated, damaged cartilage gradually degrades, and the progression of osteoarthritis is inevitable [2] (Figure 12.1). With the emergence of tissue engineering, the prospect of replacing the damaged cartilage with cartilaginous tissue constructs has drawn much interest. However, lab-generated cartilaginous tissue to date has been functionally inferior to natural cartilage, being unable to match the mechanical strength and complex structural organization [3].

The limited success of cartilage tissue engineering approach so far may be due to the lack of zonal structure. The structure of an organ is often closely related to its function [4]. Although macroscopically homogeneous, the noncalcified region of articular cartilage is organized into three distinct zones: superficial, middle, and deep [5] (Figure 12.2). Chondrocytes reside in each zone exhibiting zone-dependent morphology [5–9], varying molecular expression [10, 11], and different responses to environmental stimuli [12]. Isolated chondrocytes have also been reported to retain some zonal memory and behavior [13–15], highlighting the significance of the zonal organization.

Recapitulating the zonal characteristics of articular cartilage is therefore an important goal in cartilage tissue engineering. Developments in the past several years reflect a growing interest in using superficial, middle, and deep zone chondrocytes to engineer zonal constructs that mimic the natural cartilage architecture [15–17]. Some additional challenges are faced in engineering cartilaginous constructs with zonal properties when compared to forming homogeneous constructs. In this chapter, we address these challenges and present procedures for zonal chondrocyte isolation, zonal cartilaginous construct fabrication, and evaluation of zonal properties.

12.2 Materials

12.2.1 Reagents/supplies

- Biopsy punch (3.5–8.5 mm)
- Sterile surgical scalpels
- 0.2-μm syringe filter
- 100-μm cell strainer
- Syringe and needle tip (18–22 gauge)
- Dulbecco's phosphate buffered saline (PBS–, Invitrogen)
- Dulbecco's phosphate buffered saline with calcium (PBS+, Invitrogen)
- Ethylenediaminetetraacetic acid (EDTA, Ajax Finechem)
- Collagenase type 2 (Worthington)
- Low D-glucose Dulbecco's Modified Eagle Medium (LG DMEM, Invitrogen)
- High D-glucose Dulbecco's Modified Eagle Medium (HG DMEM, Invitrogen)
- General media additives (for LG DMEM and HG DMEM):

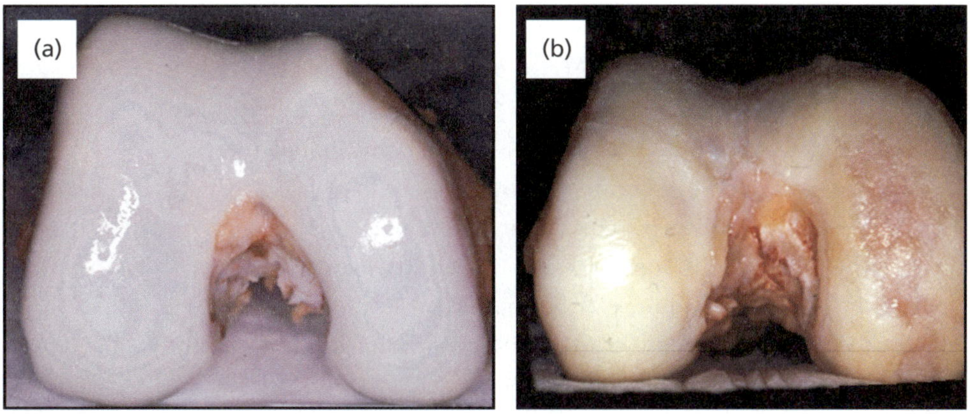

Figure 12.1 Human (a) healthy and (b) osteoarthritic articular cartilage.

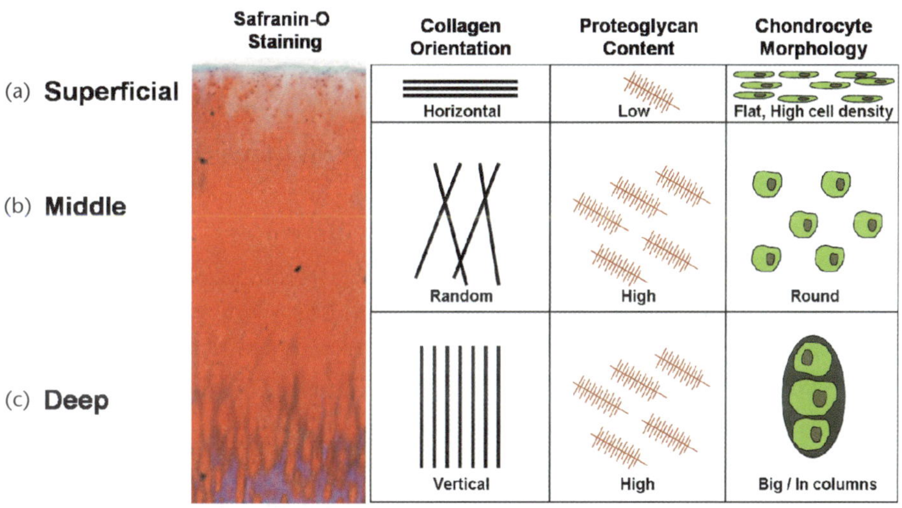

Figure 12.2 Zonal characteristics found in articular cartilage. (a) Superficial zone cartilage has horizontal (parallel to the articular surface) collagen orientation with relatively low proteoglycan content. Chondrocytes in this region show flat morphology and higher cell density compared to the other regions. (b) Middle zone cartilage has random collagen orientation, high proteoglycan content, and round chondrocytes. (c) Deep zone cartilage has vertical collagen orientation (perpendicular to the articular surface) and a high proteoglycan content. Deep zone chondrocytes show a columnar arrangement [1].

- N-(2-Hydroxyethyl)piperazine-N'-(2-ethanesulfonic acid) (HEPES, 10 mM, Invitrogen)
- Nonessential amino acids (0.1 mM, Invitrogen)
- Penicillin G sodium (pen, 50 U/mL, Invitrogen)
- Streptomycin sulphate (strep, 50 μg/mL, Invitrogen)
- L-proline (0.4 mM, P5607, Sigma-Aldrich)
- Fetal bovine serum (FBS, Hyclone)
- L-ascorbic acid 2 phosphate tri-sodium salt (ascorbic acid, WAKO)
- Bovine serum albumin (BSA, A4919, Sigma-Aldrich)
- Dexamethasone (Dex, Sigma-Aldrich)

- ITS+1 (Sigma-Aldrich)
- Transforming growth factor-β1 (TGF-β1, Sigma-Aldrich)
- 0.25% trypsin with 1-mM EDTA (trypsin-EDTA, Invitrogen)
- PRONOVA UP LVG sodium alginate (FMC BioPolymer)
- High viscosity sodium alginate (ISP)
- Sterilized filter paper (Whatman #1)
- PKH26 Red Fluorescent Cell Linker Kit (Sigma-Aldrich)
- Monensin sodium salt (Sigma-Aldrich)
- Monoclonal mouse IgG antibovine proteoglycan 4 antibody 3A4 (Professor Bruce Caterson, Cardiff University)
- R-phycoerythrin-conjugated goat antimouse secondary antibody (Invitrogen)
- UltraPure DNase/RNase-Free Distilled Water (Invitrogen)
- RNeasy Micro Kit (Qiagen)
- β-Mercaptoethanol for electrophoresis >= 98% (β-ME, Sigma-Aldrich)
- 1.5-ml DNA low binding tubes (Eppendorf)
- Agarose LE (Roche)
- SuperScript III first-strand synthesis supermix for qRT-PCR (Invitrogen)
- 0.2-ml PCR tubes (Eppendorf)
- Platinum *Taq* DNA Polymerase kit (Invitrogen)
- DNA Molecular Weight Marker XIV, 100 base pair ladder (Roche)
- QIAquick Gel Extraction Kit (Qiagen)
- Quant-iT PicoGreen dsDNA assay kit (Invitrogen)
- Express SYBR GreenER qPCR supermix universal (Invitrogen)
- 384-well PCR plates (Applied Biosystems)
- Tissue-Tek O.C.T. compound (Sakura Finetek)
- Tissue-Tek Cryomold 25 × 20 × 5 mm (Sakura Finetek)
- Menzel SuperFrost Plus microscope slides (Thermo Fisher Scientific)
- Phosphate-buffered saline solution (PBS; 10 mM Na_2HPO_4, 0.9% w/v NaCl, pH 7.5)
- Polyclonal rabbit IgG antihuman lubricin (proteoglycan 4) antibody (Abcam ab28484)
- IgG matched control antibody (Abcam ab37415)
- VECTASTAIN Elite ABC-Peroxidase kit (Vector Laboratories)
- Vector ImmPACT DAB substrate (Vector Laboratories)
- Mayer's hematoxylin (Amber Scientific)
- Crystal Mount aqueous mounting medium (Sigma-Aldrich)
- Cover slips (Paul Marienfeld)

12.2.2 Facilities/equipment

- Cell culture facility
- Osteochondral Autograft Transfer System (OATS, Arthrex)
- Sledge microtome (HM440E, Microm)

- Custom-made alginate disk mold (disk diameter: 4–6 mm, thickness: 1.5–2 mm)
- Bioprinter (e.g., BioScaffolder from SYS+ENG)
- Flow cytometer (e.g., FC500 from Beckman Coulter)
- Fluorescence microscope
- Nanodrop ND-1000 spectrophotometer (Thermo Scientific)
- Peltier Thermal Cycler PTC 200 (MJ Research)
- Applied Biosystems 7900HT Fast Real-Time PCR System, Applied Biosystems
- CM1850 cryostat (Leica Microsystems)

12.3 Methods

12.3.1 Obtaining and tracking zonal chondrocytes

12.3.1.1 Zonal cartilage harvest

Microtome sectioning [15]

1. Clamp the joint securely and remove osteochondral cylinders using the OATS perpendicular to the articular surface or using a surgical saw to obtain a relatively flat surface. Maintain an aseptic environment at all times and irrigate with PBS– supplemented with pen/strep to minimize the chance of contamination.
2. Set up a sledge microtome. Sterilize the blade of the microtome. Mount the osteochondral block on the microtome chuck with the cartilage side up. Align the block with the knife edge and section in 100–200-μm-thick sections to obtain superficial, middle, and deep cartilage. Collect slices from different zones in separate wells of a 6-well plate with PBS– containing pen/strep. Note that the thickness of the superficial, middle, and deep zones vary between regions of the body, species, and different research groups; be internally consistent.

Core sectioning (Figure 12.3)

1. Obtain full-thickness cartilage cores perpendicular to the articular surface using a biopsy punch under aseptic conditions. Punch to the calcified cartilage and remove cores by slicing along the calcified cartilage.
2. Firmly hold the cores with the forceps and gently section superficial (top 10–20%), middle (40–45%), and deep (40–45%) layers using a scalpel blade.
3. Keep the sample moist at all times using sterile PBS– supplemented with pen/strep.

Direct slicing [10, 13]

1. While holding the scalpel blade nearly parallel to the cartilage surface, gently slice out a thin strip of superficial layer cartilage (top 10–20%) starting from one edge with a continuous zigzag motion.
2. Ensure that the superficial strip being sliced out is relatively transparent and uniform in thickness. The region where the superficial layer has been removed will be slightly rougher, with less gloss compared to the untouched parts.
3. Once the entire superficial layer is removed, continue slicing down to the middle and deep layers in the same manner.

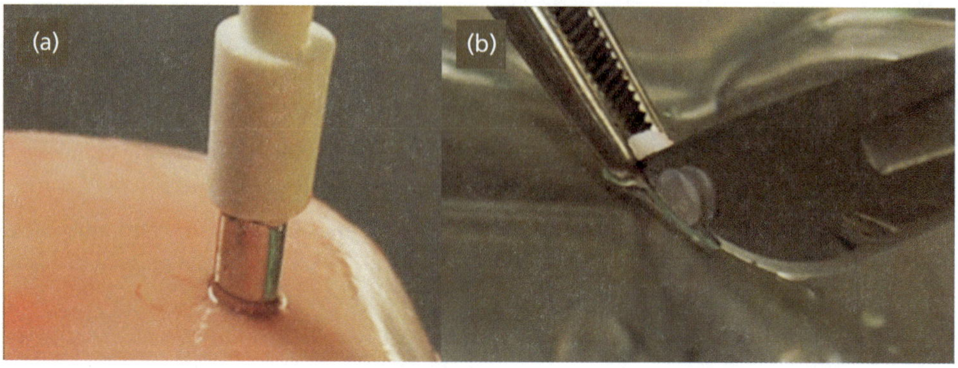

Figure 12.3 Core sectioning. (a) Full-thickness cores are taken from the articular cartilage using a 4-mm biopsy punch. (b) Cartilage cores are sectioned using surgical scalpel blade into superficial (10–20%), middle (40–45%), and deep layers (40–45%).

4. Keep the sample moist at all times with sterile PBS– supplemented with pen/strep.

Zonal abrasion [18]

1. Holding the scalpel blade perpendicular to the cartilage surface, firmly scrape the cartilage with constant force.
2. Repeat step 1 four times to fully remove the superficial zone.
3. Once all the superficial zone cartilage is taken, harvest the middle and deep layers by slicing.

12.3.1.2 Zonal chondrocyte isolation and expansion

1. Rinse the zonal cartilage with PBS– containing the Penicillin/Streptomycin antibiotic solution. Dice slices using a sterile scalpel (~1 mm^3).
2. Weigh collagenase type 2 and resuspend in LG DMEM to a concentration of 0.15%, and filter the collagenase solution using a 0.2-μm syringe filter. Warm the solution to 37°C.
3. Determine the wet weight of cartilage. Add approximately 10 mL of the collagenase solution for every gram of cartilage tissue. Place the sterile stir bar into the cup and stir in the incubator at 52 rpm for 16 hours.
4. Once digested, pass the solution through a 100-μm cell strainer into 50-mL falcon tubes and rinse three times with 20 mL of PBS–. Centrifuge the tubes at 750 × g for 5 minutes at room temperature to obtain the cell pellets. After aspirating out the supernatant, wash the cells by resuspending in PBS– and centrifuge. Resuspend in LG DMEM supplemented with 10% FBS and 0.1-mM ascorbic acid (expansion media) and count using the Trypan blue exclusion test and a hemocytometer.

Cells can be further expanded using standard protocols for monolayer cultures and cell passaging. Note that chondrocytes begin to lose their chondrogenic phenotype with the extended monolayer culture, and recovery of the differentiated state in a hydrogel is delayed with a prolonged expansion time [19].

1. Seed cells at a low density (e.g., 3,000 cells per cm^2) in tissue culture flasks.
2. Refresh with expansion media twice a week.
3. At subconfluency, wash the cell layer with PBS– to remove the serum components.
4. Treat with a thin layer of 0.25% trypsin-EDTA.
5. Stop the trypsin action with LG DMEM-10% FBS.
6. Centrifuge 700 × g for 5 minutes to form a cell pellet and resuspend the cells in LG DMEM-10% FBS.
7. Count the cells using a hemocytometer.

12.3.1.3 Cell labeling

One important issue with zonal constructs, in comparison to homogeneous constructs, is tracking the cells from each zone to establish their localization and function after the culture and/or implantation. Ideally, cells from the different zones should all be labeled with different colors such that they can be localized at the end of the experiment. For short-term (days) cultures, cells can be labeled with cytoplasmic dyes (CellTracker, Invitrogen). For longer-term (a few weeks) cultures and short-term in vivo studies, photostable quantum dots (QTracker, Invitrogen) or membrane dyes such as PKH26 (Sigma) can be used. For long-term (months) cultures and in vivo studies, cells transfected to express fluorescent proteins should be used to avoid a loss of fluorescence that is not associated with a loss of cells. Here, we provide a protocol that has been used to stain the chondrocytes for in vitro [20, 21] and in vivo [22] studies.

1. Isolate the cells using your standard cell passaging protocol (Section 12.3.1.2), and wash once with LG DMEM.
2. Resuspend the cells in 1 mL of dilution buffer (Diluent C, provided with the PKH26 kit).
3. Combine the cell suspension with 1 mL of 2× (40 μM) PKH26 in a dilution buffer and incubate for 5 minutes at room temperature, with a periodic mixing of the tube.
4. Stop the reaction with 2-mL FBS and incubate for 1 minute.
5. Wash twice with 5-mL LG DMEM-10% FBS to obtain viable fluorescent cells that can be plated or incorporated in tissue-engineered constructs. Cells will halve their fluorescence upon dividing, so it is best to keep the labeling step as close as possible to the construct formation.

12.3.2 Zonal construct formation

12.3.2.1 Cell encapsulation and alginate disk formation (Figure 12.4)

1. Make a 2% alginate solution by dissolving sodium alginate (FMC) in PBS– in a warm water bath, followed by a 0.2-μm syringe filtration.
2. Make a 102-mM $CaCl_2$ solution and sterilize. HEPES (20 mM) can be added to stabilize the pH.
3. Spin down freshly isolated or passaged chondrocytes with a known cell number at 750 × g for 5 minutes. Aspirate the supernatant and discard. Resuspend the chondrocyte pellet in 2% alginate at a desired concentration (e.g., 10^7 cells/mL alginate).

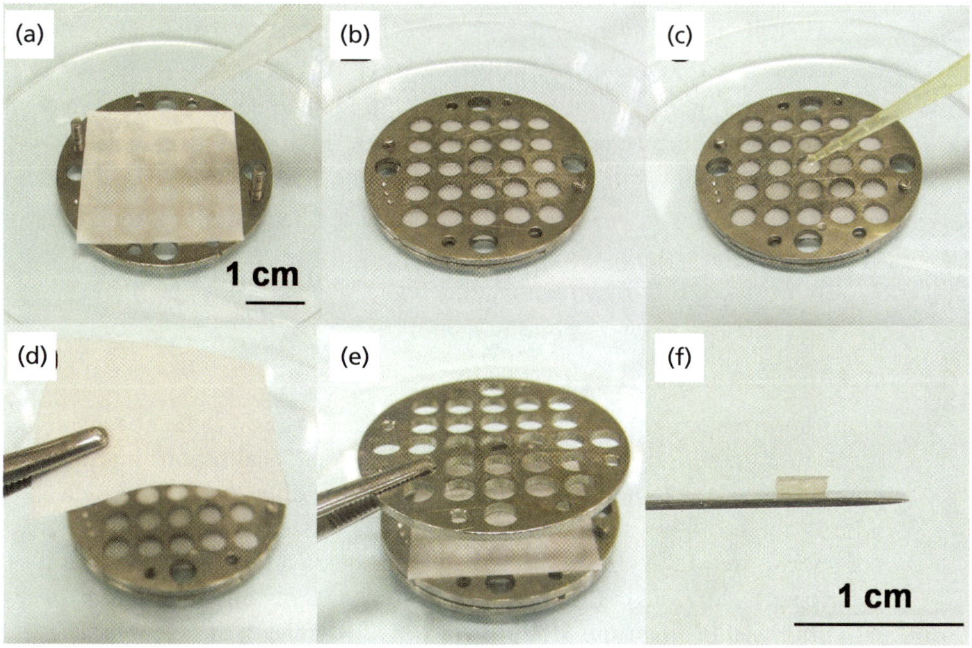

Figure 12.4 Making the alginate disks. (a) Autoclaved filter paper is soaked with 102-mM $CaCl_2$. (b) The disk mold is put directly on top of the wet filter paper. (c) The chondrocyte/alginate mixture is gently pipetted into the mold. (d) Mold is covered with filter paper soaked in $CaCl_2$. (e) The lid is fastened to the mold with screws. The mold is then immersed in $CaCl_2$ for 10 minutes. (f) The alginate disk is released from the mold.

4. Fabricate a mold by drilling holes with the desired disk diameter through a stainless steel or polysulfone sheet (1–2 mm); clean and autoclave.
5. Soak a sterile filter paper with 102-mM $CaCl_2$, and lay it under the mold.
6. Gently pipette the chondrocyte/alginate mixture into the wells of the mold, while avoiding bubble formation and ensuring that the alginate mixture does not leak through the bottom.
7. Once all the wells are loaded with the alginate mixture, cover the mold top with another filter paper soaked in 102-mM $CaCl_2$. Gently hold down the filter paper with a porous metal piece, and let it soak in $CaCl_2$ for 10 minutes to cross-link.
8. Remove the disks from the mold and transfer to a well-plate. Wash with PBS+.
9. Culture the alginate gels in a serum-free chondrogenic differentiation medium (HG DMEM, 1.25-mg/mL BSA, 10^{-7} M Dex, 1% ITS+1, 0.1-mM ascorbic acid, 10 ng/mL TGF-β1) [23, 24].

12.3.2.2 Combination of alginate disks to form layered constructs (Figure 12.5)

1. Line a Petri dish with dry sterile filter paper and wet it with a few drops of 200-mM EDTA. Filter paper should not be too wet; otherwise, a meniscus will form when an alginate disk is placed on top.
2. Transfer the zonal alginate constructs on the wet filter paper and leave for 1–2 minutes to partially dissolve the alginate disks.

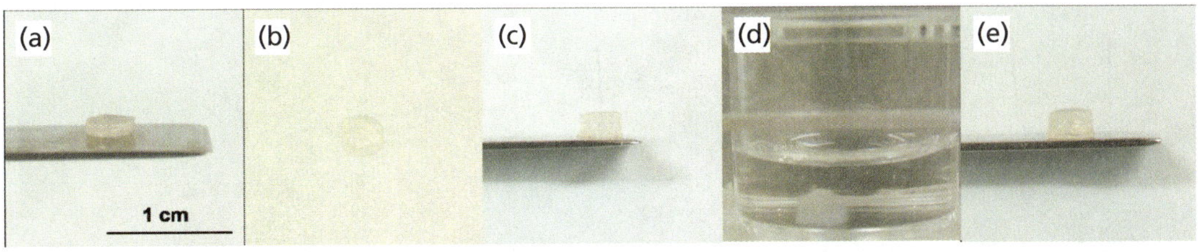

Figure 12.5 Combining alginate disks to form zonal constructs. (s) Zonal chondrocytes encapsulated in alginate disks. (b) Sterile filter paper is soaked in 200-mM EDTA and transferred to a Petri dish. Zonal constructs are put on top of the wet filter paper. (c) Zonal constructs are combined by placing the sticky (dissolved) sides together. (d) Combined construct is immersed in $CaCl_2$ for 5 minutes. (e) The constructs are rinsed briefly in PBS+ and transferred into the differentiation media.

3. On a separate Petri dish, arrange the zonal constructs together so that the sticky (dissolved) sides are put together. Cross-link the construct by immersing in 102-mM $CaCl_2$ for 5 minutes.
4. Briefly rinse the combined construct with PBS+ and culture it in a chondrogenic differentiation medium.

12.3.2.3 Cell printing (Figure 12.6)

Bioprinting technologies use computer-aided systems to produce structurally defined cartilaginous tissue constructs. Such systems can be used to print zonal cartilaginous constructs layer by layer, containing cells from different zones of the articular cartilage while maintaining their viability. One of the advantages of cell printing is the ability to fabricate hydrogel constructs with open porous structure. As a result, the thickness of the construct is not nutrient-limited to 1–2 mm.

1. Prepare the alginate solution by dissolving a high-viscosity alginate powder (10% v/v, ISP) in a culture medium at 37°C.
2. Gently mix isolated zonal cells with alginate ($1–10*10^6$ cells/mL) and avoid the formation of bubbles. Note that different families of hydrogels can be used for cell printing; these include alginates [25] as well as thermo- and photo-cross-linkable hydrogels [26].
3. Transfer the cell suspensions to 50-mL syringes and place these cartridges in the bioprinter or another three-axis dispensing system (e.g., BioScaffolder; SYS+ENG).
4. Load a scaffold model of 10 × 10 mm via the CAD/CAM software (e.g., PrimCam), which translates this information for the layer-by-layer fiber deposition by the machine. By using an inner nozzle diameter of 210 μm and varying pressure (1–2 bars) and deposition speeds (100–300 mm/min), the fiber thickness can be tailored [27].
5. Print the construct in a Petri dish and cross-link the construct for 10 minutes in 102-mM $CaCl_2$ solution.
6. Culture the constructs in a serum-free chondrogenic differentiation medium (HG DMEM, 1.25 mg/mL BSA, 10^{-7} M Dex, 1% ITS+1, 0.1-mM ascorbic acid, 10 ng/mL TGF-β1) [23, 24].

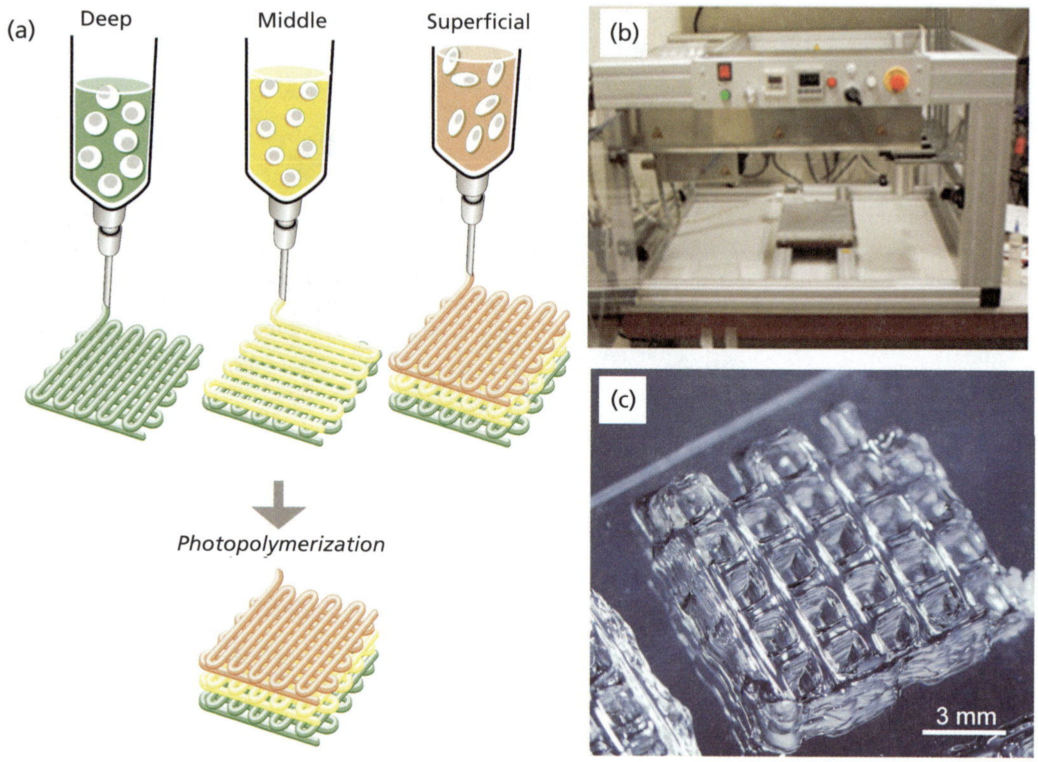

Figure 12.6 (a) Concept for printing zonal constructs where chondrocytes from the deep, middle, and superficial zones are suspended in distinct hydrogel precursors and printed using bioprinting technologies in defined geometries. Cells suspended in alginate can be loaded into the cartridges. (b) Constructs, based on CAD drawings, can then be printed using the multiple print heads of the Bioscaffolder, which contain cells from different zones. (c) Printing of multiple layers results in a thick hydrogel with defined pores throughout. (Adapted from [28].)

12.3.3 Analyses

12.3.3.1 Cell purity

Given appropriate cellular markers, flow cytometry can be used to characterize the purity of the isolated zonal chondrocytes and how these populations change with time in culture (Figure 12.7). The preferred zonal marker at this time is proteoglycan 4 (PRG4), which identifies chondrocytes from the superficial zone. However, this is a secreted molecule, necessitating special procedures for its detection by flow cytometry (see steps 1 and 3).

1. Treat cells with 10^{-7} M monensin for 16 hours prior to harvest to retain newly synthesized PRG4 in the cells.
2. Harvest the cells using your standard protocol for cell passaging (Section 12.3.1.2).
3. Transfer = 10^5 cells to a 1.5-ml tube and centrifuge 400 × g for 5 minutes to form a cell pellet. Keep the number of cells constant for all samples. Include cells from each zone for PRG4 staining and IgG controls.
4. Fix and permeabilize your cells. One simple method for this is to add 1-ml ice-cold methanol to each tube and mix with a pipette. Incubate samples at 4°C for 15 minutes on a rocker plate.

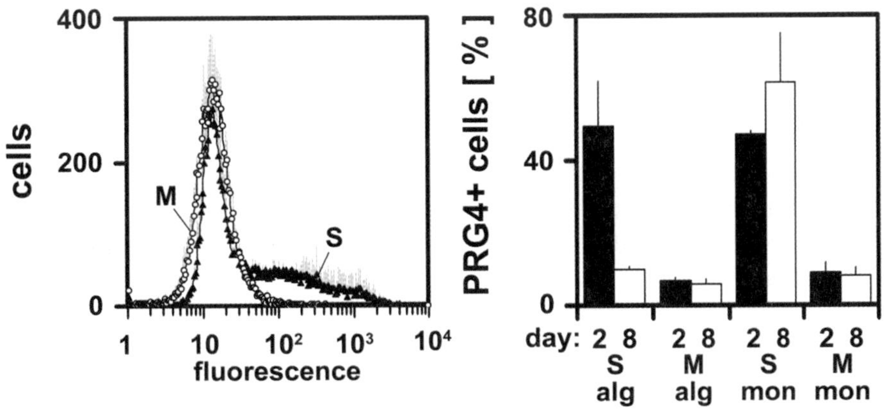

(a) (b)

Figure 12.7 Proteoglycan 4 (PRG4) expression by bovine chondrocytes from the superficial (S) and middle (M) zone during alginate (alg) and monolayer (mon) culture. (a) Flow cytometric analysis of monensin-treated cells for PRG4 on day 2 of monolayer culture ($n = 2$, mean ± SD). (b) Percentage of PRG4-expressing cells ($n = 4$, mean ± SEM), determined by immunocytochemistry, at days 2 and 8 of an alginate and monolayer culture (**p < 0.01, ***p < 0.001). (Reprinted from [29].)

5. Centrifuge the samples at 400g for 5 minutes and decant supernatant.
6. Add 1 ml of primary antibody (for 10^6 cells) in cold PBS-3% BSA to each sample, and incubate for 50 minutes at 37°C on a rocker/shaker. For bovine chondrocytes, the primary antibody 3A4 (Professor Bruce Caterson) can be used at a 1:2,000 dilution.
7. Centrifuge the samples for 5 minutes at 400 × g, decant the supernatant, and wash the cells twice with PBS-3% BSA.
8. Resuspend cells in 1 ml of a fluorescent-conjugated secondary antibody, diluted to the manufacturer's specifications in PBS-3% BSA, and incubate for 50 minutes at 4°C on a rocker/shaker.
9. Centrifuge the samples for 5 minutes at 400 × g, decant the supernatant, and wash the cells twice with PBS-3% BSA.
10. Resuspend the cell pellet in PBS-3% BSA.
11. Analyze 10,000 cells on a flow cytometer such as FC500 Flow Cytometer (Beckman Coulter), with appropriate filters for your secondary antibody.
12. You will likely end up with a bimodal distribution of cells representing the PRG4-positive and PRG4-negative fractions [~50% positive for superficial chondrocytes, Figure 12.7(a)]. Determine the percentage of positive cells using your flow cytometry analysis software (e.g., CXP Analysis), or by exporting the histograms and analyzing in Excel.

12.3.3.2 Cell localization

Fluorescence microscopy can be used to localize cells that have been labeled (Section 12.3.1.3) in constructs after in vitro culture or in vivo implantation. This can give an estimate of cell retention and migration of the cells within the construct. Such information is important in establishing the efficacy of zonal cartilaginous constructs. Additionally, immunofluorescence techniques could be used to colocalize specific molecules with cells from specific zonal origins. This protocol is based on [22].

1. Label the cells (e.g., superficial chondrocytes) using PKH26 (Section 12.3.1.3).
2. Encapsulate the labeled (and unlabeled chondrocytes, e.g., middle/deep) cells in alginate disks and culture for 2 weeks in a chondrogenic differentiation medium (Section 12.3.2.1), changing the medium twice a week.
3. Combine the zonal constructs together (Section 12.3.2.2) and culture in a differentiated medium for an additional 4 weeks.
4. Snap-freeze and section the construct (Section 12.3.3.3, *Tissue sectioning*). Counterstain the cell nuclei using 0.01-mg/mL Hoeschst 33258.
5. Visualize the PKH26-labeled cells under the fluorescent microscope.

12.3.3.3 Matrix localization

Immunohistochemical methods can be used to identify zonal marker proteins in constructs and to determine their spatial distribution within the matrix [30].

Tissue sectioning

1. Wash the alginate gels for 30 minutes in PBS+.
2. Incubate the gels for 40 minutes in a solution containing equal parts of PBS+ and Tissue-Tek O.C.T. compound.
3. Transfer gels into an appropriate volume of the O.C.T. compound in Tissue-Tek Cryomolds and incubate for 40 minutes.
4. Freeze the embedded gel in liquid nitrogen.
5. Cut 5-μm cross-sections with a microtome.
6. Collect the sections on microscope slides (e.g., Menzel SuperFrost Plus; Thermo Fisher Scientific).

The immunohistochemistry methods shown in the following section are for the analysis of the superficial zonal marker PRG4 [31]. However, there are additional zonal markers that can be evaluated using a similar protocol including clusterin [32] for the superficial zone, and CILP [33] and COMP [34] for the deeper zones.

Immunohistochemical analysis of the proteoglycan 4 expression on frozen sections

1. Fix the frozen sections in 100% cold acetone for 15 minutes. Note that cryosections should be used fresh within 2 weeks after cutting.
2. Block nonspecific binding of the antibodies by treating the samples with 2.5% normal horse serum (e.g., VECTASTAIN Elite ABC-Peroxidase kit) for 20 minutes.
3. Dilute the polyclonal rabbit IgG antihuman lubricin (proteoglycan 4) antibody (1:200) and the polyclonal rabbit IgG isotype control antibody (1:1,000) in PBS.
4. Incubate the sections with either the lubricin antibody or the isotype control antibody for 1 hour at room temperature in a humidified chamber.
5. Wash the sections for 5 minutes with PBS.
6. Apply a biotinylated secondary antirabbit IgG antibody (e.g., VECTASTAIN Elite ABC-Peroxidase kit) to the sections for 30 minutes.
7. Wash the sections for 5 minutes with PBS.
8. Incubate with an avidin and biotinylated horseradish peroxidase complex reagent (e.g., VECTASTAIN Elite ABC-Peroxidase kit) for 30 minutes in a humidified chamber.

9. Wash the sections for 5 minutes with PBS.
10. Apply a 3,3′ diaminobenzidine substrate (e.g., Vector ImmPACT DAB Substrate) for up to 5 minutes. Note that the formation of the brown chromogens on the sections should be monitored under the microscope to optimize the incubation time if necessary.
11. Rinse with tap water for 5 minutes.
12. Counterstain the cell nuclei in sections with Mayer's hematoxylin for ~1 minute. Note that incubation time should be optimized on noncritical samples.
13. Wash under running tap water.
14. Seal the stained sections with an aqueous mounting medium (e.g., Crystal Mount, Sigma-Aldrich) and cover slips (Paul Marienfeld). For long-term storage, stained sections should be dehydrated in a graded ethanol series and mounted in a synthetic resin (e.g., DPX, Sigma-Aldrich).
15. Capture the images with a camera mounted on a microscope (e.g., QImaging MicroPublisher 3.3 RTV, QImaging on an Olympus BX41 microscope).

12.3.3.4 Gene expression

Cells from the different zones in cartilage express zone-specific marker proteins [35]. Quantitative real-time reverse transcriptase-polymerase chain reaction (qPCR) can be used to determine expression levels of messenger ribonucleic acid (RNA) encoding specific zonal marker proteins in zonal constructs. The following methods have been optimized to determine gene expression levels in alginate constructs containing between $0.1–1.0{*}10^6$ cells [36].

RNA extraction, quantification and quality control

1. Dissolve the alginate constructs in 1-ml buffer (containing 10-mM HEPES, 50-mM EDTA, 150-mM NaCl) at 37°C for 10 minutes.
2. Spin the suspension at 700 × g for 5 minutes, remove the supernatant and resuspend the tissue pellet in one volume of lysis buffer (RNeasy Micro Kit; 300 μL sufficient for a hydrogel with $1.0–5.0{*}10^5$ cells) supplemented with 1% v/v β-ME.
3. Disrupt the remaining cell matrix aggregates using a plastic pestle or similar. Note that samples could also be snap frozen in liquid nitrogen at this point to help disrupting the tissue and/or for short-term storage at –80°C, if necessary.
4. Homogenize the tissue lysate by passing through a 20-gauge needle (or by using other adequate methods).
5. Mix the lysate with one volume of 70% ethanol (molecular biology grade) and transfer the samples (including possible precipitates) immediately into RNeasy MinElute spin column placed in a 2-ml tube.
6. Follow the manufacturer's instructions of the RNeasy Micro Kit when proceeding with column deoxyribonucleic acid (DNA) digestion, RNA cleanup, and RNA elution.
7. Determine the quantity and quality of the extracted RNA by spectrophotometry. We commonly use a Nanodrop ND-1000 spectrophotometer, which does not require the dilution of the RNA samples. High-quality RNA will show an A_{260}/A_{280} ratio of above 2.0 and A_{260}/A_{230} ratio of above 1.8.

8. To further assess the quality of the extracted RNA, electrophorese 1 μL of an RNA sample in a 1.5% agarose/Tris-acetate-EDTA (TAE) gel for 30 minutes at 100V. Note that quality RNA is defined by the presence of two distinct 28S rRNA and 18S rRNA bands, with the former at least twice as intense as the latter.

First-strand complementary DNA (cDNA) synthesis

1. Transfer equal amounts of total RNA into PCR tubes and adjust the volume with UltraPure water (= 1 μg total RNA in a total volume of 8 μL). We recommend including a water-only no template control (NTC), which should be processed as a normal sample up to the final qPCR. The amplification of a PCR product in the NTC will indicate contaminated RT-PCR chemicals and other unspecific PCR reactions.
2. Add SuperScript III first-strand synthesis supermix (including SuperScript, RNaseOUT, 2.5-μM oligo (dT), 2.5 ng/μL random hexamers, 10-mM $MgCl_2$ and deoxynucleoside 5′-triphosphates (dNTP)) and mix for 10 minutes.
3. Heat the reaction mixture for 30 minutes at 50°C and for 5 minutes at 85°C in a thermal cycler and chill briefly on ice.
4. Add 2U/μL *e. coli* RNase H (SuperScript III kit; 1 μL in a 20-μL reaction) and incubate at 37°C for 20 minutes.

Primer design

1. Design forward and reverse primers using adequate software (e.g., Primer Express version 2.0; Applied Biosystems; see Table 12.1) or select suitable primer sets from the literature. Note that the following parameter settings should be used to define acceptable primer sets: minimum primer melting temperature (T_m) of 57°C, maximum of 63°C and optimal T_m of 60°C, with no more than 2°C difference in T_m between primers; GC content between 45–55%; primer length between 18–25 bases; amplicon length between 75 and 200 base pairs. All primer sets should be designed to be intron spanning or, where possible, placed on an intron-exon-border. Primer specificity should also be confirmed with BLASTN (NCBI) against the human genome (all assemblies). In addition, primers should be tested for secondary structures using appropriate software (e.g., IDT Scitools Oligoanalyzer 3.1; Integrated DNA Technologies).

Generation of DNA standards from gene-specific PCR amplicons

1. For each gene, transfer equal volumes of a standard PCR master mix (containing 1 U Platinum *Taq*, 1.5 mM $MgCl_2$, 0.2 mM of dNTP mix, 0.2-μM sequence specific forward and reverse primers and 1-μL cDNA template in a total volume of 50 μL) in 0.2-μL PCR tubes.
2. Perform standard PCR reactions in a thermal cycler (e.g., Peltier Thermal Cycler PTC 200; MJ Research) with the following temperature cycling conditions: 94°C for an initial 2 minutes, then 35 cycles of 94°C for 30 seconds, 55°C for 30 seconds, and 72°C for 30 seconds.
3. Separate the PCR products by electrophoresis at 100V for 45 minutes on a 2% agarose/TAE gel.

Table 12.1 List of Primers Used in qPCR of Zonal-Specific Markers

Gene Symbol (Primer Source)	Sequence (5'→3')	GenBank Accession Number	Amplicon Position
ACAN	F: GCCTGCGCTCCAATGACT	NM_001135	739-844
(Primer Express)	R: TAATGGAACACGATGCCTTTCA		
CILP	F: GCAAAAGCATCCTGAAGATCAC	NM_003613	993-1107
(Primer Express)	R: GGAGTCTCTGCCCTCACAAAC		
CLU	F: CTATCTGCGGGTCACCACG	NM_001831	1331-1402
[37]	R: ACCACCTCAGTGACACCGGA		
COL10A1	F: ACCCAACACCAAGACACAGTTCT	NM_000493	201-264
[38]	R: TCTTACTGCTATACCTTTACTCTTTATGGTGTA		
PRG4	F: GAGTACCCAATCAAGGCATTATCA	NM_005807	3431-3510
(Primer Express)	R: TCCATCTACTGGCTTACCATTGC		

4. Visualize the PCR products with ethidium bromide under ultraviolet light. Note that a DNA molecular weight standard should be included on the gel to confirm the approximate size of the PCR products.
5. Excise the band of each transcript from the agarose gel using a sterile scalpel blade.
6. Purify PCR amplicons from agarose using a gel extraction method (e.g., QIAquick Gel Extraction Kit, Qiagen).
7. Quantify the PCR products with the Quant-iT PicoGreen dsDNA assay kit. We found that amplicon concentrations are commonly very low (2–20 ng/μL), which is why standard spectrophotometry at 260 nm cannot be used for quantification.
8. Convert the yields to absolute cDNA transcript copy numbers based on a molar mass of 660 g/mol for 1 base pair DNA and the Avogadro constant.

qPCR

1. Transfer equal volumes of a SYBR-green qPCR mix containing forward and reverse primers (each at 200 nM final) in a 384-well plate. Note that PCR reactions can be easily scaled up to accommodate a 96-well format.
2. Add equal volumes of diluted cDNA in at least duplicates for each sample. Note that we recommend using cDNA equivalent to 5–10 ng of total RNA per 10-μL PCR reaction. Serial diluted standards (e.g., purified PCR target amplicons) covering at least 5 logs of amplicon copy number should be included to carry out the absolute quantification of cDNA copy numbers.
3. Follow a three-step cycling protocol for PCR amplification with an initial 5-minute incubation at 50°C to activate heat-labile uracil DNA glycosylase, followed by a 2-minute denaturation at 95°C and 40 cycles of 95°C for 15 seconds and 60°C for 30 seconds in a 384-well, format-enabled, real-time PCR system (e.g., Applied Biosystems 7900HT). Note that all real-time reactions should include a postamplification melt curve analysis to determine the melting temperature of the amplified PCR product, indicating the amplification of a single product of the correct sequence.
4. Analyze real-time curves in a semi-log view with the PCR system software (e.g., ABI Sequence Detection System software version 2.3) by setting the baseline to accommodate the earliest amplification plot and selecting threshold values in the

log-linear phase of the PCR cycle. The cycle number determined by the software is directly proportional to the amount of a starting cDNA transcript. A PCR reaction is considered to be 100% efficient if the standard curve with the quantity of the gene standard in log view plotted against the C_T value shows a slope of –3.31. PCR reactions with standard curve slopes between –3.1 and –3.6 are generally acceptable. New primer sets or changes in the PCR conditions must be optimized for ideal efficiency first before being applied into a laboratory routine.

5. Calculate the cDNA copy number for each reaction by direct comparison to the known standards for each gene, which are run concomitantly. In the absence of a standard, relative expression levels can be calculated by using the comparative cycle threshold (C_T) method (User Bulletin #2: ABI PRISM 7700 Sequence Detection System, Applied Biosystems).
6. Normalize the target gene expression for each sample to a housekeeping gene (e.g., 18S rRNA F: 5′-GATCCATTGGAGGGCAAGTCT-3′; R: 5′-CCAAGATCCAA CTACGAGCTTTTT-3′).

The SYBR green dye system has been chosen in our qPCR protocols as it presents a more flexible and cost-efficient method than TaqMan probes. However, special care must be taken during the optimization of any primer set when using SYBR green. The dye binds to any double-stranded DNA in the PCR reaction and will therefore also detect unspecific amplifications.

12.3.3.5 Biomechanical properties

Depth-dependent mechanical properties can be determined by analyzing photomicrographs taken during loading on a custom microscope-mounted loading device using image correlation techniques [39, 40]. These techniques use either phase-contrast images, as described in [41], or fluorescently-labeled cell nuclei, as described here and in [39, 41, 42].

1. Harvest the construct and treat with PBS+ including protease inhibitors. Freeze and thaw to kill cells if needed for fluorescent dye being used (e.g., propidium iodide).
2. Cut the construct diametrically and label the nuclei by immersing in PBS+ with 20-μm propidium iodide and protease inhibitors for 1 hour at 4°C.
3. Rinse the samples in PBS+ and mount in a custom confining chamber on an inverted microscope between porous platens [5].
4. Compress the sample 0%, 10%, and 20% of the initial thickness, at a rate of 0.2 μm/s, while monitoring the load. Allow to equilibrate for 30 minutes (depending on tissue geometry and tissue relaxation time needed), and take a fluorescence image using a 4× objective at each strain level.
5. Use these images to compute the two-dimensional strain (with 0% as a reference image) using image correlation software (e.g., VIC2D, Correlated Solutions, Inc.).
6. Compute the average axial strain at each depth to give a depth profile of the strain. If you wish to calculate the aggregate modulus (for confined compression), fit the equilibrium stress data at each compression level and the local strain to a nonlinear model [43].

12.4 Discussion and Commentary

Chondrocytes from the different zones have distinct roles within articular cartilage [44]. Superficial zone chondrocytes direct their biosynthetic efforts to maintain the integrity of the articulating surface, secreting the lubricating molecule PRG4, which adheres to the articular surfaces to promote near frictionless articulation of the cartilage [10]. Middle and deep zone chondrocytes show a robust production of matrix molecules and also produce zone-specific protein markers (middle zone: CILP [33], lower deep zone: Col X) [1]. These characteristics, necessary for the successful recreation of the zonal cartilage, are not maintained if a mixed cell population is used to engineer cartilage tissue.

The incongruent presence of chondrocytes originating from different zones could have a negative effect on the overall quality of the cartilaginous construct. PRG4, the superficial zone marker, has been reported to have a significant role in inhibiting construct integration in vivo [32], and constructs cultured in the presence of PRG4 had significantly less adhesive strength compared to those cultured without it [45]. Designing constructs that recapitulate zone-specific properties and functions may solve this issue and contribute to the development of tissue-engineered cartilage with improved, more native-like characteristics.

The procedures outlined in this chapter are not comprehensive in nature, but provide a foundation of experimental methods for developing and evaluating zonal cartilaginous constructs. While alginate hydrogels are described in this chapter, several other hydrogel systems including agarose [16], and poly(ethylene glycol) (PEG) [46, 47] have also been used for zonal construct formation. These alternative hydrogels require different conditions for cross-linking (change in temperature or UV light exposure), and thus the methods of Section 12.3.2 do not apply, although the other methods in Sections 12.3.1 and 12.3.3 remain important. Methods to fabricate zonal constructs using various biomaterials to be enhanced and the specific microenvironments required for the optimal in vitro culture of zonal chondrocytes need further investigation. Finally, zonal constructs must be evaluated alongside homogeneous constructs (using the methods detailed in Section 12.3.3) as well as standards of care, such as microfracture, chrondrocyte implantation, autograft, or allograft, following implantation in vivo to determine their potential for clinical use.

Troubleshooting Table

Problem	Explanation	Potential Solution
Construct properties are similar between zones.	Native cartilage did not have zonal structure (e.g., OA cartilage).	Verify structure using histology. Isolate cartilage from different region.
	Initial isolation was not pure.	Check purity using flow cytometry. Use a different method for zonal harvest.
	Cells have dedifferentiated and are not redifferentiating.	Reduce the cell expansion. Use a different medium for redifferentiation. Use a different material for construct formation.
Cells are mixed between layers.	Layers were not fully formed.	Cross-link longer or with a higher-strength cross-linker.
	Cells are migrating.	Increase the polymer content/cross-link density.
Cells were labeled but cannot be found.	Dye has faded.	Use a higher concentration of dye or a different class of dye. Keep samples in the dark to avoid photobleaching. Reduce the duration of the study.
	Cells have died.	Perform a viability study and adjust parameters such as cross-linking time, concentration, and media content.
	Cells have been lost from defect.	Increase mechanical properties of the construct. Choose a different site for implantation. Cover the implant with a membrane.
Construct delaminates	Poor integration strength between layers	Increase the cross-link density between layers. Use an alternative adhesive such as fibrin glue. Use a different material for construct formation.

12.5 Summary Points

1. Zonal chondrocytes can be harvested using microtome sectioning, core sectioning, direct slicing, and zonal abrasion. Since cartilage thickness can vary between species, histological assessment is recommended.
2. Chondrocyte labeling prior to encapsulation can help to determine the cell localization and distribution within the zonal construct in vitro and in vivo.
3. Custom-made molds are commonly used to form hydrogel-based constructs. However, novel cell printing technologies are also being used to make cartilaginous constructs as they can generate highly controlled 3D zonal architecture with different zonal chondrocytes in each layer.
4. The distribution of the zonal chondrocytes, the production and deposition of zone-specific markers (e.g., PRG4 and CILP), and the depth-dependent mechanical properties are some of the important assessment criteria of zonal cartilaginous tissue. These qualities can be evaluated using short-/long-term chondrocyte labeling, immunohistochemical staining, real-time qPCR of zonal markers, and mechanical characterization at a subtissue length scale.
5. Different types of hydrogels have been used to engineer zonal cartilaginous tissue. The application of other biomaterials/scaffolds (such as nanofiber mesh) in zonal cartilage tissue engineering is currently under investigation in our lab to develop cartilaginous tissue constructs with improved functionality.

References

[1] Buckwalter, J. A., and H. J. Mankin, "Articular Cartilage: Tissue Design and Chondrocyte-Matrix Interactions," *Instr. Course Lect.*, Vol. 47, 1998, pp. 477–486.

[2] Buckwalter, J. A., "Articular Cartilage Injuries," *Clin. Orthop. Relat. Res.*, Vol. 402, 2002, pp. 21–37.

[3] Steinert, A. F., et al., "Major Biological Obstacles for Persistent Cell-Based Regeneration of Articular Cartilage," *Arthritis Res. Ther.*, Vol. 9, No. 3, 2007, p. 213.

[4] Poole, C. A., "Articular Cartilage Chondrons: Form, Function and Failure," *J. Anat.*, Vol. 191, Pt. 1, 1997, pp. 1–13.

[5] Grande, D. A., et al., "Cartilage Tissue Engineering: Current Limitations and Solutions," *Clin. Orthop. Relat. Res.*, Vol. 367, Suppl., 1999, pp. S176–S185.

[6] Clar, C., et al., "Clinical and Cost-Effectiveness of Autologous Chondrocyte Implantation for Cartilage Defects in Knee Joints: Systematic Review and Economic Evaluation," *Health Technol. Assess.*, Vol. 9, No. 47 2005, pp. *iii–iv*, *ix–x*, 1–82.

[7] Mithoefer, K., et al., "The Microfracture Technique for the Treatment of Articular Cartilage Lesions in the Knee. A Prospective Cohort Study," *J. Bone Joint Surg. Am.*, Vol. 87, No. 9, 2005, pp. 1911–1920.

[8] Niikura, T., and A. H. Reddi, "Differential Regulation of Lubricin/Superficial Zone Protein by Transforming Growth Factor Beta/Bone Morphogenetic Protein Superfamily Members in Articular Chondrocytes and Synoviocytes," *Arthritis Rheum.*, Vol. 56, No. 7, 2007, pp. 2312–2321.

[9] Simon, T. M., and D. W. Jackson, "Articular Cartilage: Injury Pathways and Treatment Options," *Sports Med. Arthrosc.*, Vol. 14, No. 3, 2006, pp. 146–154.

[10] Schumacher, B. L., et al., "A Novel Proteoglycan Synthesized and Secreted by Chondrocytes of the Superficial Zone of Articular Cartilage," *Arch. Biochem. Biophys.*, Vol. 311, 1994, pp. 144–152.

[11] Buckwalter, J. A., and H. J. Mankin, "Articular Cartilage: Degeneration and Osteoarthritis, Repair, Regeneration, and Transplantation," *Instr. Course Lect.*, Vol. 47, 1998, pp. 487–504.

[12] Brittberg, M., et al., "Treatment of Deep Cartilage Defects in the Knee with Autologous Chondrocyte Transplantation," *N. Engl. J. Med.*, Vol. 331, 1994, pp. 889–895.

[13] Aydelotte, M. B., R. R. Greenhill, and K. E. Kuettner, "Differences Between Sub-Populations of Cultured Bovine Articular Chondrocytes. II. Proteoglycan Metabolism," *Connective Tissue Research*, Vol. 18, No. 3, 1988, pp. 223–234.

[14] Frenkel, S. R., et al., "Chondrocyte Transplantation Using a Collagen Bilayer Matrix for Cartilage Repair," *J. Bone Joint Surg. Br.*, Vol. 79, No. 5, 1997, pp. 831–836.

[15] Klein, T. J., et al., "Tissue Engineering of Stratified Articular Cartilage from Chondrocyte Subpopulations," *Osteoarthritis Cartilage*, Vol. 11, No. 8, 2003, pp. 595–602.

[16] Ng, K. W., G. A. Ateshian, and C. T. Hung, "Zonal Chondrocytes Seeded in a Layered Agarose Hydrogel Create Engineered Cartilage with Depth-Dependent Cellular and Mechanical Inhomogeneity," *Tissue Eng. Part A*, Vol. 15, No. 9, 2009, pp. 2315–2324.

[17] Waldman, S. D., et al., "The Use of Specific Chondrocyte Populations to Modulate the Properties of Tissue-Engineered Cartilage," *J. Orthop. Res.*, Vol. 21, No. 1, 2003, pp. 132–138.

[18] Darling, E. M., J. C. Hu, and K. A. Athanasiou, "Zonal and Topographical Differences in Articular Cartilage Gene Expression," *J. Orthop. Res.*, Vol. 22, No. 6, 2004, pp. 1182–1187.

[19] Benya, P. D., and J. D. Shaffer, "Dedifferentiated Chondrocytes Reexpress the Differentiated Collagen Phenotype When Cultured in Agarose Gels," *Cell*, Vol. 30, No. 1, 1982, pp. 215–224.

[20] Chawla, K., et al., "Tracking Chondrocytes and Assessing Their Proliferation with Pkh26: Effects on Secretion of Proteoglycan 4 (Prg4)," *J. Orthop. Res.*, Vol. 24, No. 7, 2006, pp. 1499–1508.

[21] Chawla, K., K. Masuda, and R. L. Sah, "Tracking Chondrocytes and Assessing Their Proliferation with Carboxyfluorescein Diacetate Succinimidyl Ester (Cfda, Se): Effects on Cell Functions," *Tissue Eng. Part C Methods*, 2009, *in press*.

[22] Chawla, K., et al., "Short-Term Retention of Labeled Chondrocyte Subpopulations in Stratified Tissue-Engineered Cartilaginous Constructs Implanted In Vivo in Mini-Pigs," *Tissue Eng.*, Vol. 13, No. 7, 2007, pp. 1525–1537.

[23] Jakob, M., et al., "Specific Growth Factors During the Expansion and Redifferentiation of Adult Human Articular Chondrocytes Enhance Chondrogenesis and Cartilaginous Tissue Formation In Vitro," *J. Cell Biochem.*, Vol. 81, No. 2, 2001, pp. 368–377.

[24] Welter, J. F., L. A. Solchaga, and K. J. Penick, "Simplification of Aggregate Culture of Human Mesenchymal Stem Cells as a Chondrogenic Screening Assay," *Biotechniques*, Vol. 42, No. 6, 2007, pp. 732, 734–737.

[25] Cohen, D. L., et al., "Direct Freeform Fabrication of Seeded Hydrogels in Arbitrary Geometries," *Tissue Eng.*, Vol. 12, No. 5, 2006, pp. 1325–1335.

[26] Fedorovich, N. E., et al., "Evaluation of Photocrosslinked Lutrol Hydrogel for Tissue Printing Applications," *Biomacromolecules*, 2009.

[27] Fedorovich, N. E., et al., "Three-Dimensional Fiber Deposition of Cell-Laden, Viable, Patterned Constructs for Bone Tissue Printing," *Tissue Eng. Part A*, Vol. 14, No. 1 2008, pp. 127–133.

[28] Klein, T. J., et al., "Strategies for Zonal Cartilage Repair Using Hydrogels," *Macromol. Biosci.*, Vol. 9, No. 11, 2009, pp. 1049–1058.

[29] Klein, T. J., et al., "Tailoring Secretion of Proteoglycan 4 (Prg4) in Tissue-Engineered Cartilage," *Tissue Eng.*, Vol. 12, No. 6, 2006, pp. 1429–1439.

[30] Schuurman, W., et al., "Zonal Chondrocyte Subpopulations Reacquire Zone-Specific Characteristics During In Vitro Redifferentiation," *Am. J. Sports Med.*, Vol. 37, Spuul. 1, 2009, pp. 975–1045.

[31] Schumacher, B. L., et al., "Proteoglycan 4 (Prg4) Synthesis and Immunolocalization in Bovine Meniscus," *J. Orthop. Res.*, Vol. 23, No. 3, 2005, pp. 562–568.

[32] Khan, I. M., et al., "Cartilage Integration: Evaluation of the Reasons for Failure of Integration During Cartilage Repair. A Review," *Eur. Cell Mater.*, Vol. 16, 2008, pp. 26–39.

[33] Lorenzo, P., M. T. Bayliss, and D. Heinegard, "A Novel Cartilage Protein (Cilp) Present in the Mid-Zone of Human Articular Cartilage Increases with Age," *J. Biol. Chem.*, Vol. 273, No. 36, 1998, pp. 23463–23468.

[34] Ekman, S., et al., "Ultrastructural Immunolocalization of Cartilage Oligomeric Matrix Protein (Comp) in Porcine Growth Cartilage," *Calcif. Tissue Int.*, Vol. 60, No. 6, 1997, pp. 547–553.

[35] Klein, T. J., et al., "Tissue Engineering of Articular Cartilage with Biomimetic Zones," *Tissue Eng. Part B Rev.*, Vol. 15, No. 2, 2009, pp. 143–157.

[36] Leong, D. T., et al., "Absolute Quantification of Gene Expression in Biomaterials Research Using Real-Time Pcr," *Biomaterials*, Vol. 28, No. 2, 2007, pp. 203–210.

[37] Tureci, O., et al., "Cascades of Transcriptional Induction During Dendritic Cell Maturation Revealed by Genome-Wide Expression Analysis," *FASEB J.*, Vol. 17, No. 8, 2003, pp. 836–847.

[38] Daouti, S., et al., "Development of Comprehensive Functional Genomic Screens to Identify Novel Mediators of Osteoarthritis," *Osteoarthritis Cartilage*, Vol. 13, No. 6, 2005, pp. 508–518.

[39] Schinagl, R. M., et al., "Video Microscopy to Quantitate the Inhomogeneous Equilibrium Strain within Articular Cartilage During Confined Compression," *Ann. Biomed. Eng.*, Vol. 24, No. 4, 1996, pp. 500–512.

[40] Wang, C. C., et al., "Optical Determination of Anisotropic Material Properties of Bovine Articular Cartilage in Compression," *J. Biomech.*, Vol. 36, No. 3, 2003, pp. 339–353.

[41] Schinagl, R. M., et al., "Depth-Dependent Confined Compression Modulus of Full-Thickness Bovine Articular Cartilage," *J. Orthop. Res.*, Vol. 15, No. 4, 1997, pp. 499–506.

[42] Klein, T. J., et al., "Depth-Dependent Biomechanical and Biochemical Properties of Fetal, Newborn, and Tissue-Engineered Articular Cartilage," *J. Biomech.*, Vol. 40, No. 1, 2007, pp. 182–190.

[43] Kwan, M. K., W. M. Lai, and V. C. Mow, "A Finite Deformation Theory for Cartilage and Other Soft Hydrated Connective Tissues—I. Equilibrium Results," *J. Biomech.*, Vol. 23, 1990, pp. 145–155.

[44] Wong, M., et al., "Zone-Specific Cell Biosynthetic Activity in Mature Bovine Articular Cartilage: A New Method Using Confocal Microscopic Stereology and Quantitative Autoradiography," *J. Orthop. Res.*, Vol. 14, No. 3, 1996, pp. 424–432.

[45] Schaefer, D. B., et al., "Lubricin Reduces Cartilage—Cartilage Integration," *Biorheology*, Vol. 41, No. 3-4, 2004, pp. 503–508.

[46] Sharma, B., et al., "Designing Zonal Organization into Tissue-Engineered Cartilage," *Tissue Eng.*, Vol. 13, No. 2, 2007, pp. 405–414.

[47] Kim, T. K., et al., "Experimental Model for Cartilage Tissue Engineering to Regenerate the Zonal Organization of Articular Cartilage," *Osteoarthritis Cartilage*, Vol. 11, No. 9, 2003, pp. 653–664.

CHAPTER

13

Cartilage and Synovial Joint Regeneration by Cell Homing in Bioprinted, Anatomically Correct 3D Scaffolds

Chang Hun Lee and Jeremy J. Mao

Columbia University Medical Center, Tissue Engineering and Regenerative Medicine Laboratory, and Fu Foundation School of Engineering and Applied Sciences, Department of Biomedical Engineering, New York, NY, Corresponding author: Jeremy J. Mao, address: Columbia University Medical Center, 630 W. 168 St. PH7 East, New York, NY 10032, phone: 212-305-4475, fax: 212-342-0199, e-mail: jmao@columbia.edu

Abstract

Cartilage regeneration requires 3D scaffolds to accommodate structural and mechanical strength, as well as diffusion and gas exchange needs. To date, few scaffolds have satisfied these conflicting needs. This chapter describes a novel, anatomically shaped 3D composite scaffold that enabled functional regeneration of the entire articular cartilage surface of a synovial joint condyle, leading to weight-bearing and locomotion in a small animal (rabbit) model. Polycaprolactone and hydroxyapatite were comolten and deposited layer-by-layer into image-reconstructed anatomical shape and dimensions of a synovial joint condyle with repeating internal units of microstrands and interstrand microchannels. Growth factor-loaded hydrogel was infused into the scaffold's microchannels to promote articular cartilage regeneration by endogenous cells. This first in vivo demonstration of synovial joint regeneration by endogenous cell homing into prefabricated, anatomically correct scaffolds without cell transplantation validates 3D bioprinting as a meritorious approach for the regeneration of complex tissues by either cell transplantation or cell homing approaches.

Key terms arthritis, bone
cartilage, regenerative medicine,
TGFβ, tissue engineering

13.1 Introduction

Fabrication of 3D objects used to be a high-end industrial endeavour, but is becoming a technology platform that can be pursued by individual laboratories. Following a 3D architecture that is usually generated by a computer-aided design (CAD), rapid prototyping devices generate the actual 3D object by depositing successive layers of materials of choice via solidification of melts, layer photopolymerization, or bonding of particles using either laser beam induced sintering (selective laser sintering) or special binders [1–3]. Given that 3D printing enables rapid prototyping in a faster, a more affordable, and an easier manner, it offers great potential for manufacturing products including, but not limited to, footwear, houseware, automobile, dental, and medical industries. As recently highlighted in the mass media, customized footwear fitting your own feet will potentially be available in the near future by 3D printing technology. The relevance of 3D printing to regenerative medicine is represented by an emerging interest in designing and fabricating scaffolds for tissue regeneration [4–6].

Arthritis is a worldwide pandemic. With advancing human life span, osteoarthritis is anticipated to escalate as one of the chronic diseases of ageing process. The structural breakdown of cartilage and bone of the synovial joint is a healthcare burden [7, 8]. Currently, synovial joints with late-stage osteoarthritis are surgically replaced by a synthetic prosthesis of metal, plastic, and/or ceramics. Current prosthetic joints, despite a well-documented clinical success, are associated with severe drawbacks including wear and tear, aseptic loosening, and a limited lifespan. In relatively younger patients, the current total joint arthroplasty is limited and suffers from substantial difficulties associated with secondary surgeries such as scar tissue formation and a lmited host tissue availability [9]. Commercially available, biologically based therapies including the autologous chondrocyte transfer or mosaicplasty are designed for focal cartilage lesions, rather than as a substitute for total joint prosthesis, and yet are associated with drawbacks such as incomplete integration, suboptimal conformity of cartilage surface, altered cartilage phenotype, and donor site morbidity. To date, there are no biological substitutes for the entire synovial joint condyle.

Previous works have reported tissue-engineered grafts for the entire synovial joint condyle using cells and bioscaffolds in experimental models [10–16]. Stratified layers of cartilage and bone structures with dimensions of the human temporomandibular joint (TMJ) condyles or phalangeal condyles have been formed ectopically in vivo from several cell sources such as a single population of a bone marrow–derived mesenchymal stem (MSCs) [10, 12, 15, 17] or differentiated chondrocytes and osteoblasts [18, 19]. However, these tissue-engineered grafts for the entire synovial joint have been limited in the dimensions that may not be applicable for large joints including the knee and hip. Scaling up tissue-engineered grafts is one of the essential requirements to meet the clinical implantation for synovial joint replacement, but it is associated with the challenges of vascularization and cell survival. Regenerating tissue over 100–200 μm exceeds the capacity of nutrient diffusion and waste removal, and thus requires a vascular supply [20, 21]. Accordingly, it has been proposed that increasingly refined internal structures such as interconnected pores enhance angiogenesis and tissue regeneration [22–24]. However, this hypothesis has yet to be rigorously tested in vivo.

In this chapter, we describe procedures to fabricate 3D anatomically shaped bioscaffolds in an in vivo model for cartilage and synovial joint regeneration. The anatomic contour and internal porous structures were designed and reconstructed using a layer deposition with rapid prototyping. A 3D computer model with anatomical parameters was generated to include sequences of layers, which were then used to construct an entire anatomically shaped and dimensioned synovial joint condyle. A composite of polycaprolactone-hydroxyapatite (PCL-HA) was then dispensed layer-by-layer to fabricate synovial joint condyle scaffolds with repeating internal units of microstrands and interstrand microchannels. A transforming growth factor beta 3 (TGFβ3)-loaded hydrogel was infused onto the microchannels of the PCL-HA scaffold as an articular cartilage layer. The fabricated, anatomically shaped bioscaffolds surgically replaced synovial joint condyles in a rabbit model. Up to a 4-month postoperative follow-up showed the regeneration of the entire synovial joint condyle consisting of articular cartilage that integrated to a vascularized and mineralized subchondral bone. Given that no cells were transplanted, we submit that the homing of innate cells into the bioprinted bioscaffolds is responsible for the regeneration of complex tissues, including the presently exemplified synovial joint condyle.

13.2 Experimental Design

The 3D architecture of a synovial joint in a patient can be obtained by computer tomography (CT) or magnetic resonance imaging (MRI). To practice this concept, we laser-scanned a humeral joint condyle of a skeletally matured rabbit at a 12.7-μm resolution (Berding, Loveland, Ohio) to build a 3D CAD model. A composite of polycaprolactone (PCL) and hydroxyapatite (HA), which has physical properties and a biodegradation rate suitable for bone regeneration [25–28], was melted to deposit, layer-by-layer, the anatomically shaped and dimensioned synovial joint scaffold by CAD design. Interlaid strands and interconnecting microchannels had diameters of 400 μm in the cartilage portion, not only to mimic its avascular environment but also to entrap the TGFβ3-loaded hydrogel layer. High-density collagen gel (4 mg/mL) was selected to deliver TGFβ3 to accommodate cartilage regeneration by guided innate cells as the matrix degrades. The overall dimension of the anatomically shaped synovial joint condyle is several orders of magnitude greater than the capacity of nutrient diffusion and waste removal in the range of 100–200 μm [20, 21]. Accordingly, the 200-μm microchannels were designed as conduits for cell recruitment and angiogenesis in the subchondral bone portion. By a 4-month in situ implantation, the TGFβ3-mediated replacement joints fully resumed functions including weight-bearing and locomotion. Cartilage tissue regenerated and constituted the articular surface of scaffolds with TGFβ3 delivery. The quality and quantity of the regenerated articular cartilage and subchondral bone were evaluated by radiography, histomorphometric analysis, immunofluorescence, and biomechanical testing.

13.3 Materials

- 3D Bioplotter system (EnvionTec, Germany) (Figure 13.1)
- 3D axis dispensing system: working area XYZ: 300 × 300 × 120 mm; resolution in XYZ: 50 μm; speed: 1 to 100 mm/s
- Base plate (XY): 400 × 400 mm with controlled basement heating up to 100°C

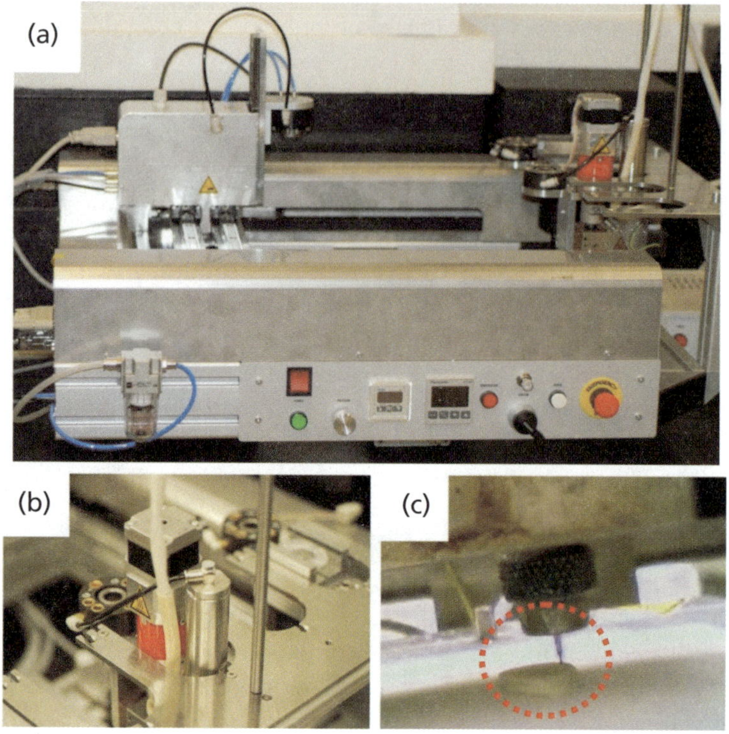

Figure 13.1 Fabrication of anatomically correct bioscaffolds with internal microstructures. (a) Bioplotter system for layer-by-layer fabrication of bioscaffolds. (b) A composite of polycaprolactone and hydroxyapatite (PCL-HA) was molten into dispensing cartilage. (c) The material was then dispensed through a fine metal needle following the layer path created by 3D anatomical data as well as internal microstructures.

- Controlled cartridge can be heated up to 300°C
- Automatic pressure control up to 10 bars
- Two types of dispensing heads: High-Temp & Viscous Dispensing-Head (HTV-Dispense-Head) and Low-Temp & Viscous Dispensing-Head (LTV-Dispense-Head)
- Import of dispensing path per layer by CAD/CAM-Bioplotter-SW
- Polycaprolactone (M_n ~ 80,000, Sigma)
- Hydroxyapatite (Powder, Sigma)
- 27G steel encapsulation needle (DL Technology, LLC, Haverhill, Massachusetts): inner/outer diameters: 0.2 mm/0.508 mm
- Transforming growth factor beta 3 (TGFβ3) (R&D systems)
- Hydrochloric acid (HCl) (Sigma)
- Bovine serum albumin (BSA) (Sigma)
- Bovine collagen type I (R&D systems)
- Sodium hydroxide (NaOH) (Sigma)
- Phosphate buffered saline (PBS) (Invitrogen): 1× and 10×
- Lab oven (Fisher Scientific)
- Paraffin
- Sterile dH_2O

13.4 Methods

13.4.1 Bioplotting PCL-HA scaffolds for synovial joint condyle tissue engineering

1. Prepare 3D volumetric data that defines the outer shape of scaffold.
    - The embedded software imports .DXF (AutoCAD drawing exchange format) or .STL (Stereolithography) file.
    - The 3D data file can be prepared by processing CT or MRI images using commercialized medical CAD programs (e.g., MIMICS, 3D Doctors).
    - The 3D CAD model of the scaffold should be an integral solid of which the body is entirely surrounded by surface objects without a void surface.
    - The size of the 3D CAD model should not exceed the provided working area ($300 \times 300 \times 120$ mm).
    - The 3D CAD model may need to be aligned as considering the depositions of material layer-by-layer as increasing Z. Basically, layers in lower Z are to be larger than layers in higher Z to maintain the stability during the dispensing process.
    - The 3D CAD model may be simplified as considering the dispensing resolution (50 μm).
2. Set the dispensing parameters:
    - Applied air pressure: 3.5 bars
    - Temperature: 120°C for cartilage and 40°C for the basement plate
    - Feeding rate XY (Fxy): 120 mm/min
    - Thickness of each layer: 0.16 mm (80% of the needle inner diameter)
    - Strand distance XY: 0.6 mm for bone layers: 200-μm microchannels, 1.0 mm for cartilage layers: 400-μm microchannels; thickness of bone and cartilage can be adjusted by specific needs
    - Dispensing pattern of layers: predefined 0° to 90°; 0° to 90° setting will create rectangular microchannels and other patterns from 0°~ 135° or arbitrary can be selected for specific needs
3. Place weight-measured PCL in the cartilage of HTV-Dispense-Head, heat up to 200°C, and wait for 3–5 minutes until all materials are melted.
4. Measure the weight of the HA powder (25 wt% of PCL) and mix it thoroughly with the molten PCL by stirring for more than 30 minutes.
5. Set the cartilage temperature down to 120°C and wait for 10–15 minutes until it is cooled down.
6. Import a 3D model data file and construct a dispensing path set of each layer by applying a predetermined parameter set.
7. Run the machine. The PCL melt will be dispensed following the layer paths constructed by 3D data. Once the polymer strand comes out from the heated cartilage, it will be cooled down and solidified. The shape of the 3D scaffold will be formed by depositing layers.
8. The process time varies from several minutes to hours as the complexity of the internal structure, the area of layers, and the thickness of scaffold.

13.4.2 Infusing TGFβ3 in a collagen gel into the microchannels of a PCL-HA scaffold

1. Prepare a paraffin mold with the anatomical shape of articular cartilage.
    - Place the paraffin in a 60°C oven and wait until it is melted.

- Tightly wrap the articular surface of the PCL-HA condyle scaffold with aluminum foil.
- Dip the wrapped articular surface into the paraffin melt and cool it down at room temperature.
- Repeat the above step several times to obtain a mechanically stable mold for the articular surface.
- Carefully separate the paraffin mold from the PCL-HA scaffold.

2. Reconstitute TGFβ3 at 20 μg/mL in sterile 4 mM HCl containing 1 mg/mL BSA.
3. Prepare a neutralized collagen solution as following (per 1 mL of final solution):
   - Place on ice the following: collagen, sterile 10× PBS, sterile distilled water (dH_2O), and sterile 1N NaOH.
   - Mix 100 μL of 10× PBS with 28 μL of 1N NaOH.
   - Add 72 μL of dH_2O containing total 10 ng of TGFβ3; the TGFβ3 solution prepared from step 2 can be reconstituted again in regular PBS or dH_2O to meet the final concentration of 10 ng/mL.
   - Add 800 μL of collagen and pipette up and down to mix.
4. Place the paraffin mold on a flat surface.
5. Pipette a predefined volume of the collagen solution containing the TGFβ3 prepared from step 3 into a sterile articular surface mold.
   - The volume of collagen solution is to be determined by the desired thickness of the collage gel layer on the selected articular surface area.
   - For a rabbit humeral condyle, 100 μL is the optimized volume for a 500-μm-thick gel layer.
6. Carefully put a PCL-HA condyle scaffold upside down on the paraffin mold.
7. Incubate in 37°C for 1 hour for the cross-linking of collagen.
8. Carefully separate the paraffin mold, keeping the collagen gel layer intact.

13.5 Results and Interpretation

Bioprinted, 3D anatomically shaped scaffolds with modularized internal microstructures can be fabricated by layer deposition. For example, a rabbit-shaped humeral condyle scaffold was fabricated with PCL-HA (80:20 wt%) [Figure 13.2(c)], from the volumetric CAD model reconstructed from 3D laser scans [Figure 13.2(b)]. These bioscaffolds with internal microstructures can be readily adopted for the tissue engineering of a broad range of tissues in vitro or in vivo. Cells and/or growth factors can be

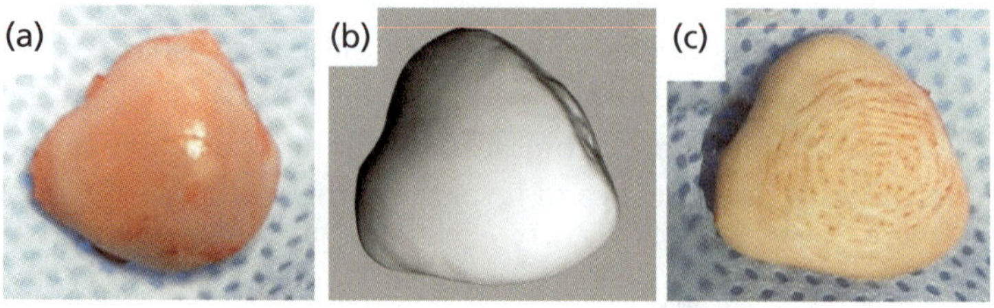

Figure 13.2 Replacement of animal forelimb joint with an anatomically correct bioscaffold. Fabricated polycaprolactone and hydroxyapatite (PCL-HA) scaffold that replaced the rabbit forelimb joint condyle. (a) The native rabbit forelimb (shoulder) condyle of a cadevaric rabbit humeral joint. (b) The 3D anatomical contour was reconstructed and used to fabricate (c) an anatomically shaped and dimensioned PCL-HA scaffold.

readily delivered in the microchannels or micropores of these 3D bioprinted scaffolds. In this chapter, we found that 3D bioprinted scaffolds enabled the functional regeneration of synovial joint condyles by cell homing and without cell transplantation. Upon the resection of the native synovial joint condyle, the defect was replaced with anatomically shaped bioscaffolds with or without TGFβ3 delivery. We found that the operated rabbits initially limped with little use of the operated forelimb, but resumed locomotion and weight-bearing by ~3 weeks following surgery (Figure 13.3). Upon a 4-month postoperative follow-up, the articular cartilage regenerated and constituted the articular surface in both TGFβ3-free and TGFβ3-infused scaffolds [Figure 13.4(a, b), respectively]. However, TGFβ3 infusion induced a full-layer articular cartilage regeneration; in contrast, only isolated areas of articular cartilage regenerated without TGFβ3 infusion. Histomorphometric analysis confirmed that articular cartilage regeneration was pronounced upon hydrogel-infused TGFβ3 delivery [Figure 13.4(d)], in contrast to poor cartilage regeneration without TGFβ3 delivery [Figure 13.4(c)]. For subchondral bones, a mineral deposition was found on the surface of microchannels formed by PCL-HA strands (200 μm) with or without TGFβ3 delivery [Figure 13.4(e, f)]. Given no cell transplantation, all regenerating cartilage and bone tissues are host-derived. These findings suggests that modularized bioscaffolds with micronchannel repeats may serve as a prototype for regenerating complex tissues, by either cell homing or cell transplantation approaches. More importantly, the present observation of the regeneration of complex tissues, including avascular cartilage and vascularized bone, suggests that cell homing may be sufficient for tissue regeneration in some, but not all, cases. It is further specu-

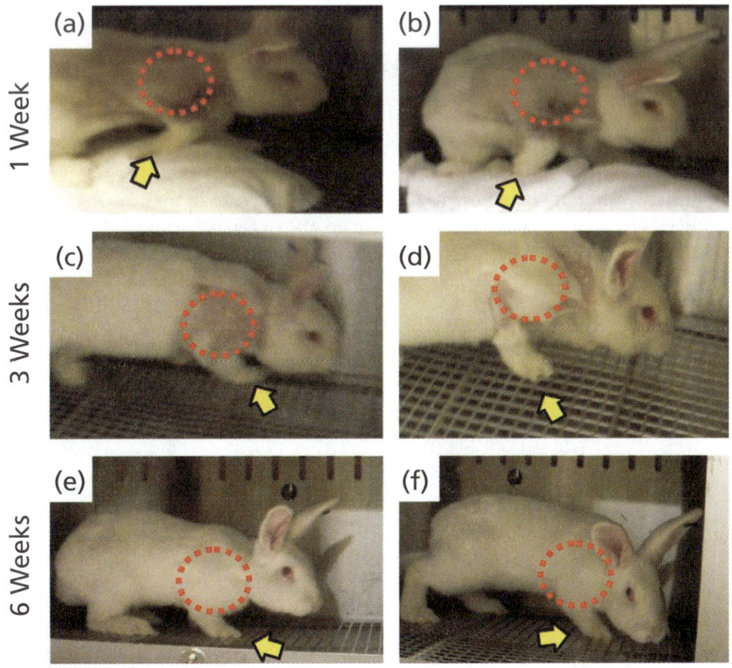

Figure 13.3 Animal with the right forelimb joint replaced by anatomically correct bioscaffolds resumed weight-bearing and locomotion. (a, b) By 1 week postsurgery, the representative rabbit limped with little use of the operated right forelimb. (c, d) By ~3 weeks, the representative rabbit begun to resume locomotion and weight-bearing with all limbs, including the operated forelimb. (e, f) By ~6 weeks, all rabbits that had received bioengineered joint replacements were able to walk virtually as unoperated, normal rabbits. Circle: operated right forelimb; arrow: ground contact point.

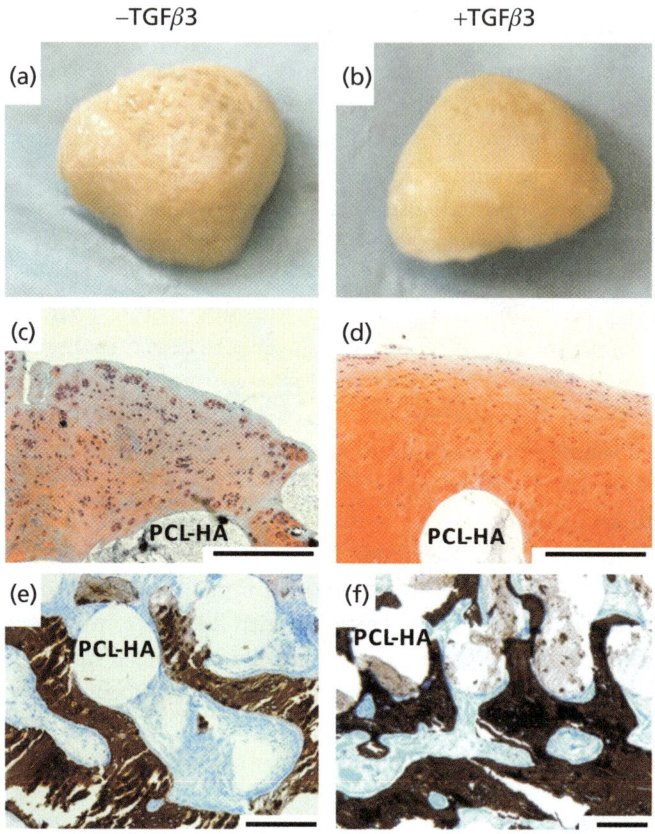

Figure 13.4 Regeneration of articular cartilage and subchondral bone in animal forelimb joint replaced by bioscaffolds. Upon retrieval of in vivo implanted joint replacement constructs at 4 months postoperative, the articular cartilage regenerated in both (a) a TGFβ3-free scaffold and (b) a TGFβ3-infused scaffold. (c) Safranin O (SO) staining revealed chondrocyte-like cells clustered in TGFβ3-free scaffold samples with suboptimal cartilage regeneration. (d) Regenerating articular cartilage in the representative TGFβ3-infused scaffold sample was notably substantial in comparison to the representative TGFβ3-free scaffold sample (c). Delivered TGFβ3 in the scaffold's microchannels led to thoroughly distributed chondrocyte-like cells, substantially more intense SO staining, and more pronounced articular cartilage that regenerated above the scaffold's superior surface (d). Von Kossa staining indicates mineral deposition in microchannels of both (e) TGFβ3-free scaffold and (f) TGFβ3-infused scaffold samples. Scale: 200 μm.

lated that the delivery of TGFβ3 enhanced cartilage regeneration by regulating homing and the differentiation of stem/progenitor cells.

13.6 Discussion and Commentary

The functional regeneration of large and complex tissues or organs including the synovial joint is an important milestone in regenerative medicine. Knowledge from previous work on the regeneration of large, vascularized structures suggests that modularized and microstructured bioscaffolds promote the vascularization of bioengineered tissues [29–32]. The present approach of 200–400-μm repeats in microstrands and microchannels of bioscaffolds is partially based on the existing challenge of diffusion and vascular supply in regenerating tissues. The rationale for 400-μm interstrand microchannels in articular cartilage is that cartilage is devoid of a vascular supply, whereas 200-μm interstrand microchannels were evidently sufficient for generating a vascularized subchondral bone. Our in vivo data revealed the functional regeneration of articular cartilage and a subchondral bone that allowed the functional recovery of the synovial joints. Remarkably, all regenerating tissue was derived by cell recruitment from the host, rather than cell transplantation. These findings suggest that the modularized scaffolds with microchannel repeats in the range of a few hundred microns are sufficient for the regeneration of large tissues, although precise physical attributes, such as microchannel diameters, likely differ among various tissues. We anticipate that similar approaches will energize the field of regenerative medicine and tissue engineering towards the regeneration of large and complex tissues and organs.

Troubleshooting Table

Problem	Explanation	Potential Solutions
Discontinuous dispensing of polymer strands	Mainly caused by low temperature of cartilage or blockage of dispensing needle	Increase the cartilage temperature. Clean the dispensing needle. Lower the feeding rate (Fxy).
Collapsed scaffold during layers deposition	May occur when underlying layers are poorly solidified upon deposition of the following layers	Decrease the cartilage temperature. Decrease the temperature of collecting plate. Add a pause (~0.5 second) in between dispensing layers.
Poor bonding between layers	Mainly caused by too quick solidification of either underlying layers or dispensing strands	Increase the cartilage temperature. Increase the temperature of collecting plate. Lower the feeding rate (Fxy)

13.7 Application Notes

The 3D bioprinting approach outlined in this chapter represents a generic method to fabricate anatomically shaped scaffolds with modularized internal microarchitecture. As highlighted in this chapter, we bioengineered the stratified layers of articular cartilage and subchondral bone with a spatial control of the internal microstructure and the regional delivery of a cell homing molecule, TGFβ3. The internal microarchitecture can be controlled and modified spatially within a bioscaffold to accommodate the biological needs for the regeneration of various tissues and organs. We have recently bioprinted softer biomaterials for adipose tissue regeneration [33]. Accordingly, bioprinting with 3D layer-by-layer fabrication may include the regeneration of multitissue interfaces in large tissues and organs.

13.8 Summary Points

1. We describe procedures to fabricate 3D anatomically shaped stratified scaffolds with modularized internal microstructure for the regeneration of complex tissues such as synovial joint condyles.
2. The dispensing parameters provided in this chapter are predesigned for engineering repeat units of 200–400-μm microstrands and interstrand microchannels. The in

vivo outcome of the regeneration of a synovial joint condyle and functional recovery indicates that successful adoption of several engineering parameters in the regeneration of complex tissues. The internal microarchitecture can be readily modified to satisfy specific needs for the regeneration of other complex tissues and organs.

3. TGFβ3 delivery via high density collagen gel into the proximal microchannels of the 3D condylar scaffolds substantiates the regeneration of articular cartilage that is integrated with the subchondral bone.
4. The potential applications of the present approaches include the bioengineering of large and complex tissues and organs, in addition to multitissue interfaces.

Acknowledgments

We thank our colleagues whose work has been cited, and those whose work cannot be cited due to space limitation, for their work that has inspired our thinking process. We are grateful to members of Tissue Engineering and Regenerative Medicine Laboratory for their dedication and hard work. We thank Ms. Qiongfen Guo and Ms. Kening Hua for their administrative and technical assistance. This work is funded by the NIH/NIBIB grant R01EB002332 to Jeremy J. Mao.

References

[1] Giordano, R. A., et al., "Mechanical Properties of Dense Polylactic Acid Structures Fabricated by Three Dimensional Printing," *Journal of Biomaterials Science*, Vol. 8, 1996, p. 63.

[2] Holman, R. K., et al., "Surface Adsorption Effects in the Inkjet Printing of an Aqueous Polymer Solution on a Porous Oxide Ceramic Substrate," *Journal of Colloid and Interface Science*, Vol. 247, 2002, p. 266.

[3] Landers, R., et al., "Rapid Prototyping of Scaffolds Derived from Thermoreversible Hydrogels and Tailored for Applications in Tissue Engineering," *Biomaterials*, Vol. 23, 2002, p. 4437.

[4] Cohen, A., et al., "Mandibular Reconstruction Using Stereolithographic 3-Dimensional Printing Modeling Technology," *Oral Surg. Oral Med. Oral Pathol. Oral Radiol. Endod.*, 2009.

[5] Lee, K.W., et al., "Fabrication and Characterization of Poly(Propylene Fumarate) Scaffolds with Controlled Pore Structures Using 3-Dimensional Printing and Injection Molding," *Tissue Eng.*, Vol. 12, 2006, p. 2801.

[6] Mrosek, E. H., et al., "Porous Tantalum and Poly-Epsilon-Caprolactone Biocomposites for Osteochondral Defect Repair: Preliminary Studies in Rabbits," *J. Orthop. Res.*, 2009.

[7] Kraus, V. B., "Pathogenesis and Treatment of Osteoarthritis," *Med. Clin. North Am.*, Vol. 81, 1997, p. 85.

[8] Lawrence, R. C., et al., "Estimates of the Prevalence of Arthritis and Selected Musculoskeletal Disorders in the United States," *Arthritis Rheum.*, Vol. 41, 1998, p. 778.

[9] Haydon, C. M., et al., "Revision Total Hip Arthroplasty with Use of a Cemented Femoral Component. Results at a Mean of Ten Years," *J. Bone Joint Surg. Am.*, Vol. 86-A, 2004, p. 1179.

[10] Alhadlaq, A., et al., "Adult Stem Cell Driven Genesis of Human-Shaped Articular Condyle," *Ann. Biomed. Eng.*, Vol. 32, 2004, p. 911.

[11] Alhadlaq, A., and J. J. Mao, "Tissue-Engineered Neogenesis of Human-Shaped Mandibular Condyle from Rat Mesenchymal Stem Cells," *Journal of Dental Research*, Vol. 82, 2003, p. 951.

[12] Alhadlaq, A., and J. J. Mao, "Tissue-Engineered Osteochondral Constructs in the Shape of an Articular Condyle," *J. Bone Joint Surg. Am.*, Vol. 87, 2005, p. 936.

[13] Grayson, W. L., et al., "Engineering Custom-Designed Osteochondral Tissue Grafts," *Trends Biotechnol.*, Vol. 26, 2008, p. 181.

[14] Mao, J. J., "Stem-Cell-Driven Regeneration of Synovial Joints," *Biol. Cell*, Vol. 97, 2005, p. 289.

[15] Martin, I., et al., "Osteochondral Tissue Engineering," *J. Biomech.*, Vol. 40, 2007, p. 750.

[16] Moutos, F. T., L. E. Freed, and F. Guilak, "A Biomimetic Three-Dimensional Woven Composite Scaffold for Functional Tissue Engineering of Cartilage," *Nat. Mater.*, Vol. 6, 2007, p. 162.

[17] Troken, A., et al., "Tissue Engineering of the Synovial Joint: The Role of Cell Density," *Proc. Inst. Mech. Eng. [H]*, Vol. 221, 2007, p. 429.

[18] Isogai, N., et al., "Formation of Phalanges and Small Joints by Tissue-Engineering," *J. Bone Joint Surg. Am.*, Vol. 81, 1999, p. 306.

[19] Weng, Y., et al., "Tissue-Engineered Composites of Bone and Cartilage for Mandible Condylar Reconstruction," *J. Oral Maxillofac. Surg.*, Vol. 59, 2001, p. 185.

[20] Jain, R. K., et al., "Engineering Vascularized Tissue," *Nat. Biotechnol.*, Vol. 23, 2005, p. 821.

[21] Koike, H., et al., "Enhanced Angiogenesis and Improvement of Neuropathy by Cotransfection of Human Hepatocyte Growth Factor and Prostacyclin Synthase Gene," *FASEB. J.*, Vol. 17, 2003, p. 779.

[22] Hollister, S. J., "Porous Scaffold Design for Tissue Engineering," *Nat. Mater.*, Vol. 4, 2005, p. 518.

[23] Langer, R., and D. A. Tirrell, "Designing Materials for Biology and Medicine," *Nature*, Vol. 428, 2004, p. 487.

[24] Lutolf, M. P., and J. A. Hubbell, "Synthetic Biomaterials as Instructive Extracellular Microenvironments for Morphogenesis in Tissue Engineering," *Nat. Biotechnol.*, Vol. 23, 2005, p. 47.

[25] Kweon, H., et al., "A Novel Degradable Polycaprolactone Networks for Tissue Engineering," *Biomaterials*, Vol. 24, 2003, p. 801.

[26] Marra, K. G., et al., "In Vitro Analysis of Biodegradable Polymer Blend/Hydroxyapatite Composites for Bone Tissue Engineering," *Journal of Biomedical Materials Research*, Vol. 47, 1999, p. 324.

[27] Williams, J. M., et al., "Bone Tissue Engineering Using Polycaprolactone Scaffolds Fabricated Via Selective Laser Sintering," *Biomaterials*, Vol. 26, 2005, p. 4817.

[28] Zein, I., et al., "Fused Deposition Modeling of Novel Scaffold Architectures for Tissue Engineering Applications," *Biomaterials*, Vol. 23, 2002, p. 1169.

[29] Atala, A., et al., "Tissue-Engineered Autologous Bladders for Patients Needing Cystoplasty," *Lancet*, Vol. 367, 2006, p. 1241.

[30] Liebenberg, S., et al., "Engineering Vascularized Skeletal Muscle Tissue," *Nat. Biotechnol.*, Vol. 23, 2005, p. 879.

[31] Ott, H. C., et al., "Perfusion-Decellularized Matrix: Using Nature's Platform to Engineer a Bioartificial Heart," *Nature Medicine*, Vol. 14, 2008, p. 213.

[32] Zimmermann, W. H., et al., "Engineered Heart Tissue Grafts Improve Systolic and Diastolic Function in Infracted Rat Hearts," *Nature Medicine*, Vol. 12, 2006, p. 452.

[33] Stosich, M. S., et al. "Bioengineering Strategies to Generate Vascularized Soft Tissue Grafts with Sustained Shape," *Methods*, Vol. 47, 2009, p. 116.

CHAPTER

14

Integration of Experimental and Computational Microfluidics in 3D Tissue Engineering

Manuela T. Raimondi,[1,2] Devin T. Bridgen,[3] Matteo Laganà,[1,2] Beatrice Tonnarelli,[3] Margherita Cioffi,[1,2] Federica Boschetti,[1,2] and David Wendt[3]

[1]LaBS, Department of Structural Engineering, Politecnico di Milano, Milano, Italy, [2]IRCCS Galeazzi Orthopaedic Institute, Milano, Italy, [3]Departments of Surgery and of Biomedicine, University Hospital Basel, Basel, Switzerland, corresponding author: Manuela Teresa Raimondi, address: Laboratory of Biological Structure Mechanics (LaBS), Department of Structural Engineering, Politecnico di Milano, 32, piazza Leonardo da Vinci, 30133 Milano, Italy, phone: +39.02.2399.4306, e-mail: manuela.raimondi@polimi.it

Abstract

We present an integrated system, combining computational flow analysis with a microbioreactor designed for three-dimensional (3D) scaffolds to study the effects of hydrodynamic conditions on cell behavior over time. Using appropriate staining and imaging protocols, thin cell-seeded 3D scaffolds with a controlled architecture are monitored nondestructively in time and space. Computational fluid dynamic (CFD) simulation quantifies the fluidic environment within the scaffold pores. The model geometry and boundary conditions directly correspond to the environment given by the flow channel and specific scaffold architecture. Integrating the computational and experimental data, local fluid conditions are correlated one-to-one with local cell behavior throughout the course of culture. This concept is illustrated using the microfluidic system to investigate the effect of shear stress on cell proliferation in 3D. We explore design considerations and potential applications in tissue engineering for studying the cell response in a perfused 3D environment.

Key terms bioreactor, cell proliferation, computational model, imaging, interstitial perfusion, microfluidics, shear stress, tissue engineering

14.1 Introduction

In the design of 3D porous biomaterials to serve as implants in tissue engineering, a central concern is the control of mass transport. While scaffold material properties, surface chemistry, and degradation behavior are important, the transport of gases and nutrients to cells and of catabolites away from cells is now established as the crucial factor affecting cell survival [1]. Tissue engineering may use fluid flow to respond to mass transport limitations; the cell-seeded scaffold is immersed in a culture medium, which is induced to flow through the scaffold structure in interstitial perfusion bioreactors.

In scaffold-based cartilage regeneration, the interstitial fluid flow of culture medium is believed to be particularly effective in up-regulating the biosynthesis of matrix proteins, as it results in cell membrane stretching, due to fluid-induced shear, and in the convection-enhanced transport of solutes [2]. Under interstitial perfusion, a simple means of increasing mass transport to cells would be to increase the medium flow rate. High flow rates induce high shear stresses on cells, which may be harmful instead of beneficial at all stages of tissue growth. We address the issue by establishing quantitative relationships between the field variables of the fluid dynamic field imposed to cells, and the cell response within the 3D tissue.

Flow around constructs in a bioreactor may be computed in terms of flow fields, shear stresses, and oxygen profiles, through the use of a computational fluid dynamic (CFD) model [3]. Incorporating flow through the scaffold in an interstitial-perfusion configuration complicates the situation by establishing a velocity scale that is related to the actual fluid velocities in the scaffold, which are not experimentally accessible and are thus impossible to measure. This complex problem is investigated by the use of detailed pore-scale CFD simulations of fluid and the solute transport in tissue engineering scaffolds [4–8]. CFD numerical techniques are able to capture flow, pressure, and concentration fields resolved at the scaffold's pore level. Calculations indicate that inappropriately designed dynamic culture environments lead to regions of harmful shear stresses or nutrient concentrations insufficient to maintain cell viability [9].

So far, attempts to calculate and control the balance of mass transport/shear stress by proper selection of medium flow rate and scaffold microgeometry have proven useful in capturing a rough understanding of the conditions favoring the initial development of engineered tissues such as bone [10] and cartilage [11–14]. These efforts have been directed towards the establishment of a quantitative correlation between levels of shear stress, obtained by averaging out the wide range of imposed shears into a single shear level value, and construct parameters such as cellularity or the change in matrix protein expression. However, the local shear stresses are widely heterogeneous [6], making correlations between shear level and effects on matrix composition very difficult to assess. A step forward in this regard would be the establishment of variable correlation as a function of spatial location. More specifically, a point-by-point correlation is generated between the local field variables calculated for the fluid dynamic field within the construct, and the biosynthetic response measured at the celularl level within the 3D construct.

The complexity of the 3D system and the associated limitations of the destructive and off-line analyses on the cellular constructs are overcome through the use of an advanced microfluidic model. This model allows nondestructive online monitoring of local parameters of the construct during perfusion culture. Microfluidic systems have rapidly gained popularity for use in cell culture, as shown by several recent examples of studying angiogenesis [15], axonal guidance [16], liver tissue engineering [17, 18], bone differentiation [19], and stem cell differentiation [20]. Microfluidic systems provide the capability to control many of the critical biochemical and biophysical factors, allow for the culture of a wide range of cell types, and can be imaged in real time at high resolution. For example, one can seed a cell type in a microchamber and examine the local response to time-dependent flows and the delivery of mechanical stimuli and growth factors. These capabilities have opened new perspectives to tissue engineering studies that were not previously possible with a conventional bioreactor system.

We have developed an integrated experimental/computational microfluidic model of in vitro–engineered cartilaginous tissue. The tissue model consists of a construct made of chondrocytes seeded on a porous 3D scaffold. The CFD simulations quantify the local shear stress distribution within the perfused scaffold microarchitecture. By using a 3D scaffold with a simple and well-defined architecture, the CFD model is dramatically simplified and more readily compared to the experimental data.CFD is used initially to help define an appropriate 3D scaffold structure, which will generate significant local variations of fluid-induced shear stress within the porous architecture when perfused. A microfluidic bioreactor is developed, allowing the online monitoring of the construct during perfusion culture. A quantitative correlation is established by the CFD simulation between the experimental data from cell cultures and the geometric configuration of the microbioreactor.

14.2 Experimental Design

The integration of computational and experimental data elucidates the effect of local shear stresses, induced by specific perfusion conditions and scaffold architecture, on local cell behavior over time under an interstitial perfusion. Specifically, we aim to quantify the proliferation of cells within defined regions of the scaffold microarchitecture. Different perfusion velocities are used to induce varying magnitudes of shear, with the local shear stress quantified by a pore-scale CFD simulation. The microfluidic model consists of a microbioreactor in which a thin 3D cellular construct, 500 μm in thickness, is cultured under an interstitial perfusion. The bioreactor allows nondestructive online monitoring of cells cultured under perfusion, drastically reducing the sample size needed to acquire statistically significant data when taking destructive time points. Confocal and fluorescent time lapse microscopy (nondestructive) is used to monitor local cell distribution within specific locations of the scaffold over the time course of the culture.

14.3 Materials

14.3.1 Solutions

- Complete medium (CM): Dulbecco's modified Eagle's medium (DMEM) (Gibco-BRL), 10% fetal bovine serum (FBS) (Gibco-BRL), 1-mM Sodium Pyruvate (Gibco-BRL), 10-mM HEPES buffer (Gibco-BRL), 1% penicillin/streptomycin/glutamine (PSG)(Gibco-BRL). Store at 4°C.

- Growth medium (GM): Complete medium with 1 ng/ml TGFβ-1 (R&D Systems) and 5 ng/ml FGF2 (R&D Systems). Store at 4°C.
- 1× phosphate-buffered saline (PBS) (Gibco-BRL). Store at 4°C.
- DAPI (Sigma)
- SYTO 13 (Sigma)
- Ethedium Homodimer 1, from LIVE/DEAD viability kit (Juro)

14.3.2 Disposables

- Glass microscope slides, 40 mm × 26 mm × 0.2 mm (Assistent)
- Platinum cured silicone tubing, 0.8 mm ID (Fisher Scientific)
- Uncoated 8-well microscopy micro slides (Ibidi)
- Coverwell microperfusion chambers (Grace Bio Labs, PC3L-0.5)
- Silicone rubber gaskets (Maagtechnic)

14.3.3 Equipment

- Roller pump (Ismatec)
- Syringe pump (Harvard Apparatus)
- Incubators set at 37°C, 5% CO_2
- Confocal microscope (LSM 710, Carl Zeiss)

14.3.4 Custom equipment

- Perfusion cell seeding system
- Microbioreactor
- 8 × 3 × 0.5 mm polystyrene scaffolds (3D Biotek)

14.3.5 Software

- Gambit (Ansys), ACIS-based solid modeler
- FLUENT (Ansys), CFD code
- SolidWorks (Dassault Systèmes SolidWorks Corp), 3D CAD design software
- Zen (Carl Zeiss), 3D reconstruction software

14.4 Methods

In this section the methods used to build an integrated experimental/computational microfluidic model to monitor local cell proliferation in relation to local shear stress are detailed. While these methods are quite specific, the general concept can be used for many different applications. Therefore, general design considerations are given in Section 14.6.

14.4.1 Microfluidic chamber design

1. The microfluidic bioreactor is designed in coordination with the specific geometry of the 3D scaffold. To ensure a strong correlation with the computational model, it is critical that the scaffold has a well-defined architecture. Rapid prototype polystyrene scaffolds with a plasma surface treatment, custom-made by 3D Biotek, are used in the proliferation experiments (Figure 14.1). The fibers are 100 μm in diameter with a pore size of 300 μm and stacked in an offset cross-hatch geometry. The overall geometry is 8 mm × 3 mm × 0.5 mm.
2. The bioreactor must be sterile while allowing easy insertion of the scaffold. It is for this reason that a sandwich design is used (Figure 14.2).
3. Once the individual bioreactor is assembled, the inlet and outlet ports are connected to the media reservoir with silicone tubing. To ensure accurate flow rates, each channel is perfused individually. The growth media can be perfused with a peristaltic pump circulating the media in a loop, or with a syringe pump for lower flow rates (Figure 14.3).

14.4.2 Computational model

1. Set up the model geometry and mesh. The ACIS-based, solid modeler Gambit is used here. Reconstruct the scaffold geometry and dimensions (Figure 14.1). Determine the existing symmetries and study only a fraction of the model to limit the computational cost (e.g., one-fourth of the model is studied here). Use a 4-node-tetrahedral mesh. Provide a number of elements and element spacing that will enable a resolution at the scaffold walls of areas smaller than a cell (<20–25 μm). Use a sufficiently fine mesh to resolve the boundary layer and the corresponding

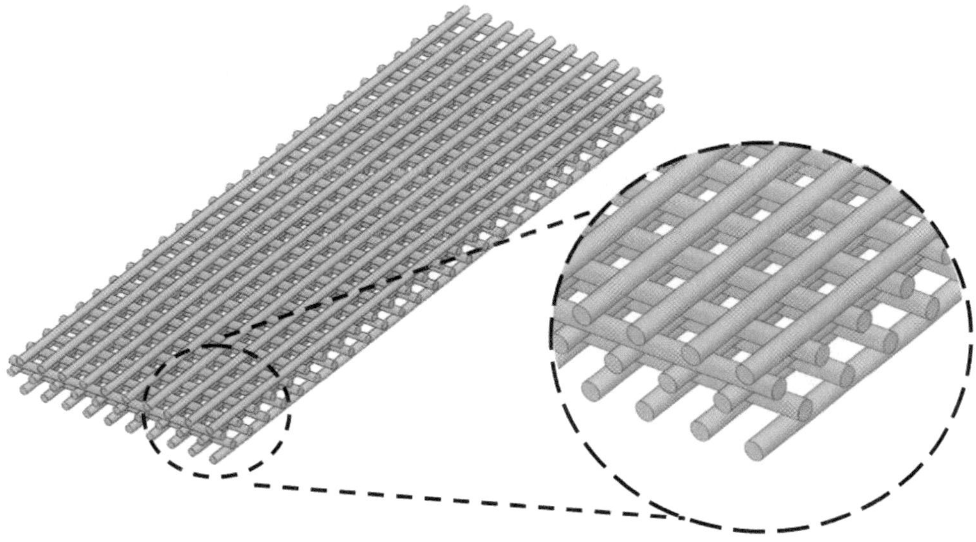

Figure 14.1 Scaffold geometry used for proliferation data. The fiber diameter is 100 μm and the pore size is 300 μm. The overall dimension of the scaffold is 3 mm × 8 mm × 0.5 mm.

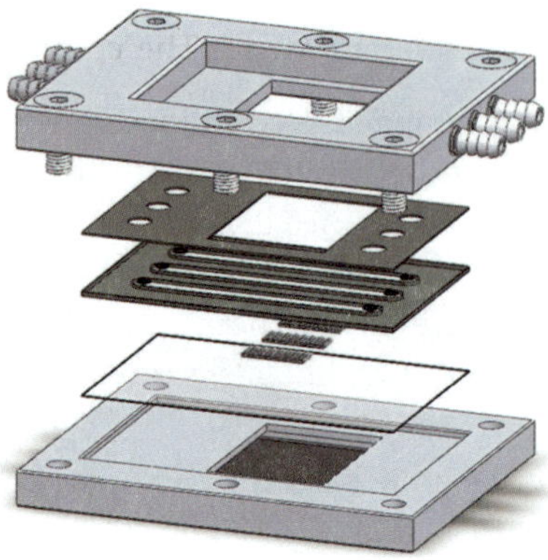

Figure 14.2 Expanded view of the microfluidic chamber. The (a) top and (f) bottom plates provide structural support and provide the pressure, using screws, to compress the assembly enough that there are no fluid leaks and sterility is maintained. It is important that they maintain a low profile so that they fit comfortably under a microscope and the objective can reach the cover slip. Our plates were custom machined out of stainless steel. The top plate contains small channels moving fluid from the threaded luer locks to the corresponding holes in the gasket below. (b) The gasket is used to ensure a tight seal between the top plate and the polycarbonate top of the flow channels. Holes on each end of the gasket allow fluid to flow from channels in the top plate, through the holes in the polycarbonate plate, and into the perfusion chamber. (c) The fluid channels are made from medical grade silicone bonded to clear, UV-transparent polycarbonate plastic. Channels in the silicone define the flow channel architecture, with fluid constrained by the cover slip and polycarbonate on the top and bottom and by the silicone on the sides. (d) The scaffolds are inserted between the cover slip and the perfusion chamber. When the top and bottom plates are screwed together, the pressure slightly compresses the silicone in the perfusion chamber, ensuring a tight fit for the scaffolds. (e) The cover slip thickness balances the structural strength with an optical efficiency when imaging, and we have found that a 0.2-mm thickness works well. This is a fragile portion of the bioreactor, and care must be taken when moving the objective of a microscope so that you do not break the cover slip. The chamber adheres to the cover slip below, providing a water-tight channel. Our design uses three 0.5-mm-thick channels per bioreactor (cat no. PC3L-0.5).

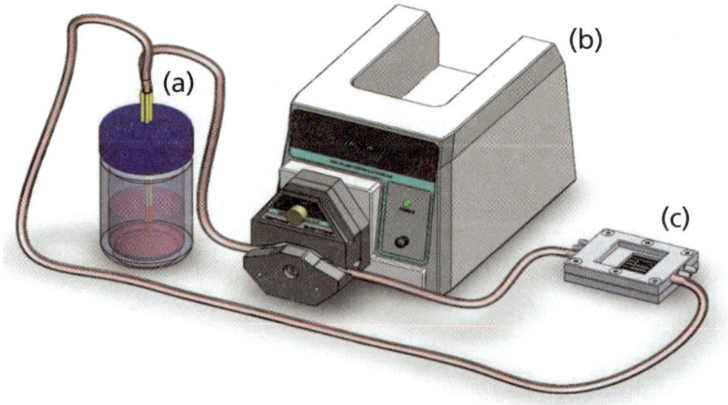

Figure 14.3 Diagram showing the full setup of the microbioreactor. (a) Culture medium reservoir. (b) Peristaltic pump. (c) Microfluidic chamber. Only one set of tubing is shown for simplicity, when in reality there are three sets per bioreactor. A filter and septum are attached to the media reservoir for, respectively, gas and media exchange.

shear stress distribution at the scaffold wall surfaces. It is also possible to discretize the fluid field with a mesh progressively refined near the scaffold walls. Here the mesh consists of 246,600 elements.

2. Set up and solve the fluid dynamic problem. The commercial finite-volume code FLUENT is used here.
   a. Set the boundary conditions. Apply no-slip boundary conditions to the solid surfaces representing the scaffold fibers under the hypothesis of rigid, impermeable walls. Impose a flat velocity profile at the inlet. The applied velocity (in the described example, 100 μm/s) will correspond to the flow rate experimentally applied through the scaffold. Apply null total stress at the outlet. Use symmetry boundary conditions for the lateral sides of the fluid domain and no-slip boundary conditions for the upper and lower surfaces of the domain.
   b. Model the fluid. Model the culture medium at 37°C as an incompressible, homogeneous, Newtonian fluid with a density equal to 1,000 kg m^{-3}. The viscosity, measured for Dulbecco's Modified Eagle Medium at 37°C, is 8.2×10^{-4} kg $m^{-1}s^{-1}$ [11].
   c. Run the simulations. The equations solved by FLUENT are the steady-state Navier-Stokes equations. Choose a segregated solver for the solution method and a conjugate gradient-based iterative solver to solve the symmetric and nonsymmetric linear systems. Here, computations are carried out on a Windows NT PC with 2-Gb RAM.
3. Analyze the results. Determine the fluid velocity magnitudes and the distribution of wall shear stress at the scaffold walls. Process wall shear stress data at the pore level to obtain the maximum, minimum, and average values, which are an estimate of the shear stress range induced at the scaffold walls.
4. Calculate the Reynolds number. Use the equation $Re = d\rho v/\mu$, where d is the hydraulic diameter, equal to 4 × fluid volume/surface area, ρ is the fluid density, v is the average inlet velocity, and μ is the fluid viscosity. Reynolds numbers are typically very low in interstitial perfusion bioreactors (e.g., here $Re = 10^{-3}$); thus, the convective terms of the fluid dynamic equations are negligible and the shear stress is linearly related to the imposed inlet flow rate. Use the calculated shear stresses to extrapolate shear stress levels for different inlet velocities.

14.4.3 Dynamic scaffold seeding

1. If not presterilized by the manufacturer, submerse the scaffolds in isopropyanol for 10 minutes, followed by three 10-minute washes and an overnight soak in DMEM at 37°C.
2. To obtain a uniform distribution of cells throughout the scaffold, cells may be seeded under perfusion in a bioreactor, as previously described [1]. It is necessary to use a low cell number, since a higher cell density could alter the scaffold pore architecture and compromise correlations to the computational model.
3. To determine the appropriate number of cells to seed, perform preliminary seeding experiments. For the 3D Biotek scaffold, having a seeding efficiency of about 10%, inject 100,000 cells per scaffold.
4. Perfuse the cell suspension through the scaffold overnight. If the fluid velocity is too high, cells may not attach to the scaffold. However, if the fluid velocity is too slow, a majority of the cells will adhere elsewhere in the bioreactor, significantly decreasing seeding efficiency. A fluid velocity of ~1,000 μm/s was used for the seeding.

14.4.4 Microbioreactor setup

1. The bioreactor is designed so that each component, aside from the scaffold, can be autoclaved.
2. While under sterile conditions, carefully take the scaffolds out of the perfusion seeding system. It is important to be gentle with the scaffolds to prevent cell detachment. Place each scaffold in CM.
3. Perform cell nuclear staining with DAPI at a concentration of 10 μg/ml. The staining protocol is as follows:
   a. Dissolve DAPI in deionized water to make a stock concentration of 5 mg/ml. Since DAPI is not very soluble, try sonicating the solution in addition to 5 minutes of vortexing.
   b. Combine 1× PBS with stock DAPI to form a 10 μg/ml solution.
   c. Incubate the constructs in the solution for 90 minutes at 37°C.
   d. Wash the constructs twice with 1× PBS before resubmerging in CM.
4. Attach silicone tubing to each inlet/outlet on the bioreactor and to the media reservoir, which has already been filled with GM. If using a syringe pump, prefill the syringe and tubing with media before attaching to the bioreactor.
5. Place the glass cover slip on the top of the bottom plate of the bioreactor.
6. Place the scaffolds with stained cells into the perfusion chambers. Work quickly so that the scaffolds do not dry out.
7. Place the flow channels onto the cover slip.
8. Place the gasket onto the flow channels, taking care to align the holes for fluid flow.
9. Place the top plate on top of the gasket, insert the screws, and tighten the top plate against the bottom plate.
10. Briefly start the pump to fill the fluid channels with media, preventing the scaffolds from becoming dry.
11. Select the desired flow rate (e.g., 100 μm/s and 1 μm/s) and start the pump, creating a fluid flow through the bioreactor which perfuses the scaffold (Figure 14.4). A static control is kept in a 6-well plate with a comparable volume of media so that the nutrient supply is not the limiting factor. The final setup should look similar to that shown in Figure 14.3.

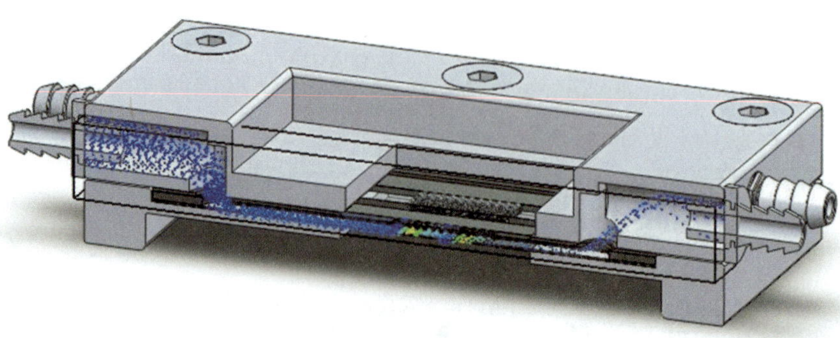

Figure 14.4 Cutaway of the microfluidic chamber. It shows the flow path of the growth media while being perfused at an average velocity of 100 μm/sec.

14.4.5 Imaging and data acquisition

1. For each desired time point, move the bioreactors to the confocal microscope. For long durations, it is advisable to use a heated environmental chamber to hold the bioreactor while taking images. A confocal microscope allows you to obtain the 3D information needed to take full advantage of the proposed design. A 10× objective with the aperture set at 1 airy unit, corresponding to an image depth of about 10 μm, is used for imaging. Using the features "tile scan" and "auto z," z-stacks in adjacent blocks are stitched together forming one large image.
2. At the final time point, an additional destructive analysis can supplement the previous data. Specifically, to look at local cell viability, the following live/dead assay protocol can be used:
   a. Stain the cell nuclei by submersing the scaffolds in 5-μM SYTO-13 Dye diluted in CM. Incubate the scaffolds for 90 minutes at 37°C, and then rinse once with 1× PBS.
   b. Stain the nuclei of the dead cells with 5-μM ethidium homodimer-1 (EthD-1), diluted in 1× PBS. Incubate for 30 minutes at 37°C, and then rinse with 1× PBS.
   c. Place the scaffolds in the 8-well microslides and submerse in 1× PBS. Image the cells.
3. Using Zen software, cells can be counted in both the high shear and low shear zones on the scaffold. It is important to have well-defined regions to compare. For the fiber-based scaffold from 3D Biotek, count the cells along a horizontal cross section of a fiber and compare it to a vertical cross section. This is described in more detail in Section 14.5.
4. To assess the total number of cells within the scaffold, detach the cells with collagenase and trypsin and manually count.

14.5 Anticipated Results and Interpretation

The results of the computational simulations allow quantification of the local flow field inside the scaffold (Figure 14.5) and the distribution of the wall shear stresses on the scaffold fibers (Figure 14.6). The local heterogeneity in the velocity and shear stress results is induced by the scaffold microstructure and the geometry of the microbioreactor channels. Therefore, with a different combination of channel and scaffold geometries, different results may be obtained. For the scaffold-microbioreactor system described here, at an applied inlet velocity of 100 μm/s, velocity magnitudes range from 0 to 370 μm/s and shear stress magnitudes range from 0 to 21 mPa.

The heterogeneous local fluid flow induces inhomogeneity in wall shear stresses, which are proportional to the velocity gradients. The lowest wall shear stresses are found at the fiber intersections, where the flow penetration is poor: the average shear stress in these areas is about 2 mPa (Figure 14.6). Conversely, the highest shear stresses are computed on the fibers oriented perpendicularly to flow, with peak values at the surfaces oriented parallel to to the top and bottom planes of the microbioreactor channels. In general, for a given scaffold, the thinner the microbioreactor channel, the bigger the difference between minimum and maximum shear stresses. Similarly, for a given

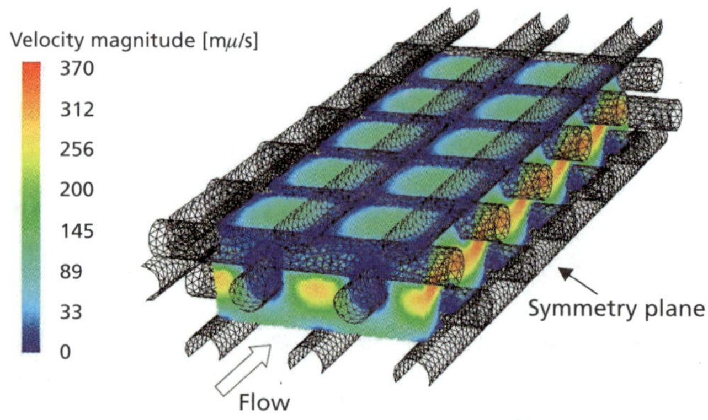

Figure 14.5 Results of CFD modeling. Calculated fluid velocity field mapped in the 3D scaffold perfused at an inlet velocity of 100 μm/s.

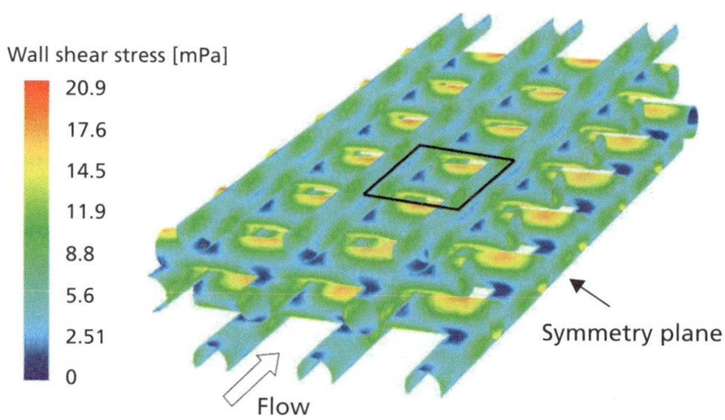

Figure 14.6 Results of CFD modeling. Calculated wall shear stress field mapped on the surfaces of the 3D scaffold perfused at an inlet velocity of 100 μm/s. The black square indicates the detail shown in the top view in Figure 14.8(b).

bioreactor chamber, the smaller the scaffold pores, the higher the expected maximum wall shear stress.

Using the given experimental protocol, a 3D reconstruction of your entire scaffold, as shown in Figure 14.7, can be obtained. Focusing on individual pores, a representative output of our method is shown in Figure 14.8. Overlapping the confocal image [Figure 14.8(a)] to the computed shear stress map [Figure 14.8(b)] gives the correlation between the computational and experimental outputs [Figure 14.8(c)]. Using this information, it is possible to clarify which specific regions would be most appropriate to compare. While a 3D reconstruction of the z stacks provides excellent qualitative data, it must be further modified for accurate quantitative analysis. It is critical that you select precisely defined voxels to compare in order to prevent bias. Each confocal image, while literally 2D, actually has a depth corresponding the the aperture size and objective used. For fibers with a circular cross section, we have found it most accurate to compare data from individual images. For example, the plane where two layers of fibers connect [Figure 14.9(a)] or the plane going through the middle of the fibers [Figure 14.9(b)] can

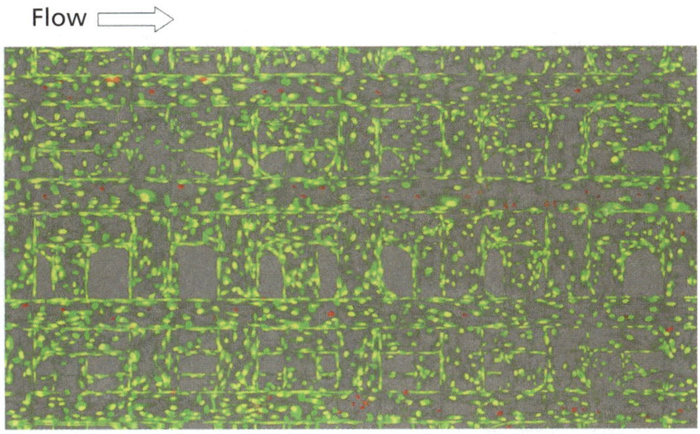

Figure 14.7 Results of confocal imaging. The 3D reconstruction of a confocal microscopy image stack using Zen software. The cells are stained with a modified live/dead assay detailed in Section 14.4.4, in which live cells stain green and dead cells stain red.

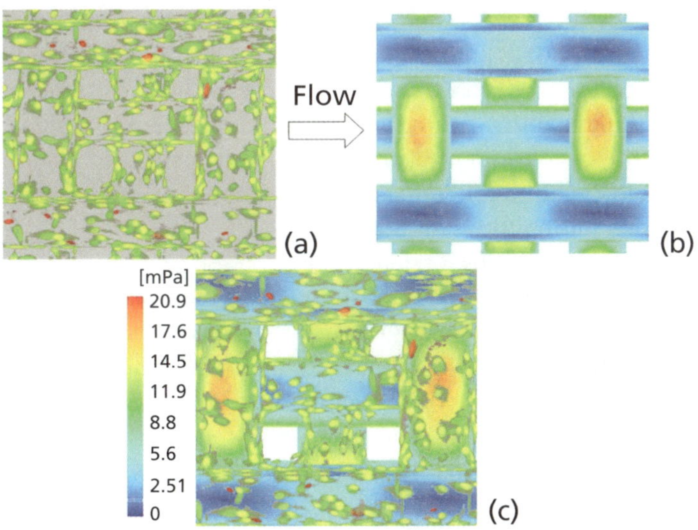

Figure 14.8 Representative output of the method. Focusing on individual pores, (a) the confocal image and (b) the computed shear stress map are overlapped to obtain (c) an image showing the point-by-point correlation between the computational and experimental outputs.

be imaged, and the number of nuclei on fibers running parallel to the flow direction can be compared with fibers running perpendicularly.

Using this microfluidic model, a 3D perfusion environment is obtained that corresponds to an accurately modeled fluid environment within the scaffold pores. By using the described microfluidic chamber, it is possible to actively monitor cell growth and behavior on the scaffold. Varying the fluid flow profile within the 3D environment, qualitative and quantitative changes in cellular activity are monitored, such as changes in cell alignment and protein expression. These changes are seen on the local level and correlated to the local fluid flow environment through the computational model.

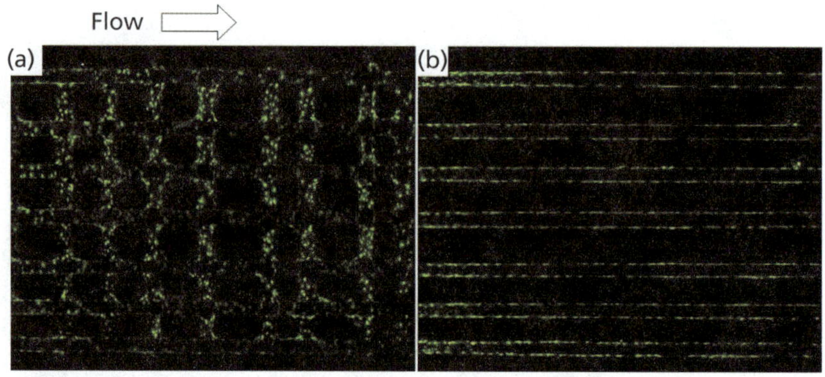

Figure 14.9 Results of confocal imaging. Cross sections, 10 μm thick, of the same scaffold from Figure 14.7. (a) The plane where two levels of fibers meet at 200 μm. (b) The cross section of fibers 250 μm deep.

14.6 Discussion and Commentary

Our target is the development of an integrated experimental/computational microfluidic model for 3D tissue engineering research. Our microfluidic model consists of a microbioreactor in which a thin 3D cellular construct is cultured under interstitial perfusion. The fluidynamics within the scaffold is quantified by a pore-scale CFD simulation, allowing the establishment of correlations between the local field variables calculated for the fluid dynamic field imposed to cells, and the biosynthetic response measured at the cell level during the course of culture.

Pioneering studies by Leclerc et al. [17, 19] established proof of concept for the scalability of the bioreactor approach to microfluidic bioreactors. However, the previous microchanneled chambers used to study the influence of shear stress on cell growth and differentiation simulated a single layer of the channel network and thus were 2D in their logic. The microfluidic model presented here accounts for 3D effects of the actual 3D scaffold structure, which is integrated in the system in several layers. This provides the benefits of controlled microfluidics with more realistic 3D cell culture and computational modeling.

When designing a microfluidic system for your experimental needs, the bioreactor and scaffold used have to be codeveloped in order to ensure accurate operation. Due to experimental constraints, we found it easier to start with design considerations for the scaffold. Fabrication methods, such as spin coating or solvent casting/particulate leaching, provide limited control of the scaffold microstructure. This prevents a realistic prediction of the fluid domain by means of geometrical computational models. The analysis of local field variables of the fluid domain does not allow a point-by-point correlation to what is seen on the actual constructs in this case, instead requiring complex statistical analysis techniques [4, 6, 21]. To ensure a strong correlation with the computational model, it is critical that the scaffold has a tightly controlled geometry. We used polystyrene scaffolds fabricated with a fiber deposition process, which maintains a tightly controlled fiber width as well as accurate fiber placement. While highly accurate and useful for our experiments, this process is limited to fairly basic cross-hatch designs. There are other fabrication methods available to generate more complex controlled microgeometries, such as stereolithography [22, 23].

We chose to use plasma-treated polystyrene as the scaffold material so that the scaffolds were transparent, allowing a greater imaging depth. It is important to be aware of how the microgeometry will affect the imaging quality as well as seeding efficiency and the shear stress profile. The cross-hatch design, with its perpendicular fibers as shown in Figure 14.4, improves seeding efficiency and maximizes the shear stress magnitude extremes. Additionally, this staggered configuration improves imaging, since the microscope does not have to look through a previous fiber layer when looking up to 400 μm in depth. The outer dimensions of the scaffold are dictated by both the microfluidic chamber and microscopy limitations. When using confocal microscopy, the typical imaging depth limit is around 300 μm. Due to the symmetry assumption used in the computational modeling, you need to be able to see at least halfway through the construct. It is for these reasons that we use a scaffold with a 500-μm thickness.

When selecting the flow rates for your bioreactor, you must first determine your upper and lower limits. The upper flow limit is generally given by the rate at which your cells are damaged or washed away. A scaffold with a different surface treatment or microarchitecture could have a higher or lower upper limit. The lower limit for fluid flow is given by a nutrient delivery to the cells and is highly dependent on both the scaffold architecture and the total cell metabolics. Monitoring outlet media with nutrient sensors, such as oxygen, would greatly assist in determining when nutrients become the limiting factor.

The cell-staining protocol is highly dependent on what cellular behavior you are trying to correlate with the fluid environment. You need to balance staining your target with maintaining normal cell behavior. Before any stain is used, you should do an assay to find the optimal exposure level, additionally checking the impact of your scaffold's autofluorescence. For example, we found that we could use DAPI up to a concentration of 10 μg/ml without affecting cell proliferation after 6 days. If you need to refresh your stain during cell culture, you can inject dye into the fluid flow during construct perfusion.

When imaging, there is a balance between image quality and the time required to take the data. We typically use a 10× objective because it has a high enough resolution for our needs and the whole scaffold can be imaged much more quickly when compared to a 20× objective. Two useful features on the LSM 710 system we used were "tile scan" and "auto Z." Tile scan has the microscope acquire a mosaic consisting of partial images, which the software reconstructs to record one complete image of the whole object. Auto Z allows the online modification of acquisition parameters for Z stacks, meaning that the gain increases with an increasing imaging depth, providing images of equal brightness at different depths. Combining z-stacks with tile scan and auto z, you can obtain a high-quality image of the entire scaffold used in the experiment, such as that seen in Figure 14.7.

The computational results determine the scaffold regions characterized by poor or strong fluid-induced mechanical stimulation (i.e., low or high shear stress at the scaffold surfaces). The computed wall shear stresses are an estimate of the shear stresses sensed by cells when adhered at the fiber walls. By using this approach, we assume that the adhered cells have negligible effect on the construct permeability and microgeometry, coherently with other studies [5–8, 24]. This hypothesis is realistic at the initial stage of the culture, from 5 days after seeding up to 2 weeks, depending on the level of cell proliferation and protein synthesis.

In fact, a high cell volume fraction alters the scaffold geometry and affects fluid flow, rendering the computational model inaccurate. Additionally, larger cell clusters with an extracellular matrix will limit the possible imaging depth. Advanced modeling techniques to predict tissue growth in 3D porous scaffolds, accounting for the fluid to structure interaction, have been developed recently [25, 26]. The development of new methods to obtain a more rigorous comparison of experimental measurements with the results obtained from modeling would open new perspectives for the validation of such predictive tools in the field of tissue engineering [27]. Our microfluidic model could potentially be used to monitor volumetric cell growth, allowing for a future dynamic flow analysis that takes into account the changing geometry of the fluid path.

Microfluidic chambers provide a highly controlled platform for acquiring data on cellular behavior under perfusion. Compared to standard culture methods with Petri dishes, microfluidics offer more control, reduced materials, real-time data monitoring, faster cell kinetics, and multiparametric analysis [28]. However, to date, systems generally look at the 2D cell culture with the exception of the 3D cell culture in gels. The methods described here provide the opportunity to combine the benefits of microfluidics with the 3D culture on various cell scaffolds. The computational modeling presented in this chapter allows the user to take full advantage of the fluid control permitted in the bioreactor.

Troubleshooting Table

Problem	Explanation	Potential Solutions
Cells disappear while in the bioreactor.	Cells are dying due to nutrient deficiencies or are being washed away due to high flow rates.	Adjust flow rate.
No fluid flow through a channel.	Misaligned gasket.	Reposition the gasket in relation to the top plate.
Fluid flow between channels.	Fluid pressure is bending the polycarbonate cover on the perfusion chamber.	Add a glass cover slip to the bioreactor between the perfusion chamber and the gasket.
3D image reconstructions look staggered.	The z distance between each image is too great.	The z-distance between images should be less than the image thickness.
Fibers show a polygonal shape after CFD meshing.	Mesh size is too large.	Refine the mesh.
Mesh has distorted elements.	The fluid domain has singularities in correspondence of the upper and lower boundaries.	Eliminate a thin portion of the fluid domain using plane intersections.

14.7 Application Notes

The microbioreactor system outlined in this chapter provides a method for real time, nondestructive data acquisition for cell culture on 3D scaffolds. The system is easily adapted to the equipment present in cell culture labs, with minimal custom components. There exist particularly important examples of applications potentially addressed by the method, in addition to the given example of cell proliferation.

1. The concept of lab-on-a-chip analysis can be applied to 3D tissue engineering with the increased control provided by computational modeling. Arbitrary combinations of environmental factors (e.g., culture media formulation and mechanical stimulation)

can be used to stimulate cells in independent culture chambers to automate analysis of cell response in actual 3D conditions. Examples are the analysis of mesenchymal stem cell (MSC) proliferation, motility, and differentiation in the context of tissue engineering of muskulo-skeletal tissue.

2. Some promising theoretical models of the multiphysic process of tissue growth [25, 26] can be validated by monitoring, in time and space, cell systems cultured in a 3D environment under perfusion.

14.8 Summary Points

1. A microbioreactor system that allows the nondestructive acquisition of data from thin 3D scaffolds with a controlled geometry has been developed. Using appropriate staining protocols, cells on the scaffolds can be monitored in real time.
2. A computational model was developed to quantify the fluidic environment within the scaffold pores. The model boundaries correspond to the environment provided by the microbioreactor system.
3. By combining the computational data with the experimental data, local fluid conditions can be correlated with local cell behavior during the course of culture, in an actual 3D culture environment.

References

[1] Wendt, D., et al., "Uniform Tissues Engineered by Seeding and Culturing Cells in 3D Scaffolds Under Perfusion at Defined Oxygen Tensions," *Biorheology*, Vol. 43, No. 3-4, 2006, pp. 481–488.

[2] Guilak, F., and C. T. Hung, "Physical Regulation of Cartilage Metabolism," in *Basic Orthopaedic Biomechanics and Mechano-Biology*, V. C. Mow and R. Huiskes, (eds.), Philadelphia, PA: Lippincott Williams & Wilkins, 2005, pp. 259–300.

[3] Williams, K. A., S. Saini, and T. M. Wick, "Computational Fluid Dynamics Modeling of Steady-State Momentum and Mass Transport in a Bioreactor for Cartilage Tissue Engineering," *Biotechnology Progress*, Vol. 18, No. 5, 2002, pp. 951–963.

[4] Porter, B., et al., "3D Computational Modeling of Media Flow Through Scaffolds in a Perfusion Bioreactor," *Journal of Biomechanics*, Vol. 38, No. 3, 2005, pp. 543–549.

[5] Singh, H., et al., "Flow Modeling Within a Scaffold Under the Influence of Uni-Axial and Bi-Axial Bioreactor Rotation," *Journal of Biotechnology*, Vol. 119, 2005, pp. 181–219.

[6] Cioffi, M., et al., "Modeling Evaluation of the Fluid-Dynamic Microenvironment in Tissue-Engineered Constructs: A Micro-CT Based Model," *Biotechnology and Bioengineering*, Vol. 93, No. 3, 2006, pp. 500–510.

[7] Boschetti, F., et al., "Prediction of the Micro-Fluid Dynamic Environment Imposed to Three-Dimensional Engineered Cell Systems in Bioreactors," *Journal of Biomechanics*, Vol. 39, No. 3, 2006, pp. 418–425.

[8] Cioffi, M., et al., "Computational Evaluation of Oxygen and Shear Stress Distributions in 3D Perfusion Culture Systems: Macro-Scale and Micro-Structured Models," *Journal of Biomechanics*, Vol. 41, 2008, pp. 2918–2925.

[9] Galbusera, F., et al., "Computational Modeling of Combined Cell Population Dynamics and Oxygen Transport in Engineered Tissue Subject to Interstitial Perfusion," *Computer Methods in Biomechanics and Biomedical Engineering*, Vol. 10, No. 4, 2007, pp. 279–287.

[10] Cartmell, S. H., et al., "Effects of Medium Perfusion Rate on Cell-Seeded Three-Dimensional Bone Constructs In Vitro," *Tissue Eng.*, Vol. 9, 2003, pp. 1197–1203.

[11] Raimondi, M. T., et al., "Mechanobiology of Engineered Cartilage Cultured Under a Quantified Fluid-Dynamic Environment," *Biomechanics and Modelling in Mechanobiology*, Vol. 1, No. 1, 2002, pp. 69–82.

[12] Raimondi, M. T., et al., "The Effect of Media Perfusion on Three-Dimensional Cultures of Human Chondrocytes: Integration of Experimental and Computational Approaches," *Biorheology*, Vol. 41, No. 3-4, 2004, pp. 401–410.

[13] Raimondi, M. T., et al., "The Effect of Hydrodynamic Shear on 3D Engineered Chondrocyte Systems Subject to Direct Perfusion," *Biorheology*, Vol. 43, No. 3-4, 2006, pp. 215–222.

[14] Raimondi, M. T., et al., "Engineered Cartilage Constructs Subject to Very Low Regimens of Interstitial Perfusion," *Biorheology*, Vol. 45, No. 3-4, 2008, pp. 471–478.

[15] Sudo, R., et al., "Transport-Mediated Angiogenesis in 3D Epithelial Coculture," *FASEB Journal*, e-pub 2009.

[16] Sundararaghavan, H. G., et al., "Neurite Growth in 3D Collagen Gels with Gradients of Mechanical Properties," *Biotechnology and Bioengineering*, Vol. 102, No. 2, 2009, pp. 632–643.

[17] Leclerc, E., Y. Sakai, and T. Fujii, "Perfusion Culture of Fetal Human Hepatocytes in Microfluidic Environments," *Biochemical Engineering Journal*, Vol. 20, 2004, pp. 143–148.

[18] Mehta, K., et al., "Quantitative Inference of Cellular Parameters from Microfluidic Cell Culture Systems," *Biotechnology and Bioengineering*, Vol. 103, No. 5, 2009, pp. 966–974.

[19] Leclerc, E., et al., "Study of Osteoblastic Cells in a Microfluidic Environment," *Biomaterials*, Vol. 27, 2006, pp. 586–595.

[20] Wu, H. W., et al., "The Culture and Differentiation of Amniotic Stem Cells Using a Microfluidic System," *Biomedical Microdevices*, e-pub 2009.

[21] Maes, F., et al., "Modeling Fluid Flow Through Irregular Scaffolds for Perfusion Bioreactors," *Biotechnology and Bioengineering*, Vol. 103, No. 3, 2009, pp. 621–630.

[22] Anderson, E. J., and M. L. Knothe Tate, "Design of Tissue Engineering Scaffolds as Delivery Devices for Mechanical and Mechanically Modulated Signals," *Tissue Eng.*, Vol. 13, No. 10, 2007, pp. 2525–2538.

[23] Melchels, F., J. Feijen, and D. Grijpma, "A Poly(D,L-Lactide) Resin for the Preparation of Tissue Engineering Scaffolds by Stereolithography," *Biomaterials*, Vol. 30, 2009, pp. 3801–3809.

[24] Spiteri, C. G., et al., "Substrate Architecture and Fluid-Induced Shear Stress During Chondrocyte Seeding: Role of Alpha5beta1 Integrin," *Biomaterials*, Vol. 29, No. 16, 2008, pp. 2477–2489.

[25] O'Dea, R. D., S. L. Waters, and H. M. Byrne, "A Two-Fluid Model for Tissue Growth Within a Dynamic Flow Environment," *European Journal of Applied Mathematics*, Vol. 19, 2008, pp. 607–634.

[26] Galbusera, F., M. Cioffi, and M. T. Raimondi, "An In Silico Bioreactor for Simulating Laboratory Experiments in Tissue Engineering," *Biomedical Microdevices*, Vol. 10, No. 4, 2008, pp. 547–554.

[27] Hutmacher, D. W., and H. Singh, "Computational Fluid Dynamics for Improved Bioreactor Design and 3D Culture," *Trends in Biotechnology*, Vol. 26, No. 4, 2008, pp. 166–172.

[28] Cimetta, E., et al., "Micro-Bioreactor Arrays for Controlling Cellular Environments: Design Principles for Human Embryonic Stem Cell Applications," *Methods*, Vol. 47, 2009, pp. 81–89.

About the Editors

François Berthiaume received a B.S. in chemical engineering from Laval University, Quebec, Canada, and a Ph.D. in chemical engineering from The Pennsylvania State University. He then became a postdoctoral fellow at the Massachusetts General Hospital, Harvard Medical School, and the Boston Shriners Hospital for Children, and remained there to join the faculty rank of assistant professor in surgery. Presently, Dr. Berthiaume is an associate professor of biomedical engineering at Rutgers University. Dr. Berthiaume has published over 100 peer-reviewed papers, reviews, and book chapters and has served on multiple grant evaluation study sections for various public and private agencies.

Jeffrey Morgan received a B.S. in biology from Syracuse University and a Ph.D. in biological chemistry from Harvard University. He was a postdoctoral fellow at the Massachusetts Institute of Technology and the Whitehead Institute. He cofounded a biotechnology company and later returned to academia as an associate professor in surgery at Harvard Medical School and the Massachusetts General Hospital, as well as a senior research scientist at the Boston Shriners Hospital for Children. Presently, Dr. Morgan is an associate professor of medical science and engineering with tenure at Brown University where he is the codirector of the Center for Biomedical Engineering. Dr. Morgan has received numerous national and international awards and patents for his research in gene therapy and tissue engineering. He has published more than 100 peer-reviewed papers, reviews, and book chapters, has edited two books, and is an inventor of 9 patents.

Index

D

The Artech House Methods in Bioengineering Series

Series Editors
Martin L. Yarmush, M.D., Ph.D.
Robert Langer, Sc.D.

Methods in Bioengineering: 3D Tissue Engineering,
François Berthiaume and Jeffrey Morgan, editors

Methods in Bioengineering: Biomicrofabrication and Biomicrofluidics,
Jeffrey D. Zahn and Luke P. Lee, editors

Methods in Bioengineering: Microdevices in Biology and Medicine,
Yaakov Nahmias and Sangeeta N. Bhatia, editors

Methods in Bioengineering: Nanoscale Bioengineering and Nanomedicine,
Kaushal Rege and Igor Medintz, editors

Methods in Bioengineering: Stem Cell Bioengineering,
Biju Parekkadan and Martin L. Yarmush, editors

Methods in Bioengineering: Systems Analysis of Biological Networks,
Arul Jayaraman and Juergen Hahn, editors

Methods in Bioengineering

3D Tissue Engineering